INDONESIAN HERITAGE

Performing Arts

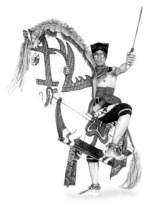

SPONSORS

This encyclopedia project was initiated and guided by the **Yayasan Dana Bakti**

with the support of the **Shangri-la Hotel**, *Jakarta.*

It was also made possible thanks to the generous and enlightened support of the following companies:

PT. Makindo
Sinar Mas Group
Bakrie Group
Bank Artha Graha
Satelindo
Telekomindo
Telekomunikasi Indonesia
Indobuildco
Indosat
Inti
Pasifik Satelit Nusantara

Plaza Indonesia Realty
Siemens Indonesia
WES Intratama Consortium
Wahana Tigamas Buana/AT&T
Konsorsium Pramindo Ikat
Artha Telekomindo
Amalgam Indocorpora
Elektrindo Nusantara
PT. Ratelindo
Komselindo

© **Editions Didier Millet, 1998**
Reprinted 1999
Published by Archipelago Press,
an imprint of Editions Didier Millet Pte Ltd,
64 Peck Seah Street, Heritage Court
Singapore 079325
E-mail: edm@pacific.net.sg
Tel: 65-324 9260   Fax: 65-324 9261

ISBN 981-3018-35-6
ISBN 981-3018-58-5 (multi-volume set)

Jakarta Office:
Buku Antar Bangsa
Menara Batavia 11th Floor Kav. 126
Jl. K. H. Mas Mansyur
Jakarta 10220 Indonesia
E-mail: bab@dnet.net.id
Tel: 62-21-574 9147   Fax: 62-21-574 9148

Printed by APP Printing Pte Ltd, Indonesia

Performing Arts

VOLUME EDITOR

Prof. Dr. Edi Sedyawati *Directorate General for Culture, Department of Education and Culture*

VOLUME EDITORIAL TEAM

Editors
Judi Achjadi
Goh Geok Yian

Designer
Joseph G. Reganit

Picture Researcher
Julianti Parani

AUTHORS

A.M. Hermien Kusmayati - *Indonesian Arts Institute, Yogyakarta*
A.M. Munardi - *Secondary School for Traditional Indonesian Music*
Bambang Murtiyoso - *Indonesian Academy of the Arts, Solo*
Deddy Luthan - *Jakarta Institute of the Arts, Indonesia*
Djatikusuma - *Member of the House of Representatives, Indonesia*
Enoch Atmadibrata - *Observer of Sundanese art forms*
Franki Raden - *Jakarta Institute of the Arts, Indonesia*
Halilintar Lathief - *Institute of Education, Ujung Pandang*
I Nyoman Sumandi - *Secondary School for Traditional Indonesian Music, Denpasar, Bali*
I Wayan Dibia - *Indonesian Academy of the Arts, Denpasar*
Jakob Sumardjo - *Institute of Education, Bandung*
Judi Achjadi - *Buku Antar Bangsa, Jakarta*
Julianti L. Parani - *Jakarta Institute of the Arts, Indonesia*
Kasim Achmad - *Jakarta Institute of the Arts, Indonesia*
Luckman Sinar - *University of North Sumatra, Medan, Sumatra*

Mahdi Bahar - *Secondary School for the Arts, Padang Panjang, Sumatra*
Philip Yampolsky - *The Smithsonian Institution, Washington D.C.*
Rahayu Supanggah - *Indonesian Academy of Arts, Solo*
Saini K.M. - *Department of Education and Culture, Indonesia*
Sal Murgiyanto - *Jakarta Institute of the Arts, Indonesia*
Soedarsono - *Indonesian Arts Institute, Yogyakarta*
Soenarto Timoer - *Department of Education and Culture (retired)*
Sri Hastanto - *Indonesian Academy of the Arts, Solo*
Sugeng Nugroho - *Indonesian Academy of the Arts, Solo*
Suka Hardjana - *Jakarta Institute of the Arts, Indonesia*
Sumarsam - *Department of Theatre, Wesleyan University, U.S.A.*
Soetarno - *Indonesian Academy of the Arts, Solo*
Tom Ibnur - *Jakarta Institute of the Arts, Indonesia*
Victor Ganap - *Indonesian Arts Institute, Yogyakarta*

ARCHIPELAGO PRESS

Contents

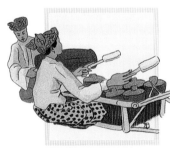

(Above) Two Javanese musicians playing the kendhang *and* bonang *(forefront) respectively.*

(Opposite) Two wayang kulit (shadow-play) puppets.

INDONESIA:
A Panorama of Performing Arts

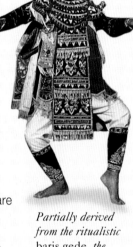

Masks from Central Java.

*T*he performing arts in Indonesia have been conditioned by socio-political situations specific to each area. Performing arts themselves are a form of cultural expression, a vehicle of cultural values, and an actualisation of aesthetic-artistic norms which have evolved over time. Acculturation processes have been instrumental in engendering changes and transformations in many forms of cultural expression, including the performing arts.

Historical Background

The history of Indonesia has a significant prelude in a string of prehistoric periods which include the Palaeolithic, Mesolithic, Neolithic, and the Bronze-Iron Ages. The first two represent a long pre-agricultural period in which hunting and food-gathering were the dominant activities within small-sized communities. Reminiscences of these activities can still be found in some of Indonesia's regional dances which contain reference to hunting.

The next phase of development, the Neolithic, is identified with the commencement of the sedentary way of life and the institution of agricultural activities. People began to live in permanent settlements, which evolved into villages. This change in the mode of living has been termed the 'agricultural revolution'. The institutionalisation of the village and the establishment of a legitimate line of descent became the basis for the development of customs and traditions which often involve art. Art forms which refer to agricultural lores and fertility rites, as well as homage to the primeval ancestor, may be considered a cultural heritage originating in this era. Examples in the performing arts are the *hudoq* dance of Kalimantan representing the warding-off of agricultural pests, and the procession of Jero Gede and Jero Luh in Bali. Jero Gede and Jero Luh are a pair of huge effigies representing the ancestral couple which are paraded from village to village. The *wayang* shadow play of Java and Bali is also hypothesised to be a creation of this age, being initially created as a depiction of the ancestors.

The Bronze-Iron Age witnessed the institutionalisation of specialised groups of people whose skills were required for the production of metal objects. Artefacts of bronze and iron were produced in abundance in this era. Economies developed beyond subsistence and the resultant exchanges of goods between families and villages generated the development of inter-village and even inter-island trading networks. Social stratification began to take form in these places.

It was on these prehistoric social bases that foreign influences entered the scene, first from India, then from the Islamic world, and finally from Europe. Each made its contribution to the development of the performing arts in Indonesia.

Partially derived from the ritualistic baris gede, *the* baris tunggal *is a modern secular dance performed for pure entertainment. Bali.*

(Below) A wayang kulit *performance at Borobudur, Central Java.*

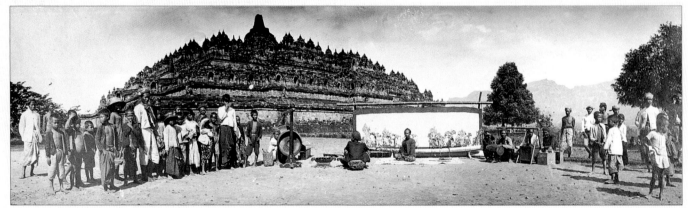

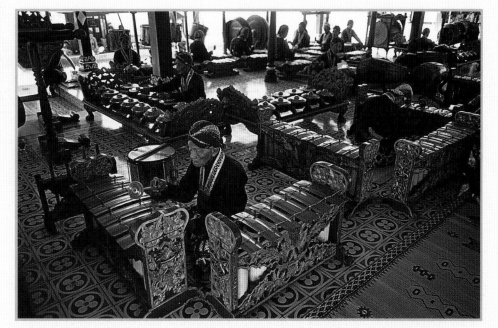

Indian cultural influence encouraged development in the aesthetics of dance and dramatic art; Islamic cultural influence introduced the idea of row- and file-dances, and drum ensembles; and the Europeans brought in the modern drama, or straight drama that did not incorporate music and dance. Chinese influence is mainly found in coastal areas.

Typology

Taking into consideration the whole range of performing arts in Indonesia, from hypothetical prehistoric forms to the most recent developments, typologies can be made using different parameters. The first is based on the number of artistic elements included in the presentation, the second on social function, and the third on whether or not the performance is a dramatisation.

Typology Based on Artistic Elements

A performance may contain 1) music only, 2) dance with music as an accompaniment or as a 'dialogue partner', 3) dramatic performance with musical accompaniment, 4) dramatic performance danced to music, 5) music-accompanied dramatic performance led/performed by a director-puppeteer using puppets to represent characters, or 6) straight dramatic play after the European model.

The last-mentioned, which is the foundation of modern Indonesian theatre art, occasionally incorporates stylistic movements and music-like elements, both emanating from the process of free composition and taking inspiration from traditional performances. Music-only performances include the *calung* in East Javanese art, the *sampek* of the Dayak of Kalimantan and the *kesok-kesok* of the Bugis people of South Sulawesi. The dance-and-music type of performance is either often performed within the framework of local ceremonies and religious rites, or may have only a secular function. Some present a 'dialogue' between musicians and dancers, such as the *gambyong* dance performance among the Javanese in which improvisation was originally the rule. Variations of the *gambyong* dance are named after the melody or song which accompanies the dance itself.

Dramatic performance with musical accompaniments is exemplified by the *drama gong* of Bali, the *ketoprak* of Java, and the *mak yong* of Riau. Traditional performances of a more classical nature constitute the fourth type. In these, characters dance out their roles, and occasionally sing, to the accompaniment of music. The great dramatic traditions of Bali and Java have even developed a characterisation system, in which the criteria for character-forming include visual aspects (make-up, mask, clothing, headdress), kinetic aspects (specific dance movements for specific characters), and auditive aspects (specific tone and sound quality for each character). The characterisation system is closely followed by the puppeteer-cum-director or *dalang,* so that a radio listener, for instance, is still able to identify the characters by the quality of the *dalang*'s auditive enactment of characters.

Typology Based on Social Function

A typology of performances can also be based on social function. Some are integral components of religious rites or ceremonies. The sacred *barong* dance-drama of Bali, in which supernatural powers are actually invoked, falls into this category, though in recent years a secular version of *barong/calonarang* dance-drama is performed exclusively for tourist entertainment. Many *barong* masks and dances are used in village-cleansing rituals and other religious ceremonies. Some performances are designed to enhance the highest position in a society, and some repertoires are 'owned' exclusively by the king's house, or the upper class, like the *bedhaya* and *serimpi* genres of the royal courts of Java and the *patuddu* and *pajaga* of South Sulawesi. The *patuddu* is considered a dance of heavenly origin brought to the royal court by an angel who married the prince. There are other dances that act as a medium for social integration, dances in which there is no distinction between performer and spectator, in which young men and women join each other in the arena. The Malay *joget* dance and the *pajogeq* of South Sulawesi are examples of such performances.

Dramatisation

A dramatised dance tells a story, while the non-representational dance does not, although it might have a set of symbolic devices to suggest special moods or character. Non-representational dances are exemplified by the *kanjet teweg* of East Kalimantan, the *alau ambek* of West Sumatra, and the *legong keraton* of Bali. They may be referred to as pure dances. The *kanjet teweg* is performed by a Dayak bride at her wedding, which tests her ability to dance elegantly on a small gong face while the secular *legong keraton* tests the skills of its preadolescent Balinese dancers.

A National Culture

Although Indonesia's national culture is still in the making, there are various cultural traits which can be identified as being 'Indonesian'. One such trait is the *Pancasila,* the state philosophy from which all Indonesians seek guidance. Another is *Bahasa Indonesia*, the national language, which typifies the conceptual formation of the Indonesian nation. In addition to these are the many art forms that typify the aesthetic expressions of the new Indonesian nation.

The Constitution of Indonesia describes national culture as arising from the minds and endeavours of all Indonesians and; it may also comprise as well the 'high points' of various regional cultures of Indonesia and incorporate foreign influences to the extent that they enhance the unity as well as humane-ness of the Indonesian nation. Several factors in real life can be identified as being related to the making of a national culture. In the performing arts, these factors are new creations, choreographies, compositions, that are neither strict continuation of an ethnic tradition, nor blind emulation of the Western example. Works by Kusbini in music, Bagong Kussudiardja in dance, and Arifin C. Noer in theatre are a few of the many examples. Western elements in fact have been incorporated, but there is a distinct Indonesian character. The 'promotion' of sub-national, ethnic forms of art as part of the national culture is also widely accepted in the country.

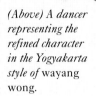

(Above) A dancer representing the refined character in the Yogyakarta style of wayang wong.

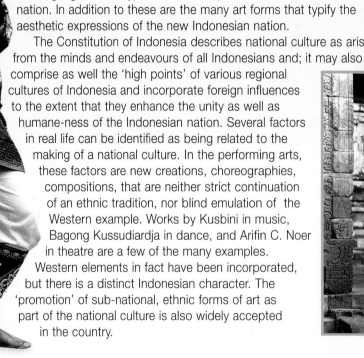

(Below) The prembon *dance-drama of Bali involves the use of masks and presents a story of which the same characters can also be found in the* topeng pajegan, *although without the storyline. This* topeng keras *character depicts a* patih *or minister.*

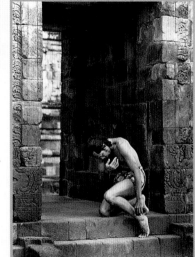

(Below) Sardono W. Kusumo is a Indonesian choreographer whose works are known worldwide. His greatest achievements have been to produce works which reflect an interesting and effective intermixture of traditional and modern elements and techniques.

Development of the Performing Arts and the National Culture

Even before the formation of an Indonesian national consciousness, each ethnic group had its own set of concepts relating to its world view, its own ethics, tastes and preferences. Differences between one group and another are very clear, and sometimes even appear to be contradictory. For instance in the performing arts, the calm and undulating Javanese dance contrasts with the dynamic Balinese dance with its staccato and syncopating rhythm; or the very different basic leg positions and steps in dances from Java-

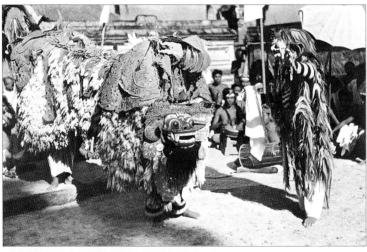

Bali, West Sumatra, Dayak Kalimantan, and coastal Malay areas. The challenge is how to make a single, new nation with such diversity.

The development of music in Indonesia is parallel to that of literature and the visual arts, which is, based on the Western model. A new class of music using the diatonic scale of Western music has emerged and developed several musical styles. This class of music has found its growth as Indonesian music and is accepted nationally. There are genres within this diatonic class such as the *keroncong*, the anthem and national heroic songs, the *seriosa*, the *langgam*, the *dangdut*, pop songs and children songs. These are regarded as Indonesian music on a national level.

The development of straight theatrical art has followed the same course. Modern Indonesian theatre came into existence using the European model, but employing the Indonesian language for its dialogue. The reference to European examples and the use of the Indonesian language in some art forms like theatre, literature and songs, have enabled these art forms to transcend ethnic boundaries, and open a new platform for the development of performing arts on a national level.

The development of dance has been more independent from Western influence. The ballet, for instance, has never become the foundation of a nationally acceptable Indonesian dance. On the other hand, the strong dance traditions from different parts of Indonesia are becoming more and more widely learned and accepted nationally.

Indonesia's cultural policy puts the formation of a national culture as a priority, while continuing to stress the need to conserve the cultural heritage, tangible and intangible. Dance, for example, gives an ideal situation, in which creativity flourishes within traditions. Even as old traditions are respected, creativity within traditions has always been recognised.

Accomplishments and Shortcomings

This same variety, diversity and vastness of the Indonesian Archipelago presents a varied assortment of performing arts of such magnitude that it would be impossible to include every example in a single volume. The Directorate-General of Culture and the various conservatoria have been the primary sources used in this book, but this has not prevented shortcomings. Unavoidably there is a predominance of Javanese and Balinese themes and a lack of photo-materials on eastern Indonesia. Moreover many performances are staged rather spontaneously and consequently go undocumented. The fact that many of Indonesia's traditional forms of dance, music and theatre are not found in this volume is hence seen as a problem of space and logistics.

As one peruses this volume, many similarities in the great variety of Indonesia's performing arts become evident. These threads of continuity are not limited to the areas represented here, but are characteristic of the entire Indonesian Archipelago. One could very well credit this to certain foreign influences that filtered through, the ebb and flow of mighty kingdoms within the Archipelago and the common roots from which all Indonesian people descend as well as the constant interaction amongst the Archipelago's inhabitants since time immemorial.

(Above) The barong ket *was used in the past as an instrument in rituals and ceremonies. The body-covering mask is said to possess tremendous power and magic which can ward off evil and natural disasters. Bali.*

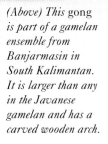

(Above) This gong *is part of a gamelan ensemble from Banjarmasin in South Kalimantan. It is larger than any in the Javanese gamelan and has a carved wooden arch.*

Temple Reliefs

The temple reliefs on Hindu–Buddhist temples in Indonesia are a very meaningful corpus of visual data that can be used to reconstruct performing arts of the 8th to 15th century, especially on the island of Java. As data they can be divided into three categories, the first being depictions of performances or scenes containing performances. This kind of relief is mainly found in Central Javanese temples, like Borobudur, Lara Jonggrang and Candi Sewu. The second group concerns theatrical conventions which are translated into many scene renderings in the reliefs. Aside from the Hindu theatrical conventions applied from the Natyasastra manuals, the narrative reliefs of Java also demonstrate the existence of original Javanese theatrical conventions analogous to that of the wayang. The last kind of data is the stories depicted which are also rendered into theatrical forms. It is assumed that the depiction of a story in a row of reliefs, especially those on the East Javanese temples, was indeed modelled after contemporary dramatic performance of the same story.

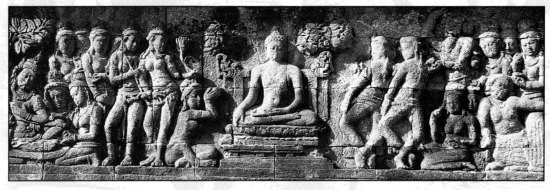

A *common feature of the temple reliefs on many Javanese temples is the rendering of scenes from stories. This relief is one of many reliefs on Borobudur (Central Java) which contain, among others, the story of Gautama before he* became Buddha. In this scene, the would-be Buddha remains deep in meditation on top of a mountain despite the lure of the seductive daughters of Mara who are sent to prevent Gautama from achieving Buddhahood.

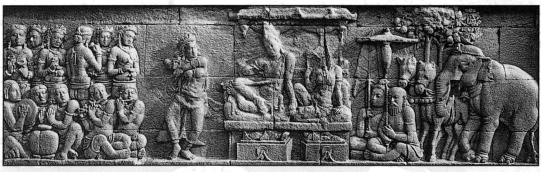

Quite a number of the narrative reliefs on Borobudur contain whole dance-poses or scenes from stories in which there is a performance of dance and music. This scene depicts a dance and music performance among high- ranking people. It is conspicuous that the dance in lofty circles depicted on the reliefs shows clear conformity to the rules of classical Indian dance expounded in the classical Hindu manual on dance and theatre.

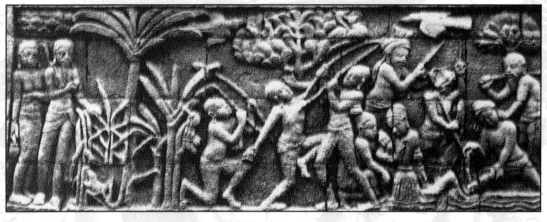

Perhaps the most significant and long-lasting influence of the Indian art of dancing is the turned-out legs in basic leg positions. This feature can be observed on these two dancing figures (left) from the Padang Lawas temples. There are also many relief panels on the balustrades of Borobudur which contain scenes which portray only dances that are not taken from any story. The above scene depicts dance among the low-ranking people.

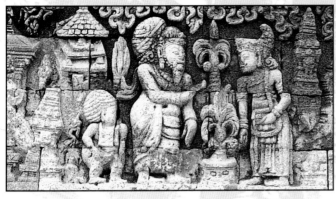

The narrative reliefs of Java demonstrate the use of original Javanese wayang *theatrical conventions in the rendering of scenes. One common convention is the use of a tree-of-life as dividing agent between scenes. Candi Tegawangi, East Java.*

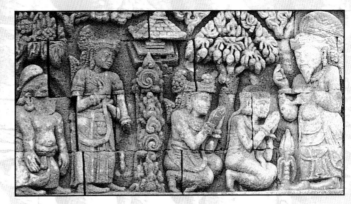

The above relief is another example of the use of the tree-of-life figure to mark a scene change. Found on Candi Tegawangi, this relief depicts a scene from the Sudamala story when Sudamala saves Parvati from assuming her demonic form as Durga.

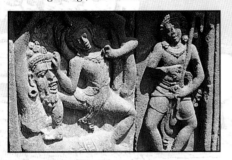

Specific gestures for specific moods prescribed in the Natyasastra are faithfully followed in many of the scenes carved in stone. These include ways to denote moods like sorrow, anger and self-esteem, as well as activities like approaching, attacking and paying homage.

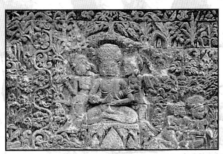

An example of reliefs depicting stories is this relief taken from Candi Surawana, East Java. The story depicted is the Arjunawiwaha. In this scene, Arjuna remained unwavering in his meditation despite the seduction of the nymphs sent by Indra to test his steadfastness.

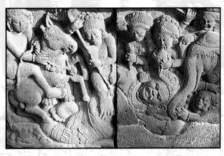

This relief is taken from the panels of Ramayana reliefs on Candi Lara Jonggrang, Prambanan, Central Java. This scene portrays the killing of Kumbakarna, the righteous brother of Rawana, the demon king, by the monkey troops led by Hanoman, the white monkey.

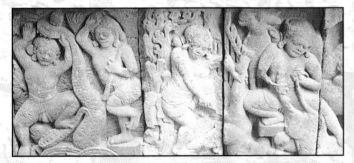

The above is another example of temple reliefs which depict a mixture of emotions such as anger and sorrow. This is a hunting or slaughtering scene in which several men are portrayed in the activity of carving up wild game. Relief from Candi Lara Jonggrang, Prambanan, Central Java.

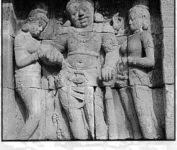

A widyadhara *and two* apsara *on the Siva temple, Candi Lara Jonggrang, Prambanan, Central Java.*

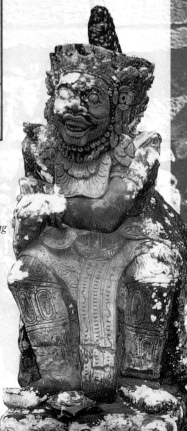

Theatrical forms and other kinds of performing arts that are popular during a certain period of time or place may sometimes be rendered in sculpture form, not just in relief. These include metal and stone sculptures of dancers and musicians. A known example is the statue of a dancer which is said to date from the early 10th century, Pura Desa, Batuan, Bali. Indonesian performing arts also develop a strong typology of characters which, though a significant departure from the Indian model of dramatic art, is a development shared by other South-east Asian theatrical traditions.

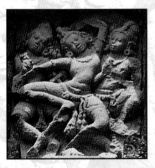

A dance scene portraying a group of three dancing apsara *from Candi Lara Jonggrang, Prambanan, Central Java.*

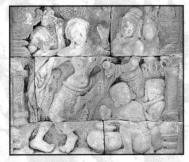

Dancer, perhaps from a high-ranking class, performing the turned-out leg style. Relief from Borobudur, Central Java.

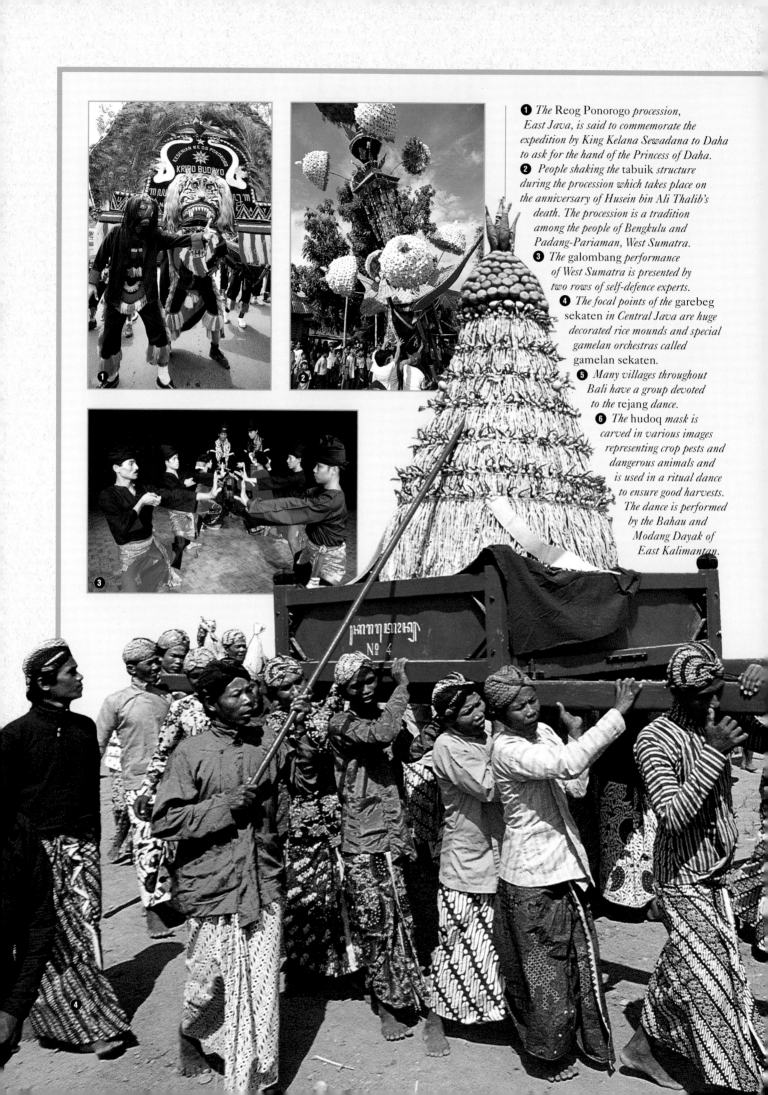

❶ *The* Reog Ponorogo *procession, East Java, is said to commemorate the expedition by King Kelana Sewadana to Daha to ask for the hand of the Princess of Daha.*

❷ *People shaking the* tabuik *structure during the procession which takes place on the anniversary of Husein bin Ali Thalib's death. The procession is a tradition among the people of Bengkulu and Padang-Pariaman, West Sumatra.*

❸ *The* galombang *performance of West Sumatra is presented by two rows of self-defence experts.*

❹ *The focal points of the* garebeg sekaten *in Central Java are huge decorated rice mounds and special gamelan orchestras called* gamelan sekaten.

❺ *Many villages throughout Bali have a group devoted to the* rejang *dance.*

❻ *The* hudoq *mask is carved in various images representing crop pests and dangerous animals and is used in a ritual dance to ensure good harvests. The dance is performed by the Bahau and Modang Dayak of East Kalimantan.*

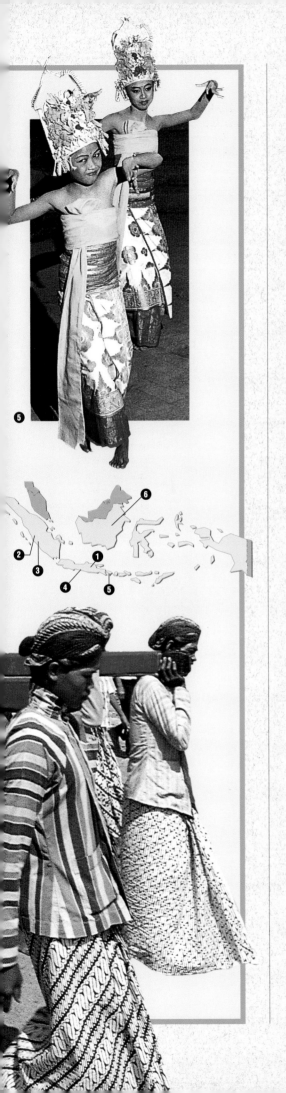

RITUAL AND PROCESSIONAL PERFORMANCES

In Indonesia, performances are often linked to ritual enactment. In some, the spirits of ancestors, deities or guardian animals take possession of human bodies and in this form, dance. In other cases, the presentation is meant to entertain spirits which have descended to Earth to join their people on some special occasion.

In the first instance, the presence of the spirits is invoked by a ritual specialist to help expel pestilence. Many of the dances performed for this purpose are native to Indonesia. Trance can be an important component: it is seen as a sign of spiritual presence. The *sanghyang* of Bali and *seblang* of East Java come under this category. *Sanghyang* performers are possessed by celestial nymphs and animal spirits whose conduct they imitate, while the *seblang* of East Java is performed as a traditional village-cleansing ritual.

Spirits of deities coming down to join a Balinese temple's anniversary celebration (*odalan*), on the other hand, enter into the bodies of wooden effigies (*pratima*); and performances of the *rejang* and *baris gede* are conducted for their entertainment, so that they will be pleased to stay a while. After the dances, the effigy is paraded in a colourful and lively procession to a bathing place some distance away for annual ritual bathing, before it is returned to the temple's innermost courtyard.

All processions have the quality of a performance. In the Javanese courts of Surakarta, Yogyakarta and Cirebon, the Prophet Muhammad's birthday is celebrated with a grand procession conveying several gigantic mounds of rice or *gunungan* to the Grand Mosque where, after prayers, they are distributed to the waiting crowd. The raucous colourful *reog ponorogo* procession in East Java is purely entertaining. The dominating feature is the heavy *dhadhakmerak* headdress, a tiger's head crowned with a huge fan of peacock feathers. The *galombang* procession greets important guests in West Sumatra. Six to twelve martial arts experts advance towards the guests in two long rows, rising and falling in wave-like movements, then part to allow the passage of a woman carrying a betel container, and two umbrella-porters. After the guest has accepted a quid of betel, the trio usher the guests into the ceremonial area.

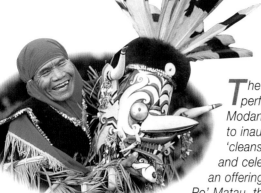

Hudoq

The hudoq is a ritual dance performed by the Bahau and Modang Dayak of East Kalimantan to inaugurate the rice-planting season, 'cleanse' the village (nguyu tahun), and celebrate harvest-time. It constitutes an offering to the rice goddess and Po' Matau, the creator of the universe. The dancers act as mediums through which prayers for a bountiful harvest and the well-being of the village, and gratitude for the harvest reaped, are conveyed.

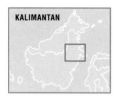

KALIMANTAN

A map showing the approximate location of the Bahau, Modang and Kenyah Dayak of Kalimantan.

(Top) A Bahau hudoq *dancer holding the mask representative of a bird pest.*

(Below) The dancers' dry banana-leaf capes swoosh as they slap their hands against their legs.

The Masks

Bahau and Modang *hudoq* dancers wear wooden masks carved in composite images of crop pests and dangerous animals. Barkcloth garments, heavily fringed with shredded banana leaves, completely cover the dancers. A feathered cap, and a wooden staff carried in the right hand, complete the costume.

Musical accompaniment is provided by gongs and the *tubun*, a small hand drum with a lizard skin (*besisi*) stretched over one end and secured with rattan binding. The dance is generally performed in a large open field by 11 dancers, each wearing a different mask. The audience encloses the dance arena.

Enactment of the Ritual

The ritual leader (*pawang*) begins by announcing the purpose of the event, followed by an invocation to the spirits to get ready to possess the dancers. Offerings are prepared for the spirits, as the *pawang* recites ritual formulae (*bememang*) before the fully costumed *hudoq* dancers.

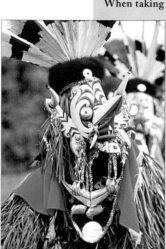

DANCE MOVEMENTS OF THE *HUDOQ*

Hand and foot movements dominate the *hudoq* dance. The body is held erect, turning slightly with each step. The arms are swung upwards to shoulder height then flung upwards, reaching as high as possible, then dropped downwards, slapping against the thighs.

Foot movements consist of stamping: with knee slightly flexed, the foot raised 30 to 40 centimetres, then stamped down forcefully to produce a sharp thudding sound. When taking a step, the raised foot is crossed over the stationary foot causing the body to sway, to the right and left. The thud of the foot followed by the slapping of hands against thighs shakes the leaf-fringed costume, making a whooshing noise. Head movements are infrequent, consisting merely of a nodding action. When the mask has a movable mouth, each nod causes it to snap shut.

The dancers move in a circle that progresses from one corner of the arena to the next until all four 'corners' have been touched. Back in the centre of the arena, they sit cross-legged (*bersila*) in a long row for the invocation, head nodding the only movement, ready to receive the possessing spirits. When this happens, they stand up, their bodies twitching, a sign that they are gradually entering a trance. They carry on the dance as already described. Finally they return to the centre, their bodies twitch again, and they sit down. The spirits have left their hosts.

Eleven dancers sit in a row in the centre of the arena. The *pawang* scatters yellow rice over their heads to signify the start of the ritual. One by one the dancers stand up and at a walking pace, in time with the music, move into a circle, arms swinging, bodies swaying, feet stamping, and then they return to the centre where the spirits possess their bodies. Once entranced, they resume dancing. The *pawang* now conveys information to the possessing spirits through endlessly recited magic formulae. The spirits are asked to nurture the plants, keep harmful pests away and protect the villagers.

The *pawang* then approaches the dancers and asks the spirits to return to their homes in the forests, mountains, four corners of the earth, caves and other places. The dancers return to the centre of the arena where they are brought back to consciousness by the *pawang*. Removing masks and costumes, they join the watching crowd. The ritual has concluded.

In another scenario, the ritual ends when two dancers wearing human masks (*hudoq punan*) suddenly appear and chase the 11 dancers out of the village, with everybody present joining in the chase. The ritual lasts between an hour and a day.

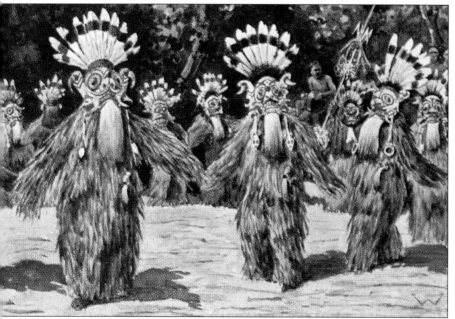

Hudoq Kita'

Hudoq kita' performances amongst the Kenyah Dayak are also related to the rice-cultivation cycle. The costume consists of a long-sleeved shirt and sarong, and a mask. Wooden masks represent human beings and are embellished with ornate curlicues and arabesques projecting from the 'ears'. They are so big that they cannot be fixed to the head, but are held by hand in front of the face. There are two kinds of masks — wooden and beaded. The two wooden masks are worn by male dancers but represent a male and a female. This pair leads the procession of dancers, with the male always in front. Only the two dancers in wooden masks go into trance. The dancers behind them wear a box-like mask that fits over the head, with a beadwork panel curtaining the face. The dancers stand in a row. These dancers represent the rice goddess.

Enactment of the Ritual

The *hudoq kita'* can be held in the yard of the longhouse, or on the long porch (*usei*). Onlookers form an enclosure in the yard or on the porch. The *pawang* enters the prepared space, to recite the magic formulae invoking the spirits. Offerings of chicken and special cakes are prepared. The *sampe'*, a three-stringed lute, is plucked and the gongs struck, producing a harmony that leads the dancers into the ritual arena. The wooden-masked dancers proceed and when they have reached the centre, the *pawang* calls for the entrance of the beaded-masked dancers.

The dancers stand in a row. As the *pawang* repeats the formulae, he touches the dancers individually and each one begins to move, following the rhythm of the *sampe'* and the gongs. The dancers continue their rhythmic movements as the *pawang* recites the messages to be conveyed to the spirits.

As their trance deepens, the pair in wooden masks move away from the others. Their movements become more assertive and agitated; hand-slapping and foot-stamping become more forceful. At the climax, music and dancing cease. The beaded-masked dancers move out to encircle those in wooden masks, where they are instructed by the *pawang* to relay the messages to the spirits possessing these

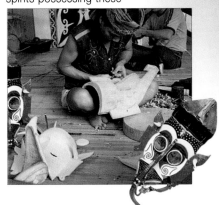

dancers. When this has been accomplished, the music recommences and the possessed dancers resume leadership of the procession.

They circle the arena several times, then line up in the centre and, continuing their rhythmic motions, sit down. The *pawang* approaches and brings the two possessed dancers back to consciousness by touching them. He then leads everybody out, one by one. When the arena is finally empty, the music stops. The ritual concludes with a communal feast.

Foot Movements

To step forward, one foot is raised a few centimetres off the ground and crossed over the other, resting momentarily on it before completing the step. In this way, the dancers shift their bodies slowly forward as the ring of dancers turn, until the wooden-masked leaders move into the centre where their foot-stamping becomes more vigorous. At this point, the *sampe'* rhythm quickens, followed by accelerated dance movements.

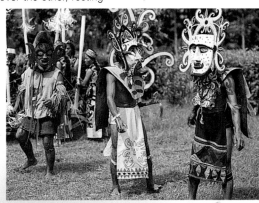

⮤Carving a hudoq *mask is one of the activities that take place on the long verandah (*usei*) of the Dayak longhouse.*

⌄The wooden masks in the hudoq kita' *represent human personalities and are decorated with ornate curlicues.*

The number of dancers in beaded masks is unlimited, the only requirements being ability and experience. They follow in single file behind the wooden-masked dancers.

HUDOQ KITA'
Movement is extremely simple. All the dancers move their heads very slightly, to the left and to the right, repeatedly. Arms are stretched forward parallel to each other, slightly bent at the elbows and slightly lower than shoulder level, moving alternately to left and right as the hands roll up and open out continuously. The torso is held erect but relaxed, and follows the direction of the foot-stamping.

The Gamelan Sekaten and Garebeg

The term sekaten *encompasses at least two related but different concepts. First, it describes festivities held annually between the fifth and twelfth days of the Javanese month of Maulud to commemorate the birthday of the prophet Muhammad. Secondly, it refers to a specific ceremonial Javanese gamelan set played at these festivities which, until the 1970s, was owned by only three royal courts: Surakarta, Yogyakarta and Cirebon (Kasepuhan).*

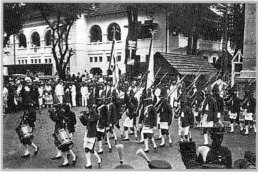

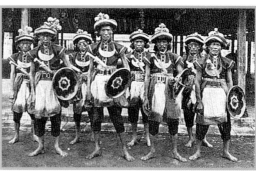

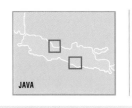

WEST AND CENTRAL JAVA

West Java
Java Sea
Cirebon ●
▲ Mount Ceremai
Danau Melahayu
▲ Mount Galunggung

Central Java
Mount Merbabu
▲
Mount Merapi ▲   Surakarta ●
Mount Lawu ▲
Yogyakarta ●

● City where Garebeg is performed   ▲ Mountain   0   20 km

Palace guards clad in traditional costumes carrying offerings to the Grand Mosque. The royal parasol is used to shelter royal regalia.

Garebeg

Garebeg is a major event involving almost all the royal family, the officials and employees of the kingdom, and the community in general. In Javanese, the word means procession, support, and an impressive and noisy event. All these are expressed in the *garebeg* ritual, which revolves around a procession of several *gunungan* (mountain-like heaps) made of rice decorated with vegetables and other foods. Hundreds of soldiers and palace employees take part in the procession, which is attended by the king and his family and watched by thousands of people.

Three kinds of *garebeg* festivities related to royal ceremonies are the *Garebeg Maulud* (marking the birth of the Prophet Muhammad), *Garebeg Syawal* (the end of the fasting month), and *Garebeg Besar* (the completion of the *haji*). Each consists of a procession that carries a pair (or its multiple) of *gunungan* from the palace to the Grand Mosque.

As the procession passes the *sitinggil* — the open pavilion where the ruler receives courtesy calls — two palace-heirloom gamelan (*Kodok Ngorek* and

Munggang) are played in its honour. Upon arrival at the mosque, prayers are said for the well-being of the community and a *selamatan* (well-wishing ritual) is held. Afterwards, everyone tries to take something from the *gunungan,* as to have a piece is believed to bring blessings.

Sekaten

The word *sekaten* is often associated with *sekati*, a measure of weight formerly used by the Javanese. It is also

(Top) The palace guards of Yogyakarta and Surakarta wear elaborate costumes in the garebeg *processions.*

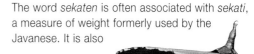

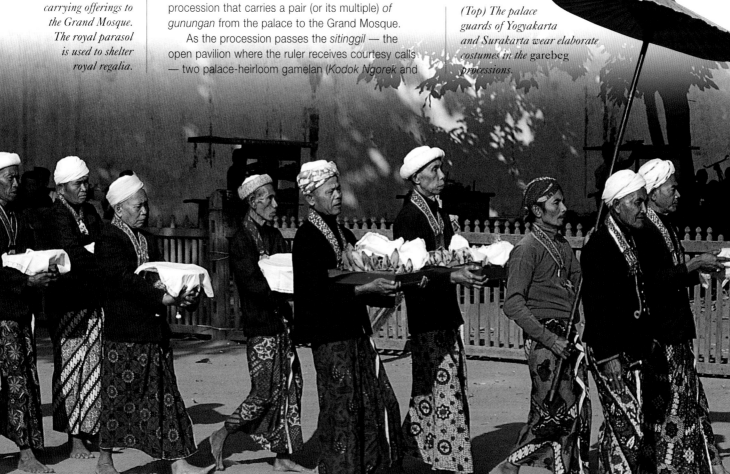

GUNUNGAN LANANG AND GUNUNGAN WADON

The *gunungan* are tokens of gratitude to God the Almighty for the abundance of food that He has bestowed upon the community. They are moulded from rice and decorated with vegetables and cakes.

The male *gunungan* or *gunungan lanang* is covered with fringes of snake beans and red chilli peppers, the top hidden under a layer of flat rice cakes that culminate in a plume of fish-shaped cakes. The more rounded female *gunungan* or *gunungan wadon* is elaborately decorated with rice cakes in a variety of shapes and colours, and bristles with bamboo skewers holding tiny cakes.

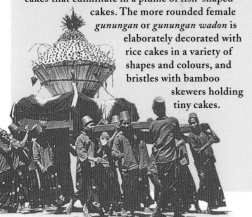

linked to *syahadatain*, meaning the two sentences of the *syahadat* or the acknowledgment of acceptance which is the primary requirement for conversion to Islam. The *gamelan sekaten* is very large and heavy, three times the size and weight of a normal Javanese gamelan.

The gamelan is seen as being part of the Hindu culture. In the transition from Hinduism to Islam in the mid-15th century, the *wali* or religious preachers cleverly used such products of the Hindu culture as means to attract people and convert them to the teachings of Islam. However, some people felt they had been coerced, and harboured a sense of *sesek ati* or resentment. Hence, the description of these gamelan as *gamelan sekati* or *sekaten*.

Gamelan Sekaten

In order to attract the people, the *gamelan sekaten* was designed to be as big and spectacular as possible, and very loud. To withstand the hard material, most hammers were made of durable material like water-buffalo horn.

The *gamelan sekaten* consists of:
● One *bonang* (set of 10 to 14 kettlegongs) played by three musicians (*pengrawit*).
● One or two pairs of *demung* (low-toned xylophones).
● Four *saron* (mid-toned xylophones) with four musicians playing the same melody.
● Two *saron panerus* (high-pitched, small *saron*), played by two musicians.
● One *bedug* (large single-headed drum) used to signal a change in tempo or speed.
● One set of *kempyang* (pairs of small kettle-gongs).
● One pair of *gong ageng* (big gongs), played by a single musician.

Repertoire

There are only three compulsory musical compositions amongst the 16 or so in the *sekaten* repertoire: *Rambu, Rangkung* and *Barang Miring*. Compositions are presented in a series (*kelompok gendhing*), each series with an opening and a closing melody. The *gamelan sekaten* uses the *gendhing ladrang* (transition melody) to move from one form of compositional structure to another.

Each presentation of *sekaten* compositions begins with a *racikan*, a melody in abstract rhythm (*balungan*), carried on by the *bonang*, with emphasis provided at certain points by the *saron*. The *racikan* is followed by a *gendhing* series presented in a normal gamelan rhythm (*dados*). Towards the end of the *gendhing* series, the tempo is accelerated, reaching a loud, fast climax (*sesek*). The presentation ends with the *suwuk*, a concluding phrase softening in tempo.

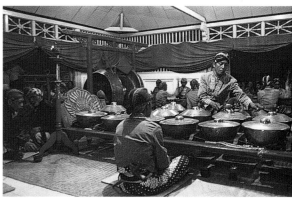

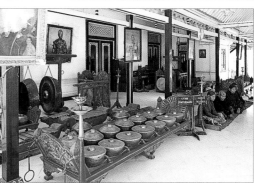

(Top and above) The palace of Yogyakarta owns two sets of gamelan sekaten, named kyahi Guntur Madu and kyahi Naga Wilaga. The gamelan sekaten set is distinguished by the larger sizes of their instruments.

PLAYING SCHEDULE OF THE *GAMELAN SEKATEN* DURING THE *GAREBEG*

	Saturday (1st day)	Sunday (2nd day)	Monday (3rd day)	Tuesday (4th day)	Wednesday (5th day)	Thursday (6th day)	Friday (7th day)
a.m.							
3 a.m.		Break	Break	Break	Break	Break	Break
6 a.m.							
Noon Prayer			**P r a y e r**				
p.m.	Gamelan A followed by Gamelan B in alternation					Break	
p.m.							

One pair of *gong ageng* (big gongs), played by a single musician.

GAMELAN SEKATEN SETS AND THEIR TONAL SYSTEMS

* = interval

	Names	Tones penunggul or bem (first-note)	*	gulu or jongga (second-note)	*	dada or tengah (third-note)	*	pelog (fourth-note)	*	lima or gangsal (fifth-note)	*	nem (sixth-note)	*	barang (seventh-note)	*
Madura	Gamelan from Sumenep now in Kedawang	244	149	266	194	297.5	116	318	204	358	175	396	171	437	191
Surakarta	Kyahi Guntur Madu (Surakarta kraton)	216	171.5	238.5	162.5	262	205.5	295	167.5	325	113.5	347	191	387.5	188
	Kyahi Guntur Sari (Surakarta kraton)	168.5	189.5	188	94	198.5	314	238	153	260	91	274	191	306	167
Yogyakarta	Kyahi Guntur Madu (Yogyakarta kraton)	201.5	63.5	209	108.5	222.5	293	263.5	117.5	292	176	316	79	338.5	302
	Kyahi Naga Wilaga (Yogyakarta kraton)	218.5	85	229.5	216	260	230.5	297	96.5	314	96.5	332	149.5	362	326
	Kyahi Munggang (Paku Alaman, Yogyakarta)	199.5	145.5	217	152.5	237	245	273	651.5	298	155.5	326	157	367	192.5
Cirebon	Sultan Anom's gamelan	262.5	158	309	180.5	343	266	400	88.5	421	134.5	455	163.5	500	208.5
	Gamelan Sekati (Kacirebonan)	292	[48]	313	[151]	314	[140]	387	[141]	420	[158]	460	[172]	508	[241]

(After Kunst, 1973)

units: cents

Wali Dances

Wali *dances are one of the most sacred of Balinese performing arts. They are all thought to be of indigenous origin, although later Hindu-Javanese elements can be seen in them, in addition to the characteristic poses, gestures and motion that make up the fundamental vocabulary of Balinese dance movement.*

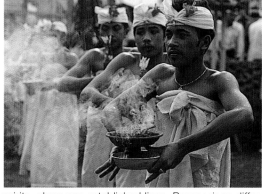

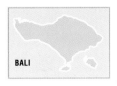

↗The memendet derives its movements and music from the baris gede *repertoire.*

Religion and Traditions

All the *wali* dances belong to the communal, village-centred aspect of Balinese culture and involve a strong element of audience participation. Trance is often present in these genres and with it, the presumption of possession by divine, and occasionally demonic, spirits. *Wali* dances are performed in connection with religious ritual, often in the context of the elaborate schedule of festivals on the Balinese religious calendar. Some are specifically associated with the traditional Bali Aga villages where many ancient Balinese traditions and practices have been maintained. All take place in the innermost courtyard of the temple.

The *Sanghyang* Dance

One of the most important genres of *wali* dances is the *sanghyang*, of which there are nearly two dozen varieties. Most are found only in remote northern and eastern mountain villages. All involve putting one or more of the dancers into trance by means of inhalation of incense smoke, and the chanting of *mantra* and prayers to enable them to receive possessing divinities (or demons). The entranced performers then interact with the audience, and sometimes with each other, dancing, mimicking animal movements and, in some localities, speaking as oracles. The performance invariably involves improvisation by the visiting

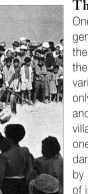

The baris gede, *also called* baris tumbak, *is a group dance performed in unison as a part of the village temple's anniversary celebration.*

spirits, along pre-established lines. Possessions differ greatly in kind and content, according to locality and the particular type of *sanghyang*. They range from the celestial nymphs of *sanghyang dedari* to the horse spirits of the *sanghyang jaran*, the boar spirits of *sanghyang celeng* and the monkey spirits of *sanghyang bojog*. All variations contain an element of ritual purification, even exorcism.

Sanghyang Dedari

Sanghyang dedari is the best known of these dances of ritual possession, and the most easily observed in Bali. The name of the dance translates roughly as 'honoured goddess nymphs' and refers to the likening of the young female dancers to the *widyadari* or demi-goddesses of Hindu mythology. Other elements of Hindu culture are difficult to trace in the genre, which is pre-eminently a product of village culture, as opposed to the sophisticated culture of the palaces.

The *sanghyang dedari* dancers are chosen from a special group of preadolescent girls of ages between 9 and 13 years old. The girls have special duties in the temple and tend to come from the priests' families.

In the past, *sanghyang* was always staged during the 'danger months', that is the fifth and sixth months of the Balinese calendar. Today, some villagers stage secular versions for tourists.

Most importantly, the *sanghyang* has been a source of inspiration for local artists in creating new dances. One famous example, the *legong* dance, has now become an important tourist attraction.

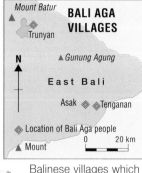

Mount Batur — **BALI AGA VILLAGES** — Trunyan — N — ▲ Gunung Agung — East Bali — Asak ◇ ◇Tenganan — ◇ Location of Bali Aga people — ▲ Mount — 0 — 20 km

Rejang Dance

Another ancient *wali* dance is the formal *rejang*. It can still be seen in many Balinese villages which have a group devoted to it. Although one of the simplest Balinese

The rejang *is of ancient origin, and amongst the Bali Aga, who retain a pre-Hindu way of life, is performed by young girls. These girls are from Bungaya, near Asak.*

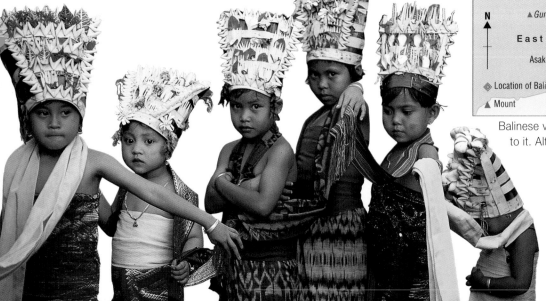

dances, the *rejang* possesses a particularly distinctive dignity and elegance. As a processional group dance, it is performed by female members of the temple congregation, and never professionally. In most villages, women of all ages take part, but in the more traditional Bali Aga villages of Tenganan and Asak in Karangasem regency, the dancers are children and teenagers.

All *rejang* dancers are dressed in formal Balinese costume, with *anteng* (breastcloth) and an elaborate headdress consisting of a gold wire frame to which are attached scores of fresh, sweet-smelling flowers. Performances are usually accompanied by the sacred heptatonic *gamelan slonding*.

Baris Gede

The *baris gede* is performed by the adult males of the village during their temple's anniversary celebration. The dancers are looked upon as the bodyguards of the visiting deities who reside for the duration in the *pratima* (effigy). They carry sacred heirloom weapons: spears, lances, shields, daggers and in some villages, vintage rifles. Each type of *baris* is named after the weapon used.

A *baris* group varies depending on the custom of the village and the number and kinds of weapons available in the village repository. The usual costume consists of a triangular headdress (*gelungan*), an apron of wide ribbons hanging from the breast (*awiran*), beautiful leggings wrapped around from knee to ankle, a lance (*tumbak*) and a dagger (*keris*) inserted into the breastband at the back. The performance is generally accompanied by the large *gong gede* ensemble.

Baris Pendet, Gabor and Mendet

The *baris pendet* is similar to the *baris gede*. Eight men, or sometimes the priests themselves, perform simple steps taken from the *baris gede* repertoire. The dance can be seen at temple festivals in Sebatu village, Gianyar

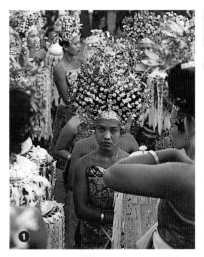

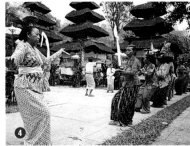

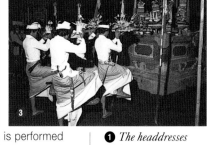

regency. Another variation, the *mendet,* is performed by a group of adult men from the temple congregation or, infrequently, by the *pemangku* or the lower-caste priests. The dancers wear their regular temple costumes but without shirts and they usually carry offerings meant for the deities. The *mendet* is a complementary dance to the *gabor*. In some areas these dances are performed in a state of trance.

The *gabor* is an elaborate dance in which groups of female dancers, usually between two and ten women, present offerings to residing deities in the *pratima*. The dance is performed as part of the celebrations in the evening of the *odalan*. The dancers are taken from the *rejang* group.

❶ *The headdresses of the Asak* rejang *dancers are adorned with golden flowers.*
❷ *The costumes of the* baris tumbak *become more elaborate with time.*
❸ *The* mendet *is performed by four men carrying ritual vessels.*
❹ *The* gabor *dance is complementary to the* baris pendet.

»*The* sanghyang dedari *dancer goes into a trance after inhaling incense smoke.*

WALI DANCES AND THEIR FEATURES

Name	occasion for holding performance	function	number of members	age group	location of dance within temple's precincts	time of day
Sanghyang Dedari	During epidemics, every fifth or 15th day of the month or holy day	To ward off disease, impending disasters or evil	Four to five preadolescent girls	Girls between nine and 12 years old	Performance begins in the *jeroan*, most holy courtyard of the temple	Usually at night
Rejang	During temple festivals	Celebrations or to ward off possible epidemics in the village	40 to 60	Women of all ages (but in Bali Aga villages, only young girls and women of the village)	Performance begins in less sacred section of the temple and is mainly conducted within the *jeroan*	Daytime, around the early afternoon
Baris Gede	During temple festivals such as the *odalan* or anniversary of temple-founding day	Celebrations	Varies from four to several dozen men usually carrying some kind of weaponry	Adult men	Performers enter from the south into the *jeroan* where the main performance is held	Afternoon, usually right after the *rejang* performance
Baris Pendet	During temple festivals	Celebrations	Eight men carrying ritual vessels filled with flowers or offerings	Adult men	Pairs of dancers dance their way to the *pelinggih* or main shrine where the offerings are laid down	Daytime

(After I Made Bandem & deBoer, 1995)

The Seblang and Gandrung of Banyuwangi

Seblang *and* gandrung *are two traditional dance performances found in the region of Banyuwangi on the eastern end of Java.* Seblang *is a ritual dance of a sacred nature, while* gandrung *is secular and social.* Seblang *is found solely in the two villages of Bakungan and Olihsari, and is considered to be the source of the less sacred* gandrung*. The* gandrung*, which has spread to almost all corners of Banyuwangi, has developed into a creative dance.*

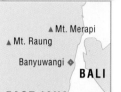

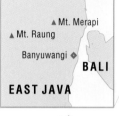

A *Sakti* Dance

Seblang is a ritual dance which is presented differently in Bakungan and Olihsari. In Bakungan, the principal dancer is a post-menopausal woman, while in Olihsari, she is a pre-pubescent girl. The movements of the dance are based on the most fundamental rhythmical power known as *sakti*. When the dancer is in a subliminal state, this natural rhythm comes to the fore. The *seblang* dancer performs in a state of trance or *kejiman*. This leads people to believe that the dance is part of the heritage of ancient worship to the gods.

Three key roles in the *seblang* are closely linked to the presence of ancestral spirits and the mythology of the supernatural world.

• *Kejiman:* The *seblang* dancer is a medium for ancestor spirits and angels. In Bakungan, the role of the dancer continues for a lifetime, and is handed down by descent. In Olihsari, a dancer performs for three years, and is selected on the basis of mystical guidance through the village elders. Without any prior training, the *seblang* dancer is able to dance graciously by the power of the spirit entering into her. Incense is burned and *mantra* or magic formulae are chanted to invoke the presence of the spirit. As the dancer falls into a trance, women begin to sing songs accompanied by the gamelan musicians (*panjak*).

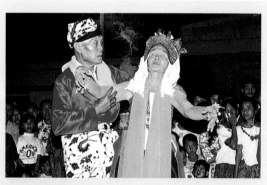

SEBLANG DANCER
The dancer wears a crown (*omprok*). In Bakungan, the *omprok* is made of fringed white cloth, while in Olihsari it is made from young banana leaves shredded into a thick fringe. A colourful arrangement of fresh flowers decorates the top of the crown.

The *seblang* in Olihsari is usually danced by a girl in her preadolescence as depicted on the left here, and in Bakungan, by a post-menopausal woman, above.

STAGE AREA
The *seblang* is performed in an open area, around a central pole with a canopy of white cloth called *payung agung* (umbrella-of-honour). An altar for offerings is set up on one side, facing the direction of the sunrise. A traditional orchestra of local musical instruments is placed at the left side of the altar or in the middle of the arena.

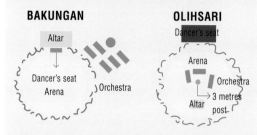

BAKUNGAN
Altar
Dancer's seat
Arena
Orchestra

OLIHSARI
Dancer's seat
Arena
Orchestra
3 metres
Altar
post

Aspects of Presentation	*Bakungan*	*Olihsari*
Dancer	old lady	young lady
Instruments	more complete	simple
Position of instruments	edge of arena	middle of arena
Singer	one person	4-6 women
Time of performance	afternoon	daytime
Month of performance	month of Besar	after Idul Fitri
Dancer's crown	made of cloth	banana leaves
Function	village cleansing	village cleansing

Assisted by an elderly woman (*pengudang*), the dancer moves to the rhythm and theme of the music and songs. The audience participates in the dancing and singing of the performance at every opportunity.

• *Ratu Sabrang*: In this part of the performance, the *seblang* dancer throws one end of her scarf in the direction of male onlookers, young men in particular. Whoever is touched by the scarf is obliged to come forward and dance with her. A song entitled *Ratu Sabrang*, which describes the bestowing of blessing by the goddess of fertility (Dewi Sri), accompanies the dancing. This act symbolises the hope that the seed selected for the fertile earth will be premium, to ensure a good harvest. The involvement of male dancers became so popular that this part of the dance was developed into the secular performance known as *gandrung*.

• *Adol Kembang:* The sale of flowers (*adol kembang*) by the *seblang* dancer, and the race at the end of the performance to get some of the flower-scented water (*toya arum*) left over from washing the dancer's face, reflect the blessings of the ancestors that bestow safety, well-being, protection and assistance. Three-pronged sticks with a differently coloured flower on each prong (*kembang telon*), referred to as *kembang dirma*, are exchanged for a contribution (*dirma*) of money by any of the spectators lucky enough to get one. The sum of money paid is voluntary; the flowers bring luck. The accompanying song is also entitled *Kembang Dirma*.

Presentation of the *Seblang*
The *seblang* is performed as a village purification (*bersih desa*) rite or a spiritual act asking for safety and well-being for the village. It is sometimes also held in gratitude for the fulfilment of a wish, such

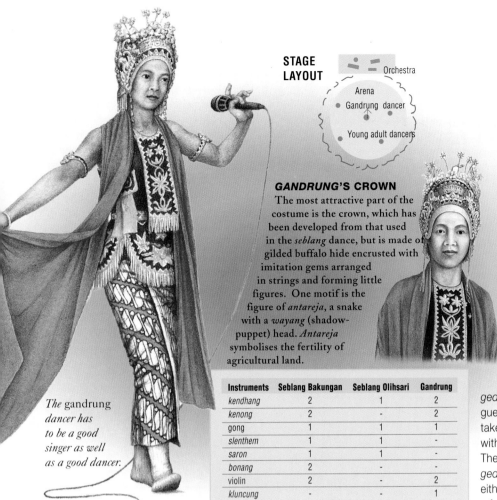

STAGE LAYOUT

Orchestra

Arena

Gandrung dancer

Young adult dancers

GANDRUNG'S CROWN

The most attractive part of the costume is the crown, which has been developed from that used in the *seblang* dance, but is made of gilded buffalo hide encrusted with imitation gems arranged in strings and forming little figures. One motif is the figure of *antareja*, a snake with a *wayang* (shadow-puppet) head. *Antareja* symbolises the fertility of agricultural land.

The gandrung *dancer has to be a good singer as well as a good dancer.*

Instruments	Seblang Bakungan	Seblang Olihsari	Gandrung
kendhang	2	1	2
kenong	2	-	2
gong	1	1	1
slenthem	1	1	-
saron	1	1	-
bonang	2	-	-
violin	2	-	2
kluncung	-	-	1

as recovery from an illness. In Bakungan, it is held in the middle of the Javanese month of Besar during the afternoon. In the village of Olihsari, the *seblang* takes place during the day until twilight during the seven days following the Idul Fitri holiday.

The *Gandrung* as a Social Dance

The *gandrung* is performed by a female dancer, also called *gandrung*, together with one to four male dancers (*pemaju*). It is very popular with the people of Banyuwangi and is staged at almost every festive event including weddings and circumcisions. The stage for the performance can be an arena, the yard, or a small platform.

Three important parts in the performance are:
- *Jejer*: The *gandrung* performs a series of movements interspersed with the singing of the song, *Padha Nonton*, playing with one or two fans in gestures of welcome (*panembrama*) as an invitation to the guests to be seated on the chairs provided. After having danced for some time, the *gandrung* sits down, but continues to entertain the guests with her song.
- *Maju Gandrung*: This part is apparently derived from the *Ratu Sabrang* dance of the *seblang* ritual performance. Led by a dancer called the *tukang*

gedhog, the guests prepare to take turns dancing with the *gandrung*. The *tukang gedhog* can be either a male or a female dancer who is well acquainted with the method of selecting guests. The male guests who dance (*pemaju*) are given the opportunity to select the kind of music they want by paying a sum of money to the *kendhang*-drummer, *pengendhang*, and by giving a tip to the *gandrung*. The *kluncing*-player, *tukang kluncing* (*kluncing* is two metal bars which are struck together to produce music; it is sometimes replaced with the triangle), directs the entire performance by gesture and song, as well as making comments to keep the atmosphere lively.
- *Seblang Subuh*: When all the guests have had their turns as *pemaju* and dawn (*subuh*) is imminent, the *gandrung* closes the programme with a dance and song entitled *Seblang Subuh*. The lyrics indicate that she must say good-bye and part with her admirers. Several songs are performed during this finale.

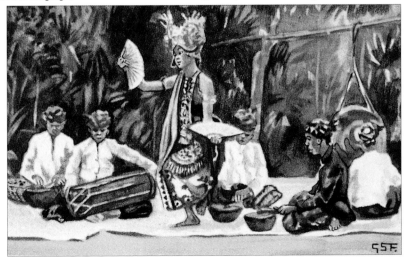

(Top) The gandrung *dancer of Banyuwangi chooses her partner by throwing one end of her scarf at a male guest. He pays a small tip for the privilege of dancing with her. The* gandrung *is derived from the more ancient and very ritualistic* seblang.

(Above) Basic movements of the jejer *that welcomes the guests to a* gandrung *Banyuwangi performance, demonstrated by an elderly master of the art.*

⌐⌐*The table shows that two violins, two* kendhang *(two-headed asymmetrical drum), a gong, two* kenong *(large kettle gong) and the* kluncing *are used to accompany the* gandrung *dance.*

«*The* gandrung *Banyuwangi is a flirting dance; the trick is for the man to get as close as possible to his partner without actually touching her, which is forbidden.*

Reog Ponorogo

*T*he reog ponorogo *is a form of popular theatre in the dance-drama category native to, or characteristic of, the Ponorogo district of East Java. It appears in all important events, such as weddings, circumcisions and commemorations of important days or festivities of a public nature.*

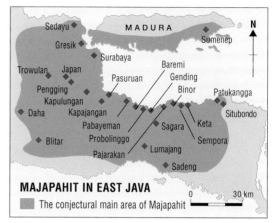

MAJAPAHIT IN EAST JAVA

The conjectural main area of Majapahit

0   30 km

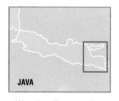

JAVA

Wengker (Ponorogo) was a dependency of 14th-century kingdom, Majapahit. This map shows the Majapahit's power centre.

» *The* singabarong *figure changes with time.*

ᴊᴊᴊ *A young woman sits enthroned on the* singabarong*'s head.*

(Below) Visnu on the shoulders of Garuda who is carrying the elixir of immortality.

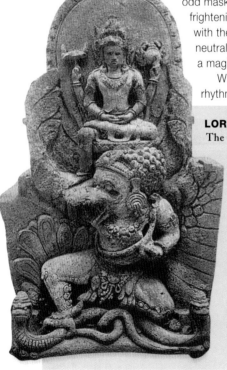

The Story

Kelana Sewandana, King of Bantarangin, sent his vizier, Bujangga Anom, to request the hand of Princess Dewi Sanggalangit of Daha. Bujangga Anom set out with a small armed escort. At the border, they were held up by an army of tigers and peacocks, subjects of King Singabarong who ruled this dense jungle. The two forces clashed; Bujangga Anom and his men were routed. Enraged, Kelana Sewandana led a bigger cavalry and infantry to avenge the insult. At the climax of the ensuing battle, when Sewandana appeared to be winning, King Singabarong advanced to challenge Sewandana to a duel. The lion (*singa*) or tiger-like Singabarong was accompanied by King Merak (peacock) perched arrogantly on his head, iridescent green tail-feathers spread wide in a threatening stance. The *singa* and *merak* soon defeated Sewandana.

Sewandana withdrew into meditation and his spiritual mentor soon materialised to tell him how to defeat Singabarong. Singabarong was to be baited with the beating of metal xylophones and a crowd of people dancing comically and wearing odd masks that were simultaneously funny and frightening. The two would be so carried away with the merry-making that they could be easily neutralised with a lash of *gendir wuluh gadhing*, a magic whip which he presented to Sewandana.

While the soldiers beat out a cacophonic rhythm on the instruments they had on hand (kettlegongs, suspended gongs, *selompret*, trumpet, and a great deal of clamourous shouting), the masked Bujangga Anom with the help of two officers wearing similar clownish attire drew Singabarong and Merak into the fun with his comical antics. The whip lashed out, and Singabarong and Merak were rendered powerless to withstand the assault that followed. In the end, the two begged forgiveness and the restoration of their powers, promising to do whatever Kelana Sewandana asked. Another lash of the magic whip and their power was restored, the battle ceased, and the entire entourage fell in behind Sewandana who then continued his journey to Daha.

All that remains of the drama today is this final procession to Daha, acting as a sort of mnemonic device to aid recollection of a memorised story.

The *Singabarong* mask

The most spectacular characteristic of the *reog ponorogo,* however, is without a doubt the '*barong*'. Representing the main character of the story, the huge tiger mask is brightly-coloured and eye-catching with its *dhadhakmerak* crown which can weigh from 30 to 50 and even 60 kilogrammes.

LORE ON REOG'S HISTORICAL BACKGROUND

The *reog ponorogo* is believed to have had its origins in a ritual invoking the protection of the local spiritual power, and the tiger (*singa*), which with the peacock (*merak*) was common to the thickly forested Ponorogo region in those days, was seen as the manifestation of that power. This story says that with time the 'wildlife' aspect became separated from the ritual, evolving into a form of entertainment, and in the 14th century became the perfect vehicle for commemorating a moment of great heroism.

Ponorogo is the name given to the East Javanese kingdom of Wengker in the late 15th century to mark its conversion to Islam; the *singabarong* peacock holds a pearl in its beak, symbolic of the prayer-beads used by Muslims. It is surmised that King Wijayarasa of Wengker wished to dramatise a heroic moment in history, and that the unusual *singabarong* figure resembles an unusual statue in the Belahan temple complex on nearby Mount Penanggungan dating from the reign of Airlangga of Kahuripan. This statue portrays the Hindu god Visnu standing on the shoulders of an erect Garuda with the bird's tail-feathers spread out behind.

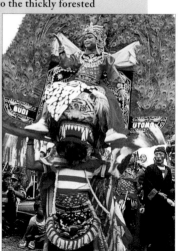

CHARACTERS AND MUSIC IN THE *REOG PONOROGO*

The central figure of the *reog ponorogo* is the *singabarong*, which is a composite of the tiger (head-mask) and peacock (crown). These two animals were once common to the Ponorogo region and perceived as living in tolerance of each other in reality; and in the *reog* theatre, they are also seen as working together to defend their territory. The *singabarong* dancer must be a very strong man, since he has to carry the weight of the heavy head-covering mask and a very tall crown of peacock feathers (*dhadhakmerak*) with his teeth or jaws. On the feathered crown sits enthroned a young man of slight frame.

The procession is led by a troop of cavalry who progress in two by two formation, like army scouts opening the road. Astride large hobbyhorses (*jathilan*) 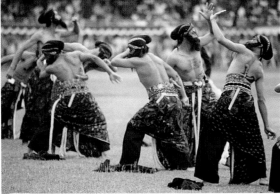 made of bamboo matting, the men clad in black costumes imitate the movements of horse-riders that are war-like and yet femininely graceful (*medoki*). Bujangga Anom, also popularly known as Bujangganong, follows with his clown-like dancing and the fearsome yet amusing countenance of his red mask, eyes bulging, nose as long as a boat's prow, thick moustache, and a mass of tangled locks as hair. *Singabarong* sways ponderously yet gracefully behind. A dashing Kelana Sewandana struts proudly behind *singabarong*, sporting kingly attire and a pretty red mask.

The musicians bring up the rear, the *kendhang* player first, carrying his instrument against his abdomen. The *ketimpung* player comes next, beating out a monotonous rhythm (*irama ajeg*) on his small drum. Behind come the *selompret* player, a *kethuk* player and a *kenong* player; then two *angklung* players flanking the *kempul* that is carried by two persons walking one in front of the other.

The loudness of the *reog ponorogo* can be heard from afar. The steady and resolute beating of the *kendhang* accompanied by the rhythms of the various metal xylophones and bamboo *angklung* and the melody-carrying trumpet make the music of the *reog* gamelan exceptional. Even more unique is that the *slendro*-tuned *kethuk*, *kenong* and *kempul* are blended with the *pelog*-tuned *selompret* producing a strange and enthralling sound that fills the air with a magical feeling — a *déja vu* of a legendary experience taken from time immemorial.

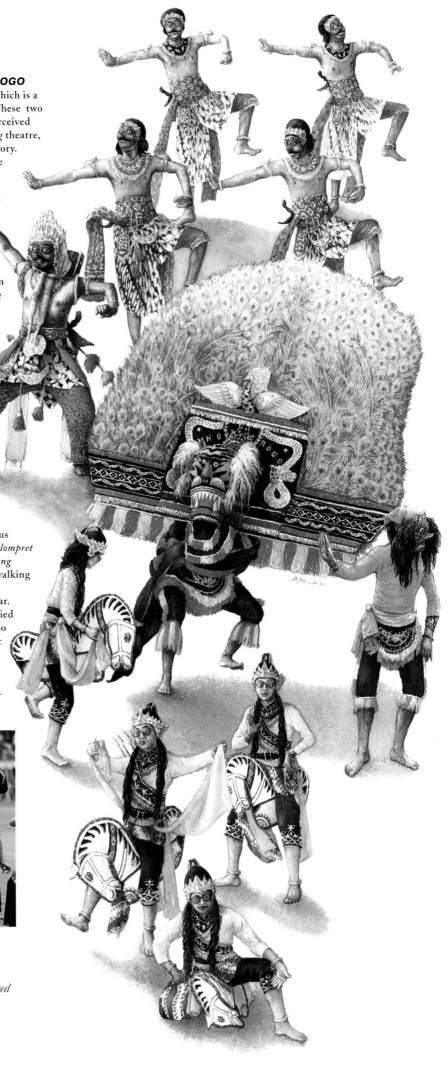

(Top) The handsome King Kelana Sewandana leading his men in their march towards the battle with singabarong.

(Above) The followers of singabarong *immersing themselves in the music and merry-making initiated by Kelana's soldiers.*

Galombang

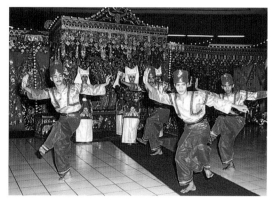

*A*lmost every Minangkabau nagari *(a political as well as territorial unit)* and urban community in West Sumatra has some sort of cultural performance dedicated to honouring important guests. Some take place as the guests are about to enter the location of the event to which they have been invited, others when they have taken their places inside. The principal element in the display is the 'art of movement' carried out to the accompaniment of music bun(ny)i-bun(ny)ian.

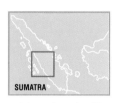

SUMATRA

》A modern-day West Sumatran wedding, showing that the galombang *continues to have a role in ceremonial life. Behind the welcoming dancers is the bridal pavilion, resplendent in gold-embroidered and sequinned velvet hangings.*

》A West Sumatran sirih *set which is often used in the* galombang *dance.*

The penghulu, *who is marked by a special heirloom scarf around his neck, accepts a quid of betel as a sign of not only his good intentions but also his appreciation for the honour being shown him.*

Galombang Performance in Minangkabau

While the art form itself is called galombang or tari galombang (tari=dance), its actual performance is known as bagalombang or main galombang (ba=the act of doing; main=play, perform). Conventionally speaking, the galombang is a symbolic demonstration of welcome for visiting personages commensurate with their status. The word galombang also refers to a series of movements made by randai actor-dancers in a circle resembling the rise and fall of ocean waves (galombang). (Randai is a local form of folk theatre in which the story is enacted through dance and narration).

The galombang takes place just before the guests enter the site. After they are seated, further honour may be shown with the performance of the tari pasambahan. The pasambahan (offering or salute) is an urban phenomenon introduced fairly recently into the Minangkabau dance repertoire. Created by a choreographer in the modern Western sense, it comes under the category of 'recreational dance'.

The galombang performance was a part of Minangkabau culture long before the birth of the independent Republic of Indonesia (17 August 1945). Closely related to the governmental structure established by Minangkabau's first ruler, Adityavarman (AD1347-1375), it evolved into a deeply embedded constituent of Minangkabau

tradition, performed to greet such personages as visiting nagari chiefs (penghulu).

The government of early days comprised the ruler and his penghulus, and an administrative apparatus. They constituted the community's most important people. Conceptually speaking, the king was head of the Minangkabau world, while each penghulu headed either a nagari (penghulu pucuk) or an individual matrilineage within a nagari (penghulu suku). Within the confines of his own nagari, the penghulu pucuk, was perceived as ruler or 'king' since the nagari had autonomous status within the greater kingdom of Minangkabau. This is reflected in the saying: adat salingka nagari, cupak sapanjang batuang (tradition encloses the nagari, a cupak spans an internode of bamboo): the validity of a regulation extends as far as the boundaries of the nagari. The law of one nagari can be very different from that of another. The institutionalisation of the welcoming dance tradition for honouring guests indicates a close relationship between the tradition and the administrative system.

Form and Implementation of Performance

The galombang performance requires considerable skill to carry out the movements according to local aesthetic standards.

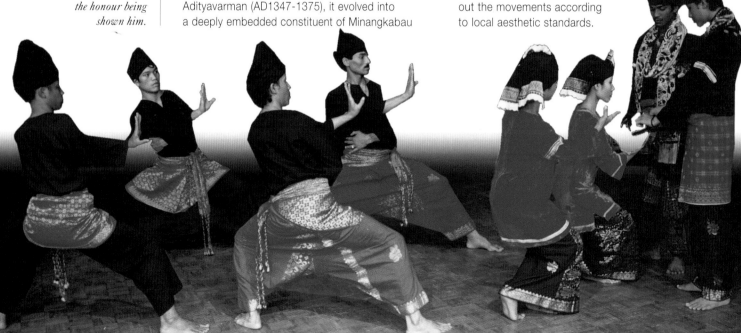

Six to 12 dancers align themselves in two long rows along the path leading to the site at which the event will take place, facing the direction from which the guests will arrive. One person is assigned to offer *sirih-pinang* (betel quid) in a ceremonial *sirih* container to the principal guest-of-honour, and one or two others to usher the guest to his seat. The musical accompaniment consists of a *gendang* (double-headed drum), *talempong* (set of kettle gongs), and *puput* (either *sarunai* [flute], *pupuik gadang* [large double reed], or *pupuik tingkolong* [ricestalk reed with *tingkolong*-leaf cone at the end]).

As the guests approach the site, they are greeted by the *galombang* dancers who move slowly and dramatically towards them, performing a series of movements that produce the effect of rising and falling waves. They stop at a distance of two to three metres from the guests. *Sirih-pinang* is offered (it is obligatory that guests take some) and the double file of dancers separates to allow the guests to pass through their ranks to the site of the main event.

The general concept of the *galombang* performance is more or less the same in all Minangkabau social units. However, variations can be discerned from *nagari* to *nagari* in both form and sequence of movement.

Galombang Performance in Pariaman

There is a host and a guest *galombang* in Pariaman. Both go into action when the guests approach the site. The host *galombang* begins; the guest *galombang* follows shortly afterwards. The two generally have an equal number of men, arranged in two pairs of rows facing each other. In front of each group is the *tukang aliah* who leads the *silek* movements.

The two groups progress towards each other in the synchronised wave-like movement of the *galombang*. When they come face-to-face, each puts on a special display of its prowess in the martial arts. As things can sometimes get out-of-hand, an arbiter, *janang*, stands ready with a *sirih* container. The moment a real fight seems imminent, he thrusts the *sirih* container between the two parties. Brought to their senses, the two *tukang aliah* salute each other under the *sirih* container held aloft by the *janang*. Each then places a red, yellow and black banner, *merawa*, across the top of the *sirih* container. In Pariaman, this signifies forgiveness and continued friendship between the two groups. Should the fight not be stopped, it continues to the beating of the *gandang tambua* (single-headed hand drum) until winner and loser emerge.

After the two parties separate or are separated, they reassemble into two long lines facing each other. Down this aisle, the host advances to fetch the guests and escort them to their places. In Pariaman, performances usually take place as a part of traditional festivities, particularly those related to the installation of a 'ruler' or *penghulu*.

Galombang Dua Baleh

One style of galombang is the *galombang dua baleh* which was created by a martial arts expert by the

MOVEMENTS IN THE *GALOMBANG*

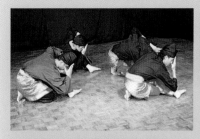
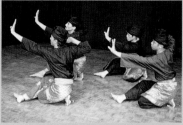
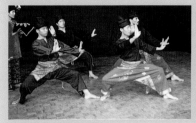
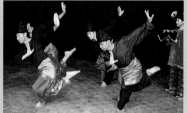

Movements are generally extracted from the local art of self-defence (*silek*), on aesthetic considerations alone. There are, in fact, three conceptual sources of movement: *silek*, nature, and symbolism. Synchronisation is controlled by a principal performer, *tukang aliah*, who calls the changes. Performers are traditionally men, who are dressed in all black loose low-crotched pants (*galembong*), loose shirt and headcloth.

name of Pandeka Tangguak in 1926. The dance was initially performed by 12 male dancers but in recent times, it can be performed by both male and female dancers.

Urban *Galombang* Performances

Variations have become more evident with urban development in West Sumatra, especially with the involvement of arts institutions as well as creative individuals. Today, modification, re-arrangement and re-creation tend to be in the hands of a single individual, as opposed to the consensus of local traditions through which the *galombang* originally developed. New sources of movement have been found in the martial arts, such as the *tari piring* (plate dance). Female performers have been introduced. A group of three women often adds elegance to the performance: one carries the *sirih* container, flanked by the other two. Behind are three men, the one in the middle carrying a yellow parasol-of-honour to shelter the *sirih* bearer. This group is positioned in the middle of the two rows of *galombang* dancers as they move towards the guests. All the performers are clothed in specific regional costume that may have been modified by the choreographer. The music may also have been reworked to conform to new concepts of harmony. This performance is called the *tari galombang* (galombang dance), to distinguish it from the traditional *galombang*. The *tari galombang* escorts the guests to their places, at which point it ends.

The movements of West Sumatran dance are sharp, forceful and definitive like those of self-defence, silek.

Tabuik

*T*he Tabuik or Tabot *is a 'miracle play' type of ritual, re-enacting the circumstances around and lamenting the death of Husein bin Abu Thalib, grandson of the Prophet Muhammad, on the battlefield at Karbala in present-day Iraq, on the 10th of Muharram in the Muslim year of 61 Hegira (AD 680). Husein died defending his hereditary right to the Shi'ah caliphate which had been seized by King Yazid of the Bani Ummayah. He was beheaded and his body chopped to pieces by Yazid's troops; his death was long mourned by the Shi'ah Muslims.*

'Fingered' poles symbolise Husein's dismembered body. As they are paraded through town, the citizens give contributions of cash and rice that will go to the needy.

(Below) The towering tabuik *structure being carried by the parade-attendants.*

The Re-enactment of Husein's Death

The *Tabuik* form of commemoration is a tradition of Bengkulu, Pariaman and Padang on the west coast of Sumatra where towering paper-and-bamboo structures representing Husein's funeral bier are paraded through town and discarded into the sea or river. This annual event takes place on the anniversary of Husein's death. The Muslim lunar year is shorter than the solar year, so the celebration advances a few days every year.

Husein's death gave rise to mythical stories in which the Shi'ah still believe. It is said that after his death, his body was miraculously flown to God in heaven on a female-headed winged-horse creature known as *buraq*, on the back of which it had been placed by a flock of angels. This event was reportedly witnessed by a Shi'ah follower who came from Cipei (Sipahi, Sepoy) in Bengal, India. Bengali Shi'ah have been visiting Indonesia's shores for many centuries, first as traders, but later as soldiers sent to

MUSICAL INSTRUMENTS

From the 1st to 4th Muharram in every *tabuik* location, the loud treble of the *dol* and *tasa* drums can be heard in the distance. The *dol* is a big hemispherical drum with a body frame made from the coconut stem or jackfruit tree trunk and covered with cowhide. The diameter of its beating surface is approximately 40 to 55 centimetres. The *tasa* is a smaller drum shaped like a shallow bowl. On the night of the 8th Muharram, a dance is performed accompanied by the playing of the *dol* and *tasa* drums and the *suling* or flute. The name of the dance is *tari uli*.

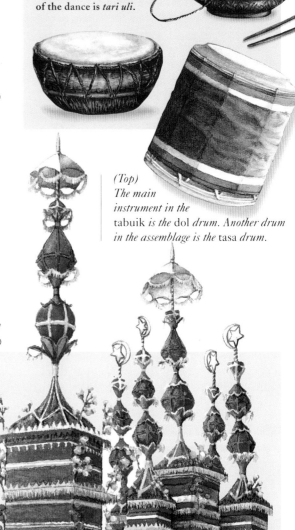

(Top) The main instrument in the tabuik *is the* dol *drum. Another drum in the assemblage is the* tasa *drum.*

TABUIK STRUCTURES

The *tabuik* can consist of two to five levels with an estimated height of 6 to 15 metres. However most have only two to three levels with a height of approximately six metres.

The body of the *tabuik* is made from bamboo framework and the stems of sago palms and wrapped around with colourful papers. The structure is further decorated with various kinds of coloured paper flowers.

A contest is held to determine which is the best *tabuik* tower built for the procession.

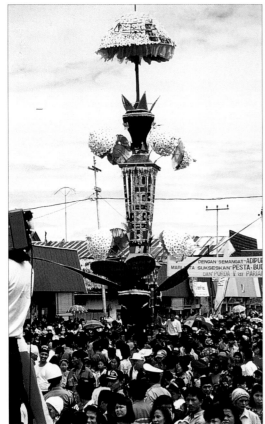

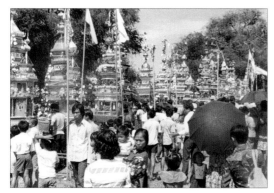

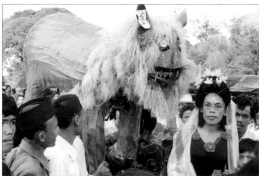

		ACTIVITIES	MUSICAL ACCOMPANIMENTS	REPRESENTATION
1 MUHARRAM	*Ma-ambiak tanah*	**Afternoon,** a final meeting held to ensure that preparations for making *tabuik* are complete. **Before 12.00 a.m.,** the tower-makers head for the nearby river where a lump of soil will be collected from the bottom. **12.00 a.m,** white incense is burned and the *dukun* prays. The soil is put in a pot, wrapped with white cloth and placed in the small tomb-like *daraga*.	The procession is accompanied by *gendang dol* and *tasa* drummers. The *gendang dol* is a large double-headed drum with cowhide membranes and is carried suspended from the shoulders by a rope. The *tasa* is a single-headed ceramic drum with a sheepskin or cowhide membrane; it hangs from the neck of the player.	The shrouded pot of earth in the *daraga* enclosure is Husein's tomb. The *daraga* enclosure itself suggests a camp or resting place for soldiers after battle or between battles.
5–6 MUHARRAM	*Manabeh batang pisang*	Several banana boles are cleanly severed from their roots with one blow of a very sharp sword, *jenawi*. Following evening players, the boles are slashed repeatedly as they are paraded through town.		Like soldiers in battle, they hack at the banana trunks with vigour, re-enacting the violent battle between Husein's followers and Yazid's troops on Karbala Plain.
7 MUHARRAM	*Mahatam*	Finger-like objects are carried high in a procession through the town, that moves slowly and solemnly like a funeral procession.	The *dol* and *tasa* drums are beaten very slowly, setting the mournful pace; this is called the *mahatam* melody.	They represent Husein's severed fingers but some say they refer to Husein's skill in handling a sword in battle.
8 MUHARRAM	*Ma-arak saroban*	The turban-parading takes place. A cloth symbolising Husein's turban is paraded through the village, borne in a wooden box (*panja*). The procession begins at midday and continues well into the night.		The purpose is to arouse sentiments that will ennoble the soul and encourage the defence of justice, as represented by Husein's fight to defend his heritage.
9–10 MUHARRAM	*Ma-oyak tabuik*	The *tabuik* is finished. It has been constructed in two separate parts, 'head' and 'body'. **4.00 a.m.** on the next day, the two are joined, and topped with Husein's 'turban'. The joining is termed *tabuik naik pangkek*, which means 'promoted' to a higher status or class. The completed funerary tower is paraded by a huge crowd who knock and shake it as they pull it here and there.	The procession is accompanied by the enthusiastic beating of the *gendang dol* and *tasa* and the endless shouting of Husein's name.	It is the re-enactment of Husein's ascension on the back of the *buraq*.

defend British holdings, particularly in Bengkulu. From here they spread northwards to other British holdings in Pariaman and Padang, West Sumatra, where the commemoration of Husein's death was soon integrated into the local traditions of the Muslim inhabitants.

In Pariaman, the *Tabuik* commemoration has several phases that are spread out over the first ten days of the month of Muharram: *Ma-ambiak tanah* (Fetching the Soil), *manabeh batang pisang* (Chopping Down the Banana Plant), *mahatam* (Carrying the Fingers), *ma-arak saroban* (Parading the Turban) and *ma-oyak tabuik* (Shaking the Tabuik).

The hacking of the banana bole replicates the manner of Husein's death. Tall thin structures symbolise his severed fingers. The pseudo-turban, paraded in a beautifully decorated box, *panja*, represents the fight-to-death in defence of his heritage.

The *tabuik* ritual is still carried out in the month of Muharram. Eight to ten towers may be made, each by a traditionally specified group of people or hamlet. At one time Pariaman was split into two factions, each making its own *tabuik*. The sense of rivalry was so strong that when the two processions met, fighting inevitably broke out, sometimes quite severe. But this no longer happens, and the *tabuik* ritual we see today has become a source of pride for the people of Pariaman, who compete in a friendly way to make the most beautiful tower.

At one stage in its development, the musical accompaniment separated into an independent form. Musical arrangers developed their own ideas, adding colour, rhythm and pattern to the *tabuik* music. The performance, too, has given inspiration to dance choreographers in creating new works based on tradition as well as classical movements. Several of these modern adaptations have been performed in festivals all over Indonesia and the world.

(Top left) The tabuik *is a popular event in West Sumatra widely attended by people from near and far.*

(Bottom left) Besides the towering tabuik *structures, other figures are also paraded,* *including this lion figure.*

(Right) The tabuik *is vigorously swung from side to side as the crowd heads towards the river. The structure is finally thrown into the river.*

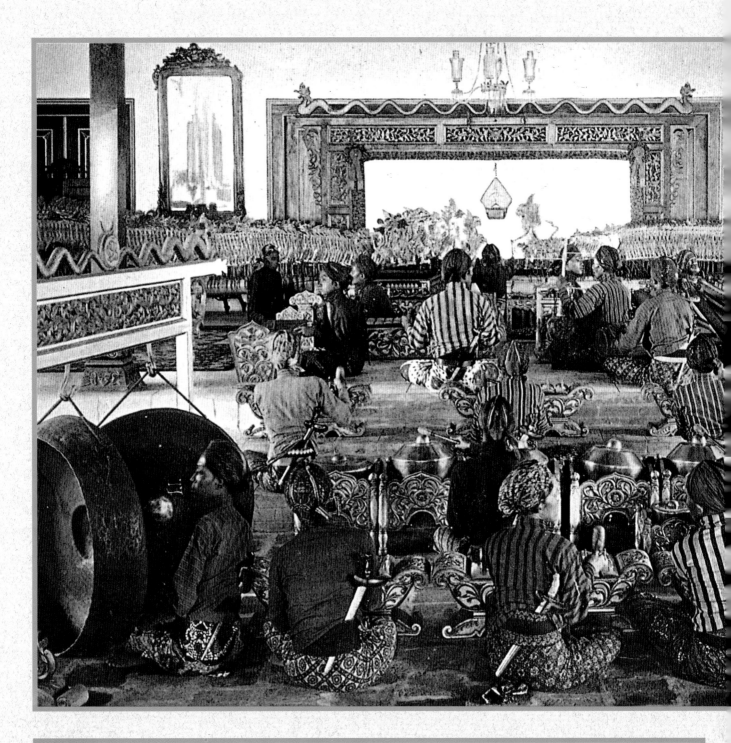

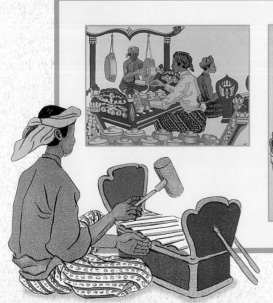

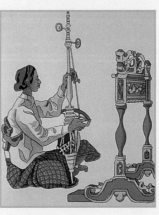

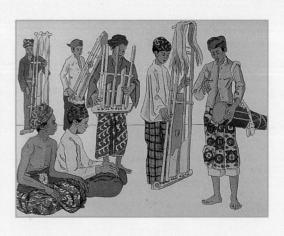

TRADITIONAL MUSICAL ENSEMBLES

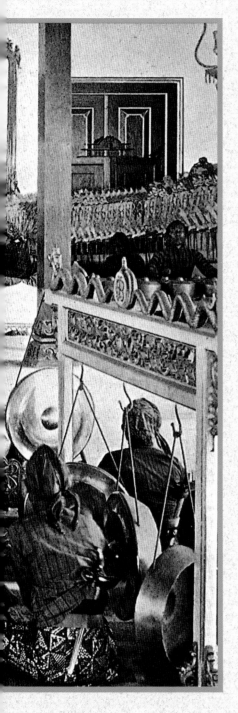

THE GAMELAN

The gamelan has two tuning systems believed to have originated in Indonesia itself: slendro *and* pelog. *Both tuning systems are basically pentatonic, differentiated by the intervals between one note and the next. All intervals in the* slendro *scale are almost equal, whereas the* pelog *tuning system is composed of small and large intervals. This creates a difference in feeling between the two.*

The tuning of one gamelan set is different from another. This however does not result from the tuner's inability to duplicate a tuning, but is due to intentional differentiation in intervals between notes in each gamelan. In Java, this difference in intervallic structure is called embat.

Indonesia's many hundreds of traditional musical ensembles can be categorised into two groups: large ensembles and small ensembles. Large ensembles consist of a large number of instruments and instrumental types with a variety of shapes, timbres and functions, while small ensembles generally have less than ten instruments of only one or two types with one or two functions.

Large musical ensembles are the product of serious work by artists through the centuries made possible by royal patronage. They dedicated themselves and their music to upholding the greatness of the king. These large ensembles belong to those areas that once formed part of major kingdoms, principally on the islands of Java, Madura and Bali.

Small ensembles belong to the world of folk music and generally predominate in rural areas as well as kingdoms lying outside Java and Bali. They are played for pure entertainment and ceremonial purposes.

Large ensembles usually consist of percussion instruments whose sound-source is made of tuned metal. The metal pieces take the shape of either keys (*bilah*) or gongs with a central boss (*pencon*), of varying shapes and sizes. Variations in thickness of material used, diversity in types of resonators and differences in playing techniques can create a wide range of rich sounds from only one type of struck (percussion) instrument. The large ensemble also contains a bowed instrument, a plucked instrument, a wind instrument and a membranophone. The human voice, both solo and in chorus, is often included as an instrument. An example of this ensemble is the gamelan.

Small ensembles may be composed entirely of bamboo instruments, such as are popular in the Banyumas region of Central Java; plucked instruments such as the *gambus* and *kecapi*, found throughout western Indonesia with a number of different names; wind instruments, such as the *saluang* and *sampelong* from West Sumatra; or bowed instruments like the *rabab darek*, *rabab pasisir* (Sumatra) and the *kesok-kesok* (Sulawesi).

Ensembles composed entirely of drums like the *rebana* (frame-drum), and *kendhang* or *gendang* (two-headed drum), are generally not tuned. This kind of music relies more on interlocking rhythms between instruments. However some of these instruments may be tuned. An example is the *gondang sabangunan* played by the Bataks of North Sumatra, which consists of a set of single-headed tuned drums called *taganing*.

Big Gong Javanese Gamelan

A gamelan ensemble consists mainly of metallophone and gong-type instruments which produce tones when struck with mallets (tabuh). A few instruments do not fall into these groups. They are a two-stringed bowed lute, a wooden xylophone, a set of drums, a plucked zither and a bamboo flute. Male and female singers also participate.

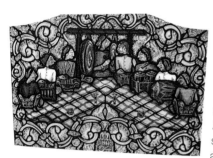

Stained glass at the Mangkunagara palace in Central Java depicting a group of gamelan players. Instruments presented in the painting include the saron, gender, demung, *gong,* kenong, bonang, *and* kendhang.

»*Gamelan-makers working on the kettlegongs meant for the* bonang *instrument.*

A copy of the treatise on Javanese gamelan music, written by K.R.T. Kertanagara in 1889.

Tuning

Most gamelan instruments are tuned to definite pitches, corresponding to two tuning systems (*laras*): the five-toned *slendro* and the seven-toned *pelog*. A complete gamelan set is actually a double set: a *slendro* gamelan and a *pelog* gamelan. Although they are never played simultaneously, they can be played alternatively within the same performance. It is not uncommon, therefore, for a single gamelan set to be owned.

Functions of the Instruments

Gamelan instruments may be classified into three major groupings:
- Instruments and vocalists that carry the melody in both simple and elaborate forms.
- Instruments that regulate musical time.
- Instruments that underline the structure of the composition (*gendhing*).

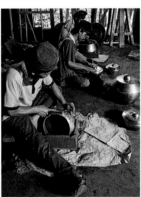

Melody

Instruments that carry the melody are divided into three broad categories. First, there are instruments that carry the melody in elaborate forms, each

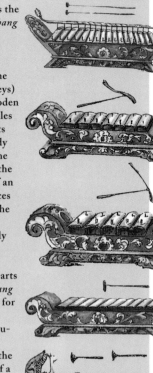

XYLOPHONES

There are various forms of xylophones, such as the *gambang gangsa, gambang kayu, saron, demung, slenthem,* and *gender.*

The *gender* (an example of a xylophone with 10 to 14 metal keys) and the *gambang* (wooden xylophone) are examples of musical instruments which carry the melody in elaborate forms. The *gender* in fact creates the fullness of sonority of an ensemble and reinforces the musical mode of the composition. The *gambang* part is usually one of the fastest. It provides a gentle and rippling sound. The parts played with the *gambang* are in parallel octaves for most of the time.

Examples of instruments in the Javanese gamelan which carry the melodic abstraction of a musical composition are the *slenthem* and *demung.* They are both low-toned xylophones.

The *peking* or *saron panerus* can paraphrase the melody by doubling or quadrupling the tempo of the *balungan.*

of which has either a leading or a supporting role in expressing the composition. The *rebab* (two-stringed bowed lute) is the melodic leader of the ensemble, especially in soft-style composition. It plays the melodic introduction (*buka*) which determines the composition structure, the tuning system and the musical mode (*pathet*) which are to be played by the ensemble. The *gender* (metallophone with 10 to 14 keys) is a leading instrument, especially the large *gender* (*gender barung*). The small *gender* (*gender panerus*) adds to the richness of the ensemble. Other instruments include the wooden xylophone (*gambang*), the plucked zither (*celempung* or *siter*), and the end-blown bamboo flute (*suling*). A female solo singer (*pesinden*) and a male chorus (*penggerong*) also fall into this group, although in a few styles of composition accompanying the *bedhaya* dances the *pesinden* may have a prominent role in expressing the melody.

The second group of instruments carries the melodic abstraction (*balungan*) of a composition. They are *slenthem* and *demung* (both low-toned xylophones) and *saron barung* (large xylophones). Each has a range of one octave. A gamelan ensemble may have one to four *demung* and two to eight *saron barung.*

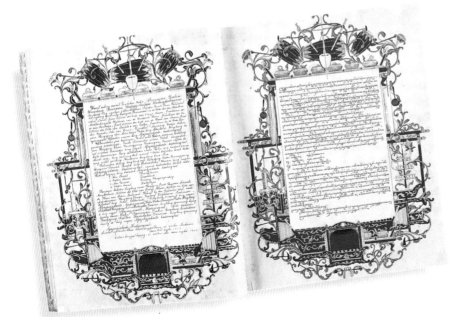

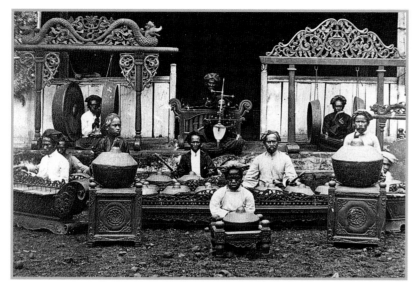

The final set of instruments function as melodic mediators between the instruments in the first two groups. They are the *bonang* (set of 10 to 14 small kettlegongs arranged in two rows) and *peking* (smallest *saron*). The large *bonang* (*bonang barung*) is one of the leading instruments in the ensemble. The anticipatory nature of its patterns provides cues in the melody for other instruments and leads the proper register of the melodic motion of the piece. Although playing twice as fast as the *bonang barung,* the role of the small *bonang* (*bonang panerus*) is not as important as that of the *bonang barung*. The *peking* can double or quadruple the tempo of the *balungan,* the melodic abstraction.

The divisions between these groups are not rigid. There are certain compositional genres or playing techniques that require one or more instruments to change their melodic functions.

Musical Time

The instruments regulating musical time consist of a set of two-headed, asymmetrical drums (*kendhang*). They set up the appropriate tempo (*irama*) for a composition, control transition between parts, and signal the end of the piece.

Based on size and musical functions, there are four kinds of *kendhang* (drum). The *kendhang ageng* (large drum) is played in those compositions or sections of compositions which have a calm or majestic feeling; the *kendhang wayangan* (medium-sized) is played for the accompaniment of the shadow-puppet play (*wayang*); the *kendhang ciblon* (small) is used to accompany dance or in 'concert' music, playing patterns associated with dance movements; and *kendhang ketipung* (the smallest) is played in combination with the *kendhang ageng*.

Musical Structure

This category consists of gong-type instruments of various sizes: *gong ageng*, *kenong*, *kempul* and *kethuk-kempyang*. They underline the formal structure of the composition. The formal structures are cyclical. The *gong ageng* marks the beginning and the end of the composition. This function is very important in maintaining a feeling of balance after

the longest structural unit. Therefore the cycle itself is called *gongan*. The *gongan* cycle is sub-divided in different ways by *kenong, kempul* and *kethuk-kempyang*.

Soft and Loud Categories

Gamelan instruments can be allocated to two different sound groups: loud and soft. Most instruments in the group carrying the melody, including the *slenthem*, are soft-sounding instruments. Others are loud-sounding.

The emphasis in using one group or the other creates stylistic differences in the playing of compositions and in gamelan ensembles. The majority of soft-style pieces are grouped in *gendhing rebab*. Other genres of soft-style pieces include *gendhing gender*, *jineman* and *palaran*. Certain *gendhing* can be performed over a range from soft to loud style. Usually small ensembles, such as *gamelan gadon* and *gamelan klenengan,* are soft-sounding.

Loud-style pieces are classified as *gending bonangan* or *gendhing soran* (loud and noisy). *gamelan bonangan* and *gamelan sekaten* are two examples of loud-sounding musical ensembles. The *gamelan monggang, kodhok ngorek* and *cara balen* also belong to this category. These last three ensembles and the *gamelan sekaten* are regarded as very sacred and archaic.

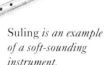

A traditional village gamelan ensemble in Bandung, West Java. The gamelan plays a crucial role in many important village festivals and celebrations.

Suling *is an example of a soft-sounding instrument.*

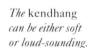

The kendhang *can be either soft or loud-sounding.*

BIG GONG ENSEMBLE
In traditional Javanese formulation, the entire gamelan orchestra is considered a precious heirloom, but some of the larger gong are reputed to possess potency on their own. ❶ Javanese gamelan player playing the big gong, ❷ the *kecer*, the *kethuk*, ❸ the gong. ❹

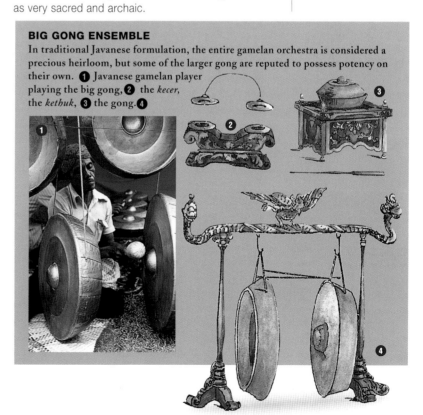

Big Gong Balinese Gamelan

The small island of Bali is the home of an astonishing variety of gamelan ensembles. Music is essential to socio-religious and cultural activities in this culture. Today, there are at least 20 different ensemble types on the island. Most are closely associated with the dramatic arts; many others are played to accompany religious ceremonies and rituals.

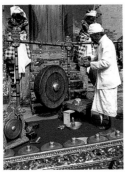

(Above) The priest performs a ritual to sanctify the gong ageng *before a performance. (Right) A Balinese* terompong *player.*

(Below) The Balinese gamelan gong gede *is composed largely of a group of* gangsa jongkok *(like the Javanese* saron*), gongs, cymbals and drums. During the feudal era, it was an important court ensemble; it is also played at the temple to accompany ceremonial* baris gede *dances.*

Root Word for 'Gamelan'

In Balinese tradition, the word 'gamelan', from the verb *gamel*, meaning 'to handle', can mean musical accompaniment (instruments, players), but it most commonly refers to the instruments as an orchestra; the players are commonly called *juru gamel*. Balinese gamelan ensembles are largely composed of percussion instruments that include metallophones, xylophones, gongs, drums and cymbals. All ensembles containing one or a pair of big gongs are usually called *gamelan gong*. The gong is regarded as a sacred instrument.

Musical Composition

There are two kinds of gamelan ensembles: those dominated by bronze instruments and those by bamboo and wooden instruments. Bronze instruments come in two main groups: xylophones with metal bars and gongs (large and small hanging gongs and kettlegongs). The metal xylophones, which are all struck with wooden mallets (*panggal*), come in two basic structural designs. In the *gender* family, bars or keys (*bilah*) are hung or sometimes laid over bamboo resonators; therefore, they produce a more shimmering, vibrating sound. In the *saron* or *gangsa jongkok* family, the bars are laid over a wooden trough, held in place with posts, and padded slightly with rubber where the metal keys come into contact with the wood; the result is a crisp, brittle sound.

Bamboo instruments encompass three groups: xylophones with bars (*bilah*) or tubes (*bambung*), flutes (*suling*), and slit-drums (*kulkul*). Some bamboo xylophones have hung bars with bamboo resonators and others, bars simply laid in a frame and arranged in order of pitch. The bamboo flutes, like the bamboo slit-drums, come in three different sizes and lengths: small (short), medium and large (long). Other important instruments in the Balinese gamelan are barrel-shaped and conical drums, cymbals and the two-stringed lute or *rebab*.

Tuning System

Balinese gamelan ensembles operate two scale systems: *pelog* and *slendro*, but only one per ensemble, except the *gamelan gaguntangan*. The *pelog* gamelan can be further classified into four-toned, and five-and seven-toned; the *slendro* gamelan, into four-toned and five-toned. Additionally, each village, each group tunes its gamelan slightly differently, so that instruments cannot be traded from one ensemble to another. Most ensembles are owned by the community, only a few by individuals.

Although female musicians have just received social recognition from the community, and the number of female gamelan groups is growing, in Balinese tradition the musicians are predominantly males. They usually organise their activities in an association known as *sekaha*. Anybody interested in playing can become a member.

Balinese gamelan music has some unique features. The instruments, especially the metal xylophones, drums and large gongs, are tuned in pairs, one of the two slightly higher than the other. In the case of metal xylophones, the lower and higher-pitched instruments are called, respectively,

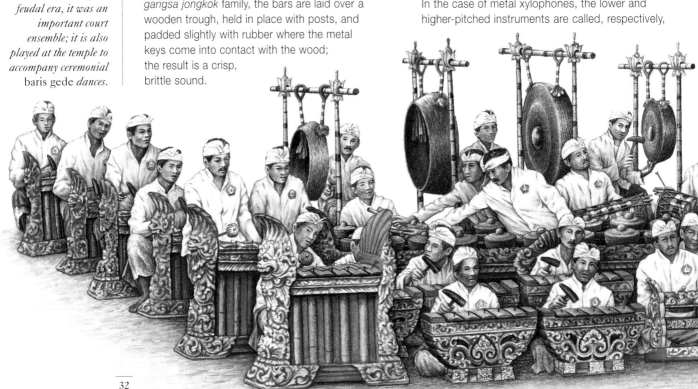

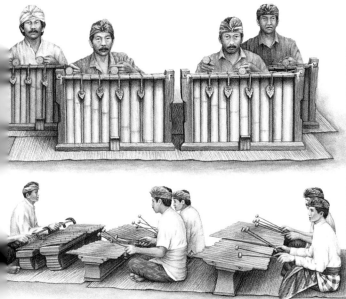

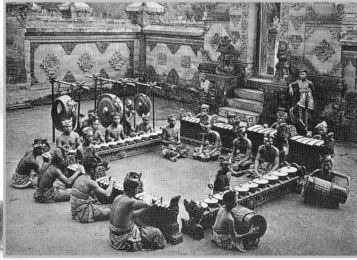

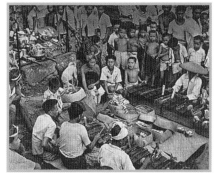

(Top) The gamelan wayang gender *is played in accompaniment to the Balinese* wayang parwa *performance.*

(Above) The gamelan gambang *consists of four bamboo- or wooden-keyed instruments (*gambang*) and two metal* saron.

pangumbang and *pangisep*; *wadon* (female) and *lanang* (male) in the case of drums and gongs. The music is generally faster and more vibrant in tone compared to, for example, Javanese music. Most Balinese ensembles produce loud, rousing music. Finally, Balinese music is dominated by interlocking techniques involving a pair of instruments of different groups.

Gamelan Types

It is believed that the richness of Balinese gamelan ensembles has developed through at least three time periods: Pre-Hindu (not to be identified only with the Bali Aga), Hindu kingdoms, and Bali within the Republic of Indonesia. Ensembles originating in the first period are relatively small in size, employ four to eight musicians and are usually composed of metal and wooden xylophones, but use no drum. Examples are the *gamelan gambang* and *gamelan slonding*, both tuned to the seven-toned *pelog* scale and both considered sacred. The *gamelan slonding* can be found in many Bali-Aga villages in Karangasem district.

Gamelan ensembles from the second period (roughly 8th to early 20th centuries) are usually larger in size with 10 to 40 musicians. These ensembles comprise metal and wooden xylophones, one or two drums, and gongs of different sizes.

New Ensembles

Gamelan ensembles of the mid-19th century to the present are physically not too different from those of the previous period. Of this group of ensembles, the *gamelan gong kebyar* is perhaps the best-known and most widespread on the island. Composed of seven pairs of metallophones of different sizes, gongs, drums, cymbals, flutes and *rebab* and employing 25 to 35 musicians, it is the standard modern concert-gamelan and accompanies stage performances, for both sacred and secular events.

Changes continue to take place in the music of Bali. The most recent innovation in Balinese gamelan music is the drum-dominated *adi merdangga* ensemble.

(Top and above right) The gamelan gong gede *is the largest ensemble on Bali, employing no less than 40 musicians. The* gong gede *accompanies the* baris gede *dance.*

(Above left) The Balinese gamelan gambang.

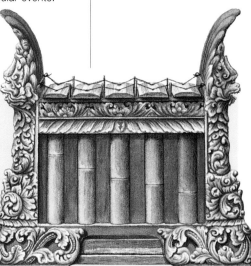

GENDER

The *gender* is played with two round-headed mallets, one in each hand. It gives tonal colour to the music. The Balinese *gender* is usually decorated with ornate designs and motifs although some *gender* can be plain. Balinese music is louder than Javanese music as the Balinese gender is struck with 'naked' wooden mallets, not padded ones.

Bamboo Music: Angklung and Calung Banyumas

Bamboo is a multi-functional plant, easily available, cheap and familiar to the people in Indonesia. In addition to providing material for house-construction, furniture, arts and crafts, food and weapons, it is also the basis of several types of music that are widely popular.

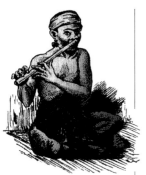

A nose flute-player from Nias, off Sumatra.

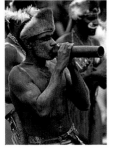

An Asmat man and his bamboo wind instrument, Irian Jaya.

An Apo Kayan woman playing a mouth organ, East Kalimantan.

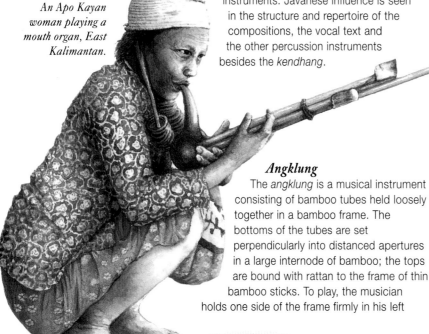

Location and Description

Banyumas, a cultural region lying on the border of Central and West Java provinces, is famous for its various kinds of bamboo music, all part of the folk music of the area. Bamboo music is often played at agricultural ceremonies to call for rain, to mark the beginning of planting seasons and at harvest time, and in family gatherings such as thanksgivings, circumcisions and weddings. It can also be played for public entertainment at various events, such as the inauguration of a building, commemoration of holidays, and art festivals.

While bamboo music is performed during traditional and family ceremonies, the orchestra itself is free from ritual attachment. As an independent form of entertainment, it does not have to be directly linked to the ritual activities that it may accompany.

The location of Banyumas, on the boundary between the Javanese and Sundanese cultures, influences the 'colour' of its music. Sundanese influence is evident in the way the instruments are played, the vocabulary of the *kendhang* (two-headed drum) playing, the vocal presentation (including the use of minor-style tones for the vocal part and the *slendro* instrument set), and the use of *angklung*-like musical instruments. All Banyumasan music employs the *slendro* tonal system (five-tone scale). Vocal arrangements often use minor tones resembling the *pelog* (seven-tone scale) or the *madenda* pitch of traditional Sundanese gamelan music, but are presented using *slendro*-tuned musical instruments. Javanese influence is seen in the structure and repertoire of the compositions, the vocal text and the other percussion instruments besides the *kendhang*.

Angklung

The *angklung* is a musical instrument consisting of bamboo tubes held loosely together in a bamboo frame. The bottoms of the tubes are set perpendicularly into distanced apertures in a large internode of bamboo; the tops are bound with rattan to the frame of thin bamboo sticks. To play, the musician holds one side of the frame firmly in his left

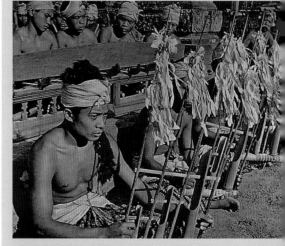

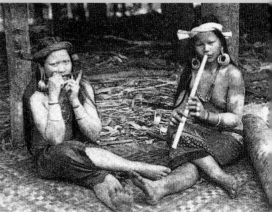

hand and shakes the instrument with his right hand that lightly holds the opposite end of the base tube between thumb and forefinger. One frame may hold three or four tubes, each producing a different note, forming an octave (*gembyang*) or any customised notes. The *angklung* is used extensively as part of several ensembles of archaic musical instruments (or those perceived as belonging to the older generation), such as the *bongkel, buncis,* and *angklung* ensembles.

a. Bongkel

The *angklung*-like *bongkel* is played by a single musician. The ensemble consists of four tubes with different *slendro*-tuned notes. To select the notes, the player merely frees from his grip the tubes that sound the desired notes, before vibrating the instrument. The *bongkel* is played for relaxation during breaks from work in the fields. It is becoming extremely rare.

b. Buncis

Buncis is the name of an orchestra composed of several *angklung*. Each is played by an individual musician while dancing. The number of *angklung* varies to suit the number of musicians either needed or available. They are complemented by a bamboo gong and a *kendhang* (double-headed drum). The musicians, who are also the dancers, wear costumes and make themselves up in what they believe to be

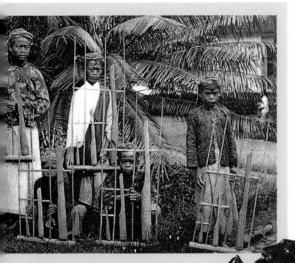

(Above) An angklung *ensemble in West Java. The* angklung *is shaken to produce sound.*

(Top left) In Bali, the angklung, *once part of the* gamelan angklung, *is no longer played.*

(Left) Dayak women playing the suling *(flute) and* genggeng *(mouth harp).*

(Right) Sculpture of a flute-player by Ida Bagus Putu, Bali.

the Dayak fashion
(the Dayak of Kalimantan),
complete with feathered headdresses, painted faces and bodies. Over short trousers they wear cloth skirt-wrappings. *Buncis* players still frequently manifest a trance-like state. *Buncis* music is played for entertainment in the field or houseyard after harvest or during celebration of certain holidays.

c. Angklung
The *angklung* ensemble consists of about 15 *angklung* hung on a *gayor* (large, bench-like frame); a *gambang* (wooden xylophone); the xylophone-like *slenthem* and *demung,* or *kenong;* large kettlegong; and the gong, all made of bamboo; as well as a set of *kendhang* (two-headed drums). This set requires three *pengrawit* (musicians). The *angklung* instrument itself can function as the melodic leader or, occasionally play a pattern interlocking with other instruments. The *angklung* orchestra can present music independently in a concert, or accompany the *lengger*, which is a type of social dance theatre where the dancers sing and (sometimes) jest with the audience.

❶ *A flute-player in the market.*
❷ *A group of children plays the* angklung. *In recent times, a festival of bamboo music for*

school children was set up in Banyumas, Central Java, to preserve this regional folk music.
❸ *A Dayak plays the* kledi *mouth-organ.*

There are several *angklung* ensembles in the Banyumas area, all in the vicinity of Purworejo, about 20 kilometres east of Purwokerto.

Calung

Calung is the youngest generation of bamboo music in the Banyumas region. It is seen as a blending of the *angklung* (bamboo) instrument with the music of the (metal) gamelan. There is no great difference between the *calung* and *angklung* orchestras in terms of instrumental use, musical repertoire, presentation or social function. The only distinction is that the *angklung* is replaced with a *gambang* (wooden xylophone), called *gambang penodos*.

Along with the development of *lengger* into a best-selling form of musical entertainment, the *calung* has evolved into a style of music that not only presents Banyumasan melodies, but also Javanese compositions from Surakarta and Yogyakarta (*gendhing wetanan* or eastern style compositions), Sundanese melodies with a Javanese flavour, pop songs, *keroncong* (an acculturation of Portuguese music and Western instruments), and *dangdut* (a blend of Indian film music, Western rock and Indonesian tastes). Several *calung* groups have even incorporated other instruments like the *siter* (zither), *suling* (bamboo flute), maracas, cymbal and tambourine, to allow the presentation of a variety of music. Different compositions with either *slendro* or *pelog* pitch, or diatonic, are still presented with *slendro*-tuned instruments in the background.

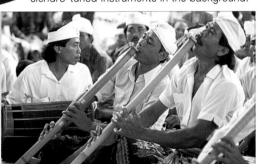

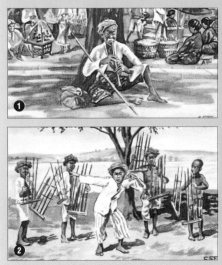

❶
❷
❸

❶ A bamboo zither from Sulawesi.
❷ A bamboo flute from Makasar, South Sulawesi. The flared end is made from a spiral of lontar leaf.
❸ A set of bamboo flutes, *suling*.

(Left) Three very long bamboo flutes form the nucleus of Bali's gamelan gambuh.

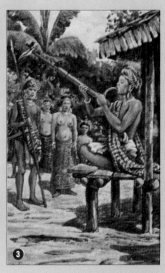

Drums

In much of the music of Indonesia, drums have an important but limited function, holding a steady beat for other musicians or dancers, or repeating a simple rhythmic pattern over and over as a framework for vocal or instrumental melody. In certain kinds of music however, drums take on a more prominent role, becoming a dominant or featured instrument in the ensemble.

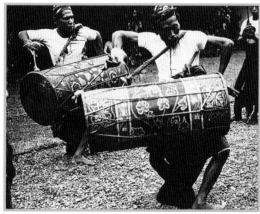

»»The kendhang belek *performance of Lombok takes two players, each with an immense drum hanging from his shoulder. Competing with each other, they effect dramatic poses while the rhythm of their drums interlock in increasing intensity until a gong is struck.*

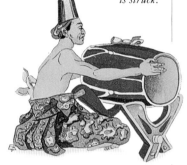

(Above): The kendhang *player.*

↗The drumming tradition is also found in the coastal groups of Kalimantan.

(Right) Balinese drummers play interlocking parts to form a rhythmic line.

Single-Headed Frame-Drum Ensemble

The most widespread form of Indonesian music featuring drums is the single-headed frame-drum ensemble. Such ensembles, containing two or three to 20 or 30 shallow, tambourine-like drums, are found in Muslim communities throughout the country, performing for family celebrations, like weddings and circumcisions, and devotional gatherings. The drums usually accompany unison male choruses singing praises of Allah or the Prophet and songs expressing Islamic precepts.

Drumming Tradition of Sumatra

North Sumatra has a particularly rich drumming tradition. The Mandailing music called *gordang sambilan*, for example, employs a battery of nine (*sambilan*) single-headed drums (*gordang*) which nearly eclipses the ensemble's melodic component, a long clarinet (*sarunai*). Three drummers, each controlling two drums, play fixed, repeating patterns to create an interlocking framework, while a fourth drummer, using the three largest and lowest-pitched drums, plays longer patterns and spontaneous variations of them. Similar ensembles are found among some of the other North Sumatran peoples. The *gondang sabangunan* ensemble of the Batak Toba looks similar but is actually quite different: a set of five drums, called *taganing*, is often played melodically by a single drummer while a sixth drum, played by a second drummer, adds low-pitched accents and rhythmic patterning. The ensemble includes gongs, to provide a fixed rhythmic

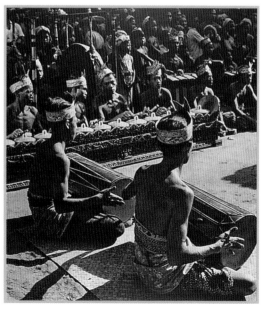

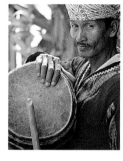

background, and an oboe-like instrument (*sarunai*), which plays the same melody as the *taganing* but in a different tuning. Tuned drum sets like the *taganing* (drum chimes) are extremely rare in the world. Outside Indonesia, the best-known examples are found in Burma and Uganda.

Another North Sumatran group, the Karo Batak, use only two drums in the *gendang lima sedalanen* ensemble. These drums are extremely small and slender — not much larger than the ears of corn they are said to resemble. When accompanying singing, they play simple, unemphatic repeating patterns, but for dance music they become more energetic. One drum, the 'mother' (*induk*), plays a fixed pattern with little variation, while the other drum called the 'child' (*enek-enek*) freely decorates and complicates.

The relationship of these two Karo drums is also found in the drumming tradition of Malay groups living in the coastal areas of Sumatra, Kalimantan and the Riau islands. In some places, the two parts are played on separate drums, as for the *ronggeng* or *joget* music of the Medan area. The two deep frame-drums are accompanied by violin, accordion (optional) and gong (optional). In other regions, the parts are played on the two heads of one long horizontal drum, as is the case in the shamanic healing ritual of the Petalangan people inhabiting the forested area of mainland Riau, Sumatra. The music for this ritual consists solely of drumming, plus occasional singing by the shaman, who also shakes an iron rattle.

Dozens of two-headed cylindrical drums, *dol*, provide the music for the Shi'ah Muslim *tabuik* or *tabot* festival celebrated in Bengkulu and West Sumatra, along with the single-headed bowl-shaped drum, *tasa* or *tansa*, that serves as a leader.

Drums in Java and Bali

Javanese and Balinese gamelan music generally makes use of double-headed drums played horizontally (*kendhang*). The diameter of these instruments is greater near one end than the other creating a rounded belly-like swelling at one end. The *kendhang* produce a wealth of sounds, from

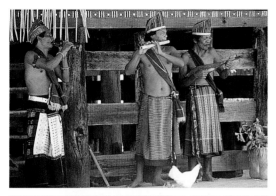

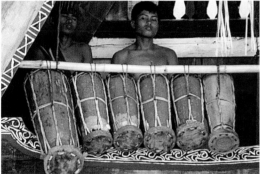

for the gamelan and cues transitions between sections or parts of a piece or score.

Drums in Lombok

The island of Lombok is rich in the varieties of arts such as music, dance and theatre. Traditional performing arts forms are still performed in few traditional Sasak villages. The Sasak traditional gamelan, *kendhang belek*, constitutes one of the few remaining forms of traditional art forms which can still be found on the island. The gamelan includes large gongs, gong chimes, drums and cymbals.

The *kendhang belek* accompanies a dance, *tari oncer*, in which two musicians play single large drums and dance together. The dancers strike dramatic poses as they dance energetically with long steps. They play rapid interlocking parts on the drums as the dance intensifies. At last with a stroke of the gong, the dance and drumming is relaxed and the music continues in a slower tempo.

(Below) The hourglass-shaped drums of Irian Jaya can be works of art.

««The gondang sabangunan orchestra of the Toba Batak includes a tuned set of five small drums (below), a larger drum, gongs and oboe-like sarunai (top).

(Below) Boy from Alor holding a moko-type drum, East Nusa Tenggara.

sharp cracks and pings to deep hums and booms. Sometimes an array of several drums may be used. In West Java amongst the Sundanese, for example, the drummer has one large horizontal drum and three or four smaller ones standing on end. In Central Javanese court gamelan music, the drummer uses two horizontal drums for certain pieces or segments of a piece, and a third for others.

Musical Structure

Drums are only one of the several principal gamelan components to have no melodic function. Instead, they play extended, clearly shaped and articulated patterns that in their contours and accents seem independent of the melody, or melodies, of the other instruments. The drum patterns may be the same length as the melody, or they may mark off segments of the melody.

Typically the drummer sets the tempo

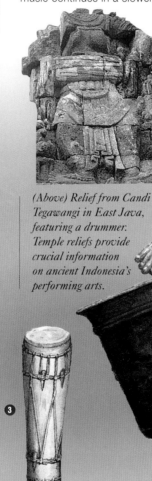

(Above) Relief from Candi Tegawangi in East Java, featuring a drummer. Temple reliefs provide crucial information on ancient Indonesia's performing arts.

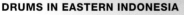

THE DRUMS ILLUSTRATED ARE NAMELY:
1. Two-toned Sumba drum
2. Medium Bugis drum (*ganrang tangnga*)
3. Hour-glass drum (*ketepong*), Kalimantan.
4. Small Bugis drum (*ganrang caddi*)

DRUMS IN EASTERN INDONESIA

Drums are the most predominant instrument in eastern Indonesian music. Hourglass, vase- and bowl-shaped, frame and barrel drums provide rhythms to announce the arrival of important persons, to announce a death, to call people to an event, to accompany dance and dramatic performances, on sacred events, and at one time to fire the battle spirit in warfare.

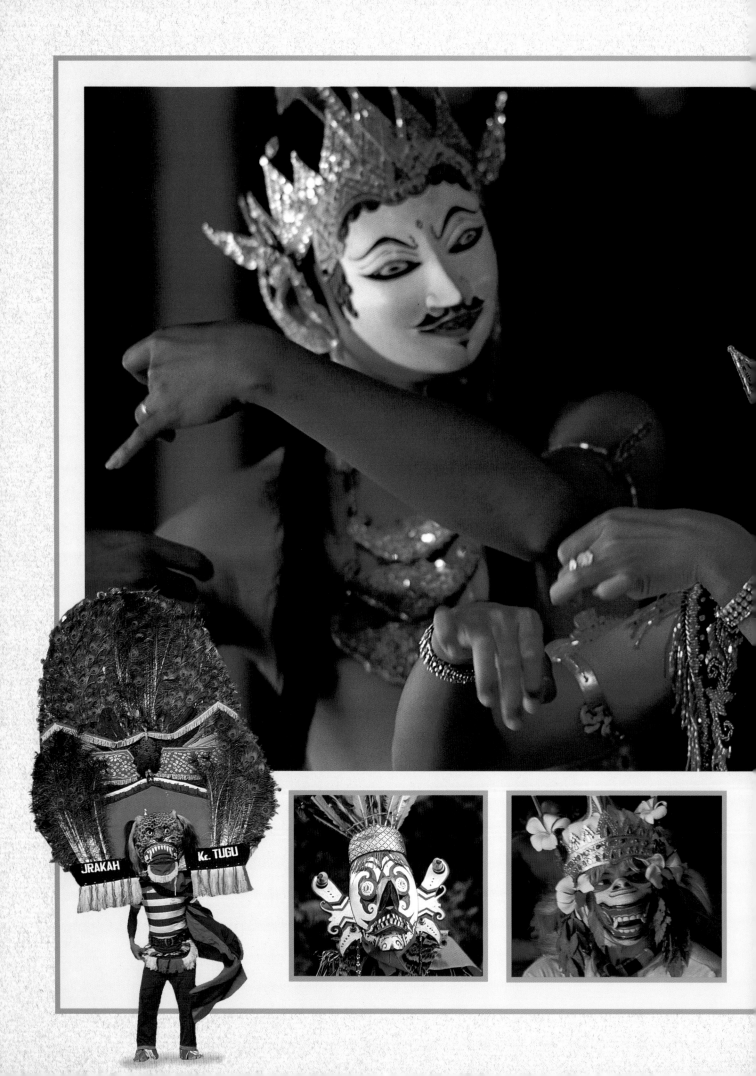

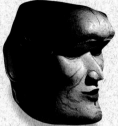

THE MASK IN PERFORMANCE

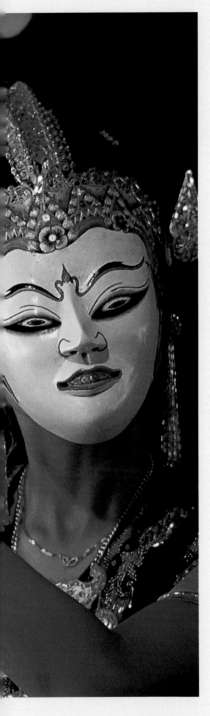

(Main picture) Two of the royal wayang wong *dancers performing a dance in the keraton of Yogyakarta. (Left to right) The* singabarong *mask from the* Reog Ponorogo *weighs up to 60 kilogrammes. The* hudoq *mask from East Kalimantan represents a species of crop pest. Sugriwa, king of the monkey troops, from the Balinese* sendratari Ramayana. *(Above right) The Balinese* Jero Luh *mask is characterised by its exaggerated facial volume.*

Masks are known to several Indonesian ethnic groups for their diverse forms and functions. They constitute a cultural product that could be as old as the tradition of its producers. A thin gold mask found in West Java is believed to have been used in prehistoric times to cover the face of a deceased person.

The main motive behind the use of masks is to represent the entire self. The mask can be defined generally as a face imitated in thin, or thinned, material, and may be described as falsification of the self. It is possible to depict an individual through a visual symbol centred on the face. Each line drawn, each feature applied is calculated to express the traits and personality of the individual it represents. The individual depicted is not limited solely to fellow man but extends both to heavenly beings with human traits and to the sub-human level.

The cultural function of a mask comprises religious and artistic facets. In the first instance, the mask constitutes a means of symbolically manifesting religious concepts, especially those related to specific mystical powers. In the latter case, the mask is a symbolic expression evoked by reaction to, and impressions of, nature and its characteristics, and certain cultural concepts portrayed through preconceived visual forms. Masks in Indonesia's many ethnic cultures initially had a religious function and it was not until later that they acquired an artistic purpose.

Indonesian masks come in three sizes: small masks which fit the face, big masks which are larger, and *barong* masks which represent great mythical characters and cover the entire body. Masks may be natural or grotesque.

The ancestral relationship of masks is discernible in the *barong landung* of Bali, performed solely in Galungan celebrations marking the change of the Balinese year. A pair of large male and female *barong*s representing an ancestral couple is paraded through the villages, accompanied by a group of people who sing and dance.

Masks representing ancestral figures can be used to invoke the ancestor depicted. They are perceived as a sign of ancestral presence. This link between man and the mystical world through the mask is generally impermanent and only valid during holy times. In the *hudoq* dance of East Kalimantan, for instance, large grotesque masks representing mystical powers are worn to frighten away destructive crop pests.

Ritualistic Mask Performances

In Indonesia, the use of animal and death masks in ritual is widespread. Masks not only act as links to ancestors but are also used to draw on mystical and supernatural powers for assistance. A ritual mask is a 'transitional object': it can transmit supernatural power, which is brought to life by performing in it.

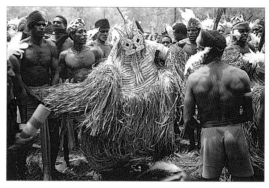

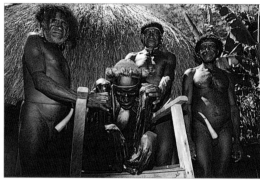

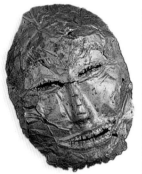

A gold thin mask believed to be used for covering the face of the dead in prehistoric times.

(Top) An Asmat jipae *mask. (Bottom) A mummified body. Dani Irian Jaya.*

(Below) Batak masks used in dances for the dead. (Bottom) Asmat skulls.

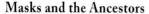

Masks and the Ancestors

A mask made of a sheet of gold was found at a prehistoric site at Pasir Angin, West Java. It is thought to have been placed over the face of a deceased person. The true purpose of this act is unknown, although it may have been carried out within the framework of a spiritual belief in the afterworld. This deed was performed by relatives, or at least closely connected persons.

Death Masks

In Irian Jaya, some death masks are related to the head-hunting tradition practised in the past. Whether the head of an enemy or an ancestor, it coalesced the power of its previous owner which could then be appropriated by carrying or wearing the head itself, or a mask modelled after the deceased, on their backs tied with a string around their necks. In the coastal area of southeastern Irian Jaya, Asmat men often carry skulls of ancestors on their backs or breasts, or use them as headrests, to keep in constant contact with their ancestors.

Asmat *Barong*-type Masks

A mask is normally designed to cover the face or the entire head, and in many places is made of wood. However, the *jipai* or *jipae* is designed to cover the whole body, except the legs. It is made in great secrecy in the men's house. The mask represents the ancestor spirit and varies in shape and material, depending upon the village and area in which it is made.

The *jipae* performance is held in connection with the *jipui pokmbu* or *pokman pokmbi* ritual which commemorates and makes contact with ancestor spirits. It takes 6 to 12 months to prepare for this event. The masked figures appear in the evening and are then pelted by the young people. Sometimes adults wield sticks at those wearing the masks. In other villages, the masks emerge from the jungle or come into sight

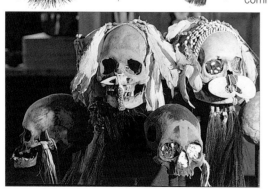

from across the river at sunrise. They dance in front of the *jeu* (men's house), are chased into the jungle, and dance again in front of the men's house. They are finally forced out of the village at dusk.

Simalungun-Batak Funeral Masks

A mask performance related to death is also found in North Sumatra. Here it is known as the *tortor toping-toping* or *tortor huda-huda* (*tortor* = dance). One group of practitioners are the Simalungun people living on the northeast end of Toba lake. A *toping-toping* performance is held on the death of a man of *sayur matuah* status (one who has led a 'perfect life', having given descent to children and grandchildren). The figures depicted by the masks (*toping-toping*) are men and women, in pairs, and a hornbill bird (*huda-huda*), all performed by men and accompanied by drums of different sizes (*gonrang bolon, gonrang sidua-dua*). The masks representing the pairs of men and women symbolise the ancestral couple heading for the world of spirits. They are guided by the hornbill bird which is portrayed by a dancer in a *barong*-type mask with an imitation hornbill's head at the top.

The funeral rite begins at the home of the deceased with a non-masked *tortor* performed by the bereaved family to pay respect to the *tondong*'s (father-in-law) family. The *tondong* then consoles his *boru*'s (daughter-in-law) family by inviting the *huda-huda* to perform. Later, the *toping-toping* dancers join in, dancing, joking, 'stealing' food and doing other foolish things to comfort the bereaved.

Barong Dances of Bali

Supernatural power is also assigned to the *barong ket* and other similar Balinese *barong* (*barong bangkal, barong macan, barong lembu, barong asu*),

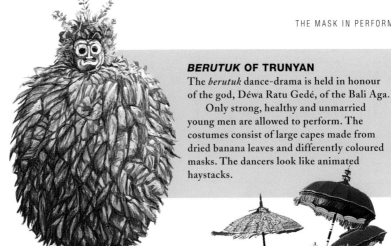

which constitute manifestations of good powers that can give protection to the entire village. Supernatural power is also found in the over-sized Rangda, a goddess-figure, invoked through a large mask with horrifying countenance, eyes bulging, tongue hanging out. Rangda's power is determined by the energies concentrated in the mask: the holiness of the wood, the might of its maker, holy letters inscribed on the inside surface, and the *taksu* or *pasupati* (supernatural strength) gained by storage in a *pura* (temple) or graveyard. The supernatural aspect is valid only in the context of the appropriate religious rite and never in secular performances that imitate it.

Another important ritual performance is the *barong landung* in which a pair of large male and female *barong* is put on and paraded from village to village. They are accompanied by a group of people who sing and dance. In each village, the pair stops at the local *balé banjar* (local assembly hall) and holds a brief performance offering advice and comedy. The *barong* pair are perceived to be the ancestral couple and are sometimes accompanied by their three 'children'.

The traditional version of the *barong* in Jakarta, *ondel-ondel*, is comparable to the *barong landung* of Bali. It may be a vestige of ancestor-worship which evolved into a secular peformance when the underlying local belief was supplanted by Islam. Representation of an ancestral couple in exceptionally large form like this is also found on Sumba, in the form of prehistoric coral-rock statues.

BERUTUK OF TRUNYAN

The *berutuk* dance-drama is held in honour of the god, Déwa Ratu Gedé, of the Bali Aga. Only strong, healthy and unmarried young men are allowed to perform. The costumes consist of large capes made from dried banana leaves and differently coloured masks. The dancers look like animated haystacks.

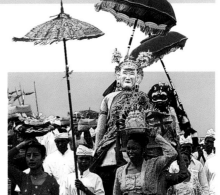

(Above) The barong landung *of Bali consists of an ancestral couple,* Jero Gede *and* Jero Luh, *who are magically protective figures.*

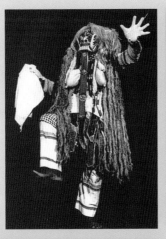 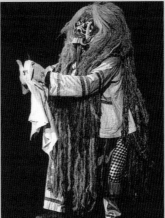

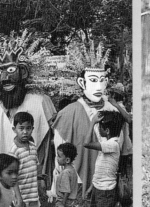 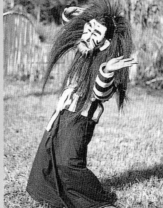

MASKS AND RITUALS

Performances with ritualistic masks bring images from the past into the present. This process is termed 'reactualisation'. Secular time is stopped and primordial mythical time is made present.

(Top row) Conforming with the force built into the mask, the Rangda mask's wearer can only be a powerful priest. Nonetheless, the supernatural aspect is valid only in the context of the appropriate religious rite and never in secular performances that imitate it. Bali.

(Bottom left) Ondel-ondel *may be a vestige of ancestor-worship which has evolved into a secular performance. Betawi.*

(Bottom right) The Batak mask dance, toping-toping, *was once performed as part of the most complete funeral ceremonies. Its presence meant that the deceased had left behind children and grandchildren, which is a perfect condition in traditional thought. The mask is made of wood. North Sumatra.*

The Mask and Characterisation System

*M*asks may have been used in prehistoric times both to represent the dead and to protect them from evil spirits. This supposition is based on the fact that there are ethnic groups within the modern Indonesian nation using masks whose origins appear to predate recorded evidence. Different kinds of masks have always distinguished different characters. This mask characterisation is consistent with that used in dance-dramas.

⟫A bondres mask characterised by its comical features and harelip, Bali.

(Below) A Balinese mask of a comical and mythical figure.

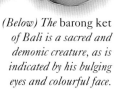

(Below) The barong ket *of Bali is a sacred and demonic creature, as is indicated by his bulging eyes and colourful face.*

Types of Mask

Masks can be divided into three broad categories: mythological creatures, stylised faces and realistic faces. The mask depicting mythological creatures, whether giant or clan emblem of mythical origin, is used as a source of protection by societies which maintain ancient forms of culture. Performances that use these kinds of masks can be found in Kalimantan, Sulawesi, Irian Jaya and Bali. In Bali, for example, the masks are considered sacred and include the *barong ket* (lion), *barong macan* (tiger), *barong bangkal* (boar), *barong lembu* (bull) and *barong landung* (giant).

The tradition of re-enacting the life-story of ancestors as a form of worship necessitated very simple systems of characterisation. An example is the *berutuk* masked drama performed among the Trunyan village people of Bali, as the climax of the *saba gede kapat lanang* ritual commemorating the anniversary of the High God. The shapes of the 21 masks used are similar; they are distinguished only by colour. Half of the masks are in white or yellow and represent female characters such as the queen of the God. The other half are characterised by dark red or dark brown masks which designate male characters such as the God himself, Betara Berutuk, the Patih (Prime Minister) and the Queen's brother.

When dramas or mask-dance plays are used to perform stories from the Ramayana, Mahabharata, Panji stories and historical tales, the characterisation becomes more intricate. In non-historical stories, the masks are carved in imitation of the *wayang kulit* (flat leather shadow) puppets' facial system.

Ramayana

According to the *Babad Dalem,* the Balinese traditional chronicle of the kings of Gelgel and Klungkung, Dalem Gede Kusambal (1772–1825) ordered his chief dancers to create a new form of dance which would use the royal collection of masks. The new genre was taken from the Ramayana and based on

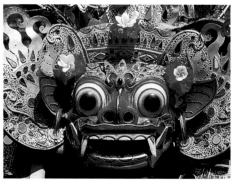

(Right) Rawana, the demon king in the Ramayana epic, who initiated the abduction of Rama's wife, Sita. (Below) The monkey troops of Sugriwa which fought on Rama and Laksmana's side in their battle with Rawana. Bali.

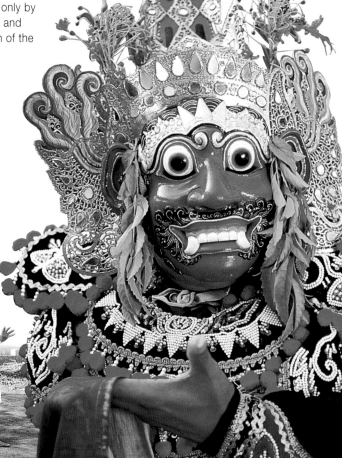

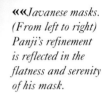

PANJI TALES

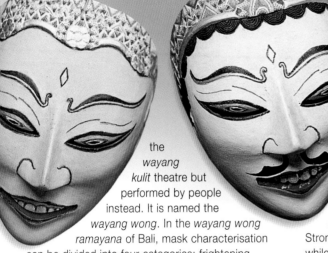

The Panji dance-drama of Central and East Java also makes use of masks. They take the facial shapes of the *gedhog wayang kulit*, which are similar to the faces of the *wayang kulit purwa*. Characterisation is effected by the shape of face, colour, and shape of eyes, nose and mouth. Evil characters like Prabu Klana Sewandana, Panji's enemy, have red masks with wide, scary eyes, prominent nose, open mouth revealing the teeth, and a big moustache. The mask for Panji, a gentleman, is very light blue with small eyes, a small nose, a partly open mouth, and no moustache. Proud refined knights such as Gunungsari, have small moustaches. Panji's amusing attendants, Bancak and Doyok, or Pentul and Tembem, have no lower jaws and are comical. Bancak's mask is white and Doyok's black.

the *wayang kulit* theatre but performed by people instead. It is named the *wayang wong*. In the *wayang wong ramayana* of Bali, mask characterisation can be divided into four categories: frightening giants, for the characters of Rawana and other giants; monkeys, for the monkey troupe; humans, for the characters of Rama, Sita, Laksmana; and comic faces, for the amusing attendants. The characters of the masks, which are made of wood, are further distinguished by colours. Evil or aggressive figures are painted dark red or reddish brown, while good characters like Rama, Sita and Laksmana are portrayed in bluish green, yellow, and white.

The Ramayana dance-drama of Central Java is also called *wayang wong*, but the masks are made of papier maché. Moreover, masks are not worn by 'human' identities like Rama, Sita, Laksmana and descendants of giants who have human characteristics, nor by Rawana himself, his son Indrajit, his brother Wibisana, his niece Trijata, or his other children. Masks are only used to portray Rawana's soldiers and the monkey soldiers under Sugriwa's leadership. The colour and shape of mask differ with each type of individual. For example, a white monkey mask identifies Hanoman; yellow (Yogyakarta) or red (Surakarta), Sugriwa; bright red, Anggada; black, Suwida; and light blue, Anila.

Mahabharata

Characterisation in the masks of the Mahabharata dance-dramas of East Java, Madura and Cirebon is also complex and based on the stylised faces of *wayang kulit* puppets. These wooden masks can be identified by colour and shape of eyes, nose and mouth, using the same system as the *wayang kulit purwa*. Basically, female characters and gentle male

characters such as Arjuna have narrow eyes, while bad characters such as Citraksi generally have big glaring eyes and a half-open mouth revealing the teeth. For female and gentle male characters, the mouth seems to smile. Strong male characters normally sport a moustache, while proud refined characters have a small moustache. The mouths of comic attendants, both in the Balinese *wayang wong Ramayana* and the Javanese masked *wayang wong*, are partly open to allow the dance-actors to speak freely.

Historical Stories

Masked dance-dramas based on historical stories are very popular in Bali, where they are normally referred to as *topeng* (mask). The masks are realistic and quite human-looking, although they represent interpretations by Balinese artists. Characterisation is similar to that of the *wayang*, which distinguishes the female, gentle male and strong male characters.

The shape of the masks is realistic, but strong characters have wide-open eyes, prominent noses, and open mouths with big moustache. Gentle male characters have small eyes, a normal nose, a partly open mouth or a closed mouth, and no moustache. Female characters do not normally wear masks, while comic attendants wear masks without a lower jaw to facilitate speech. In Bali, common people are depicted with deformities such as harelip, deformed lips and swollen nose; the masks are all made of wood. Stories from the history of Bali and ancient Java are most often performed, such as the story of Prime Minister Gajah Mada of 14th-century Majapahit for example.

«« Javanese masks. (From left to right) Panji's refinement is reflected in the flatness and serenity of his mask.

Gunungsari is the brother of Princess Sekartaji whom Panji loves.

Candra Kirana (Princess Sekartaji) is the sweetheart of Panji and a noble character.

Klana's impetuous and avaricious nature is shown in his mask.

ᴦᴦ Klana and his clown servant, Sembunglangu.

(Below) The penasar's *half-mask allows him to speak not just for himself but also for the noble characters in the Balinese* topeng *performances. Bali.*

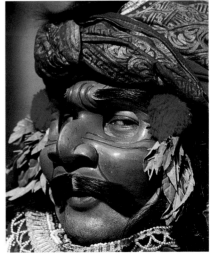

Topeng Pajegan

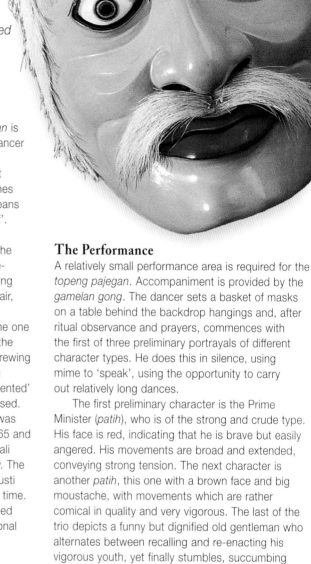

*T*he topeng pajegan *of Bali is very demanding, in terms of performance ability as well as knowledge of ritual practice and narrative sources. The* pajegan *is performed by one man who acts out a series of different characters, changing masks and making minor alterations to his costume, which he does not change, before reappearing from behind the curtain. The* topeng pajegan *is performed at rites of passage, such as weddings and toothfiling ceremonies, as well as at annual temple festivals where it takes place in the inner sanctum of the temple.*

»»»The mask of the Tua *(old man) who is the third personality to appear in the introductory dances of the* topeng pajegan.

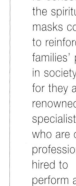

The topeng pajegan *mask-carver selects his wood carefully, requesting the permission of the tree spirit to take the wood.*

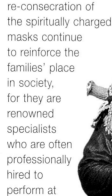

I Made Djimat picking up the penasar *half-mask from his basket of masks as he prepares to perform.*

»The topeng pajegan *performance ends with the appearance of Sidhakarya, a powerful and frightening character with a wild thatch of long white hair.*

Ritual and Traditions

The distinguishing feature of the *topeng pajegan* is that it is a ritual drama during which a single dancer portrays a story through the presentation of a succession of masked characters with different personalities. The word 'Pajegan' comes from a root word 'majeg' which means 'to do the whole thing by oneself'.

The ritual aspects of this performance are embodied in the final character who is the white-faced, buck-toothed and grinning Sidhakarya with his long wild hair, whose name means 'perfectly accomplished undertaking' or 'the one who can do the task'. He enacts the ritual of blessing that features the strewing of coins amongst the audience and the 'kidnapping' of a young child who is then 'presented' before the shrine to the gods before he is released.

According to tradition the *topeng pajegan* was first performed in Gelgel between the years 1665 and 1686, using masks that had been brought to Bali from Java as war booty in the late 16th century. The creation of the performance is attributed to I Gusti Pering Jelantik, prime minister of Gelgel at that time. The *topeng pajegan* was subsequently performed on a regular basis by selected families. Occasional public display and re-consecration of the spiritually charged masks continue to reinforce the families' place in society, for they are renowned specialists who are often professionally hired to perform at ceremonies.

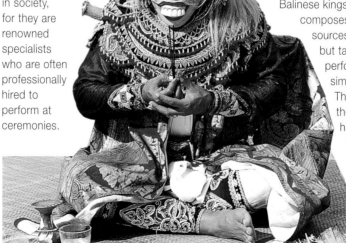

The Performance

A relatively small performance area is required for the *topeng pajegan*. Accompaniment is provided by the *gamelan gong*. The dancer sets a basket of masks on a table behind the backdrop hangings and, after ritual observance and prayers, commences with the first of three preliminary portrayals of different character types. He does this in silence, using mime to 'speak', using the opportunity to carry out relatively long dances.

The first preliminary character is the Prime Minister (*patih*), who is of the strong and crude type. His face is red, indicating that he is brave but easily angered. His movements are broad and extended, conveying strong tension. The next character is another *patih*, this one with a brown face and big moustache, with movements which are rather comical in quality and very vigorous. The last of the trio depicts a funny but dignified old gentleman who alternates between recalling and re-enacting his vigorous youth, yet finally stumbles, succumbing to the reality of his present time in life.

Then the story begins. It is always based on the traditional historical account (*babad*) of Bali that relates the semi-legendary feats of the Hindu-Balinese kings and their ministers. The dancer composes his own plays from manuscript sources according to traditional procedures but tailored to suit the particular occasion of performance. The basic story framework is similar to that employed in the *gambuh*. The dancer generally alternates between the full silent masks of noble figures with half-masks allowing speech that are worn by the clowning servant inter-preters (*penasar*) and comic peasant characters (*bondres*). Kings and noblemen convey meaning in gesture, while these attendants may speak for their masters in the Kawi language, or for themselves in Balinese. The clown-servant who appears in alternation with the other characters is often the *penasar* who is usually regarded as the descendant of the personality Semar from the *gambuh* genre. The *penasar* are represented by two characters, the *penasar kelihan* or older brother, Punta; and the *penasar cenikan* or younger brother, Widjil. The *penasar* is usually represented by Punta who wears a brown half-mask with large black moustache and bulging eyes. He sings and dances and, through his monologue, establishes the exposition of the story to follow.

The next character is the king, whose white or light green mask epitomises the refined figure. He dances an extended set-piece which demonstrates dignity, grace and beauty. Only after this lengthy solo does the king enter the specific context of the story. The king mimes alertness and indicates that he is seeing someone approach and he beckons the latter to come closer. The king exits the stage, leaving behind an invisible presence. The visitor is a messenger in half-mask who speaks alternately in Kawi for the invisible king and in high Balinese as himself responding to the king. The messenger finally departs with his orders, only to return as one of the clown-servants to expand on the story's progress and to joke and entertain.

The stage is next taken over by the *patih*, a warrior and a man of action who carries out the commands of the remote, otherworldly king. The *patih*'s mask is brown with large eyes and a fearsome moustache. Sometimes his lips are parted exposing the teeth, otherwise his lips are closed. The *patih* performs an introductory solo

dance, which is energetic and forceful yet always controlled and dignified; after which he gestures to his invisible servant to prepare for departure on their mission. A succession of comic characters (*bondres*) follow the *patih*. They belong to the lower caste and frequently represent villagers being oppressed by an enemy king. Many are marked by physical defects and wear half-masks that allow speech: the Mute, the Idiot, the Stutterer, the Cleft Palate, the Deaf, and the Flirt. They entertain an enthusiastic audience with their slapstick humour and horseplay.

The final character is the enemy king, in a yellow or red mask with moustache and large eyes. Often bestial in appearance with bared fangs, he makes a sudden entrance, talking and gesticulating excitedly. Ordering his followers to make ready, he vanishes. The *patih* returns to the stage and miming a 'hand-to-hand' battle with the enemy king, he works his way back to the curtain and table where he lifts up the mask of the enemy king to signify his defeat and the victory of the *patih*. The story comes to a close, punctuated by the appearance of the white-masked Sidhakarya and the concluding ritual.

When the entire performance is over and the ritual is completed with the appearance of Sidhakarya, the members of the audience can approach the shrine for individual prayers. The dancer puts away his masks in their basket after presenting a small offering to the god Wisnumurti, Patron of Dance, and returns to his village. In recent times, many dancers are known to compose new scripts by day and performed *topeng* plays based on them at night.

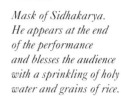

Mask of Sidhakarya. He appears at the end of the performance and blesses the audience with a sprinkling of holy water and grains of rice.

«*A collection of* bondres' *masks. They are pure clowns, marked generally by physical defects such as toothlessness, stuttering, harelip and imbecility.*

(Below left to right)
❶ *The third solo in the introductory dances is a doddering old man who sometimes forgets that he is old and is sharply reminded when his knees give out or he loses his breath.*
❷ *The* penasar *are favourites with Balinese audiences; they are the clown-attendants who speak words of wisdom.*
❸ *The handsome hero-king's performance epitomises the nobility of his character.*
❹ *The* patih *is a man of action, a quintessential warrior.*

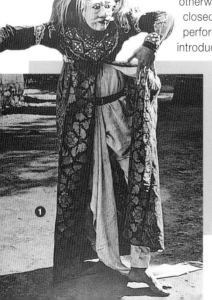

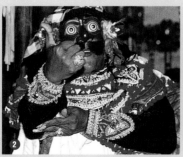

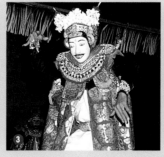

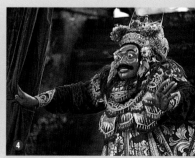

Cirebonese Topeng Play

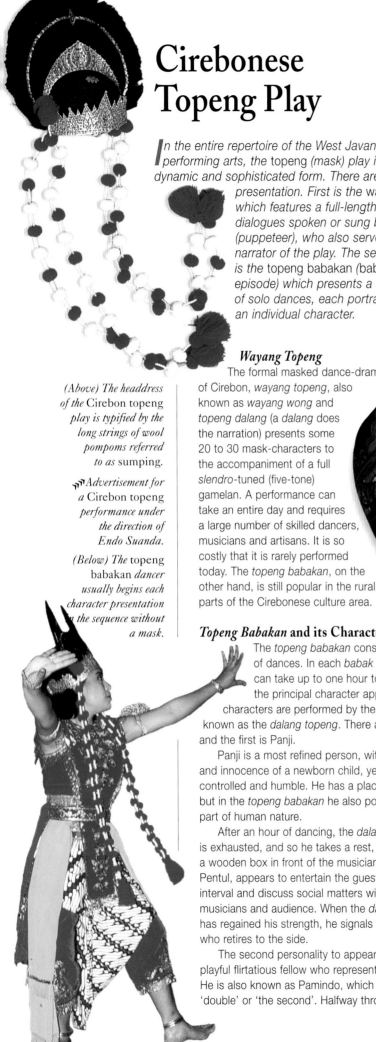

*I*n the entire repertoire of the West Javanese performing arts, the topeng (mask) play is the most dynamic and sophisticated form. There are two forms of presentation. First is the *wayang topeng* which features a full-length play with dialogues spoken or sung by a *dalang (puppeteer)*, who also serves as the narrator of the play. The second type is the *topeng babakan (babak = act, episode)* which presents a series of solo dances, each portraying an individual character.

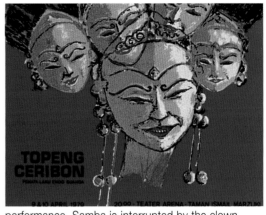

(Above) The headdress of the Cirebon topeng *play is typified by the long strings of wool pompoms referred to as* sumping.

Advertisement for a Cirebon topeng *performance under the direction of Endo Suanda.*

(Below) The topeng babakan *dancer usually begins each character presentation in the sequence without a mask.*

Wayang Topeng

The formal masked dance-drama of Cirebon, *wayang topeng*, also known as *wayang wong* and *topeng dalang (a dalang does the narration)* presents some 20 to 30 mask-characters to the accompaniment of a full *slendro*-tuned (five-tone) gamelan. A performance can take an entire day and requires a large number of skilled dancers, musicians and artisans. It is so costly that it is rarely performed today. The *topeng babakan*, on the other hand, is still popular in the rural parts of the Cirebonese culture area.

Topeng Babakan and its Characters

The *topeng babakan* consists of a series of dances. In each *babak* or scene, which can take up to one hour to complete, only the principal character appears. All the characters are performed by the same dancer, known as the *dalang topeng*. There are five in all and the first is Panji.

Panji is a most refined person, with the purity and innocence of a newborn child, yet is wise, self-controlled and humble. He has a place in history, but in the *topeng babakan* he also portrays a part of human nature.

After an hour of dancing, the *dalang topeng* is exhausted, and so he takes a rest, sitting near a wooden box in front of the musicians. A clown, Pentul, appears to entertain the guests during the interval and discuss social matters with both musicians and audience. When the *dalang topeng* has regained his strength, he signals to the clown who retires to the side.

The second personality to appear is Samba, a playful flirtatious fellow who represents childhood. He is also known as Pamindo, which roughly means 'double' or 'the second'. Halfway through the performance, Samba is interrupted by the clown Pentul who asks him who he is and what is he doing there. Samba lifts his mask slightly so that he can introduce himself. He tells Pentul that he has been invited to dance. This brief conversation introduces the performers to the audience and at the same time announces the proceedings of the performance. After this Samba continues dancing.

Next is the Tumenggung, a strong and high-ranking male character, the personification of maturity. As in the two previous scenes, the *dalang topeng* begins his performance unmasked. After finishing the first part of his performance, he takes a break, sitting near the box.

❶ *Kalana.*
❷ *Panji.*
❸ *Samba.*
❹ *Tumenggung .*
❺ *Rumyang.*
❻ *Pendem, the clown servant of Prince Panji is characterised by his comical features. He appears during intervals to entertain the audience with his slapstick humour.*

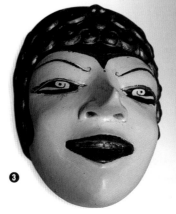
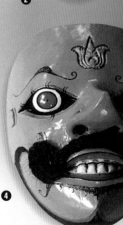

CIREBONESE TOPENG PERSONALITIES AND THEIR CHARACTERISTICS

Character	Panji	Samba or Pamindo	Tumenggung	Kalana	Rumyang
Features	White mask with delicate, downcast eyes which symbolise his refinement and humility. Thin red lips outlined in black which are curved in a sweet wistful smile.	White mask, or light pink or light blue, with gold-sprinkled curls of hair which frame the face. Downcast eyes, thin eyebrows and eyebrow-markings, an elongated turned-up nose and round cheeks. A radiant smile exposing gold teeth which is accentuated by bright red lips outlined with a thin black line.	Dark or light red in colour with large red eyes, a full moustache and a rather large, opened mouth that bares big white or gold teeth.	Dark red mask with great bulging eyes, a fierce scowl, open mouth and large protruding teeth.	Similar to Samba's mask but instead of a frame of curls, the face is surrounded by a heart-shaped hairline rendered in gold paint.
Movements	His movements are slow, very precise and graceful with tiny finger flutters, soft shoulder rolls and limited foot action.	Samba performs a highly ornamented dance with vivacious, playful and coquettish movements.	His movements are strong and forceful. Every gesture emphasises the directness, self-confidence and strength of his character.	He takes long strides with legs wide apart, his gestures are grand and full of force.	His movements nearly replicate those of Samba, but are more refined and mature.

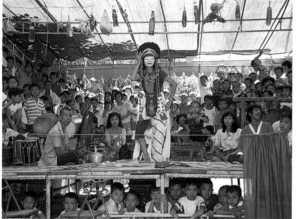

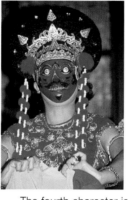

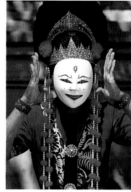

(Left to right) A temporary wooden platform is set up for a village performance of the topeng babakan. *Kalana's red mask demonstrates his quick temper, crudeness and ambition. This can be contrasted with the refined and noble character of Panji, represented by the pure white or pale-coloured mask.*

(Below) The gamelan accompaniment to the topeng babakan *performance is much livelier and the drumming more forceful than other Sundanese* wayang *dances. This energy is paralleled by the vigorous and powerful dance performed by the* dalang topeng.

Suddenly, Pentul comes on stage, boasting loudly that he is as good a dancer as the *dalang topeng*. He dons the *dalang topeng*'s headdress and asks for the same musical piece. He imitates the movements of the Tumenggung's dance, but looks so funny that the audience breaks into laughter. Unexpectedly, the music stops. The musicians call loudly to Pentul, telling him that his headdress is backwards. After fixing it, Pentul puts on a mask and recommences dancing with funny movements. The music is different and the clown stops, removes the mask and asks the musicians why the music is so strange. They tell him that he has put on the wrong mask. In disappointment, Pentul gives up and retires.

The *dalang topeng* continues the Tumenggung dance, but now he faces a counterpart, Jinggananom, who is ready for battle. This is the only scene in which a segment of story is portrayed, rather than merely a personality. He became Tumenggung Magangiraja from the kingdom of Bauwarna.

The fourth character is Kalana, who represents a greedy, evil character. In this episode, the *dalang topeng* begins without a mask. He puts on the mask when his character begins to become consumed with anger.

Rumyang comes next. He has a nature similar to that of Samba, but is more mature and refined in movement. This is the only dance which starts directly with the mask on. In performance, Rumyang represents the return to youthfulness in old age.

Masks, Costumes and Movements

The mask is carved from wood by village artisans. At the mouth of the mask is attached a split leather tongue which the dancer grips between his teeth to keep the mask on. The mask can be easily removed.

A rich variety of head movements accentuate the mask, which is the main focus of all *topeng* dances in general. There is considerable interplay between costume and dance movements, the *soder* (scarf) being flipped frequently, as are the *sumping* (long strings of wool pompoms) descending from the headdress down the cheeks. The *soder*-play is particularly evident in Tumenggeng's performance, in which he picks up the right end between toes of his right foot and kicks it behind the body with such energy that the end flips up and falls over the shoulder.

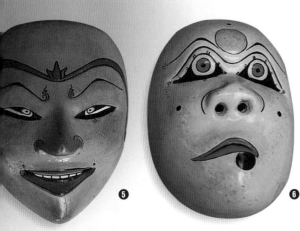

❺

❻

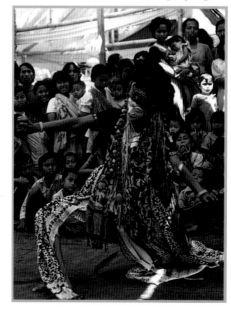

Javanese Masks from Malang and Madura

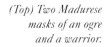

In the Malang and Madura regions of East Java, mask-dance (topeng) performances stress the role of the narrator or dalang. The dalang recites the story and conducts conversations between personalities, while dancers wearing masks play the respective roles and act out these conversations in dance movements. In Madura, these performances are called topeng dalang, showing the importance of the narrator.

Language of the Performance

The topeng dalang performance uses the Madurese language, while the wayang topeng performance is conducted in the local dialect of the Javanese language. However, these conversational languages are both rooted in ancient Javanese culture, as are the dance movements and musical accompaniment. Only two dancers playing the roles of the punakawan or comic retainers speak for themselves in the performance.

Historical Background

Malang and Sumenep on Madura were once part of the 13th-century kingdom of Singasari. A close relationship existed between the feudal administrators of Madura and Java. Before Singasari, Kadiri-Janggala in Java (11th-12th centuries) was already famous for its many literary works.

By the late 15th to the 16th centuries, the Kadiri-Janggala story became known as the story of Panji, presenting the ideal figure of Panji Inukertapati, King of Kadiri. The Madurese topeng dalang still performs the Mahabharata stories today and sometimes the Ramayana, while the wayang topeng Malang focuses on the Panji cycle. Principal differences in the two masked performance lie in language, story, kind of stage, orchestra, roles and dance styles.

Topeng Dalang Madura

The Madurese topeng dalang performance has at least 20 male performers. A performance opens with a dance by Klana Tunjungseta, a knight. He sometimes brings along four of his giant followers. The dance discloses that the god Siva has sent Klana Tunjungseta to monitor the situation on earth and the behaviour of its people. Tunjungseta's assignment is described in the subsequent play. The personalities featured in the stories are the constantly disputing

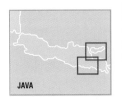

(Top) Two Madurese masks of an ogre and a warrior.

Some dance groups use a stage with backdrops that can be rolled up to display different scenes painted onto the canvas that fit in with the location of the event. On the other hand, many performances carry on without any stage props.

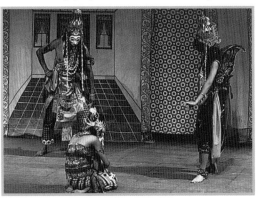

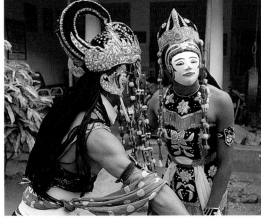

(Above) As a folk theatre, the mask-plays of Malang and Madura can be presented anywhere. The Madurese topeng play is presented here in the backyard of a house. Originally, the stage for both Malang and Madurese topeng was an open field near the village.

(Right) Long scarves draped from the waist or neck are an important dance accessory throughout Java.

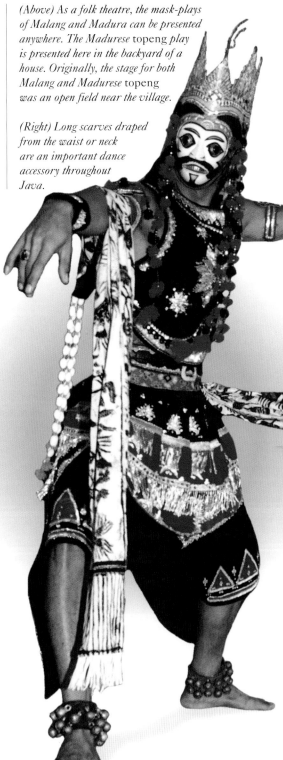

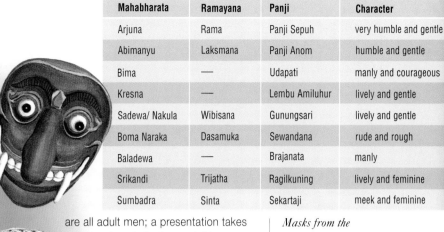

Mahabharata	Ramayana	Panji	Character
Arjuna	Rama	Panji Sepuh	very humble and gentle
Abimanyu	Laksmana	Panji Anom	humble and gentle
Bima	—	Udapati	manly and courageous
Kresna	—	Lembu Amiluhur	lively and gentle
Sadewa/ Nakula	Wibisana	Gunungsari	lively and gentle
Boma Naraka	Dasamuka	Sewandana	rude and rough
Baladewa	—	Brajanata	manly
Srikandi	Trijatha	Ragilkuning	lively and feminine
Sumbadra	Sinta	Sekartaji	meek and feminine

Masks from the
wayang topeng
Malang.
❶ *Brajanata*
❷ *Sewandana*
❸ *Buto Terong*
❹ *Ragilkuning*
❺ *Gunungsari*
❻ *Pati Sabrang*
❼ *Sekartaji*

are all adult men; a presentation takes almost a whole day or night.

The performance is preceded by the *ngremo* dance. The first *jejeran* (scene) which follows sets the background for the story. The *grebeg Jawa*, next, presents soldiers and officers leaving for war. The story climaxes with the appearance of Prabu Klana Sewandana who, with his soldiers, performs the *grebeg sabrang*. A war breaks out between the Javanese and Sabrang soldiers; however as neither party wins, it is called *perang gagal,* 'unresolved' war. Another party is introduced to complete the story or to be the arbiter.

A special dance, the *klana alus*, comes out around midnight, performed by Gunungsari, a smartly dressed nobleman, and his follower, the comic Patrajaya. During this segment of the show there are additional scenes consisting of comedic dramas based on daily rural life. Often the narrator himself performs to make the people laugh. This part can carry on until late in the afternoon or the break of dawn. Then the performers hurry to complete the story. There is a scene in which a priest gives his admonitions and another war scene which ends up in a victory for the Javanese nobleman who symbolises righteousness.

The stage for the performance is square, with a curtain at the back, behind which is the dressing room. The performers enter and leave the stage through a slit at the sides or in the middle of this curtain. Prabu Klana and Gunungsari touch and play with these slits as they dance. The narrator sits in a corner of the stage near the screen in order to be able to direct the performance. The gamelan orchestra is placed to one side. Thus, the audience can view the play from three directions.

Pandawa and Korawa. Heroic roles are represented by any one of the Pandawa brothers.

The stage is square with a backdrop of a *pendapa* (the open front hall of a Javanese mansion). Curtained doors on the right and left can be opened to let the dancers through. The narrator is hidden behind the backdrop, which has a small hole in the centre to allow him to follow the performance. The *slendro* (five-toned) gamelan set that accompanies the performance with Madurese melodies is also behind the backdrop. Only the *kendhang*-player (double-headed drum) faces the dancers.

Wayang Topeng Malang

A *wayang topeng malang* performance has the same number of performers, including 12 musicians to play the *pelog* (seven-toned) gamelan, one narrator and seven dancers who change masks during the dance to represent many different characters. Performers

Aspects	Malang	Madura
Language	Malang dialect of Javanese	High-level Madurese
Story	Panji	Mahabharata/Ramayana
Platform	Plain screen in background	Painted/moving backdrop
Gamelan	*Pelog*-tuning	*Slendro*–tuning
Function	Secular/ritual	Secular
Dance	Refined/expressive	Expressive

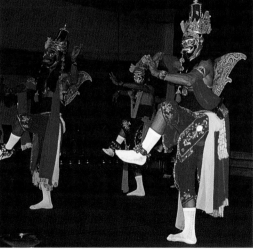

The enemy king Klana Sewandana performs the grebeg sabrang. *The* wayang topeng Malang *is designed to enliven a party. Guests, who give donations, come and go at will. Performances may also be held in connection with ruwatan rituals which release a person from bad luck.*

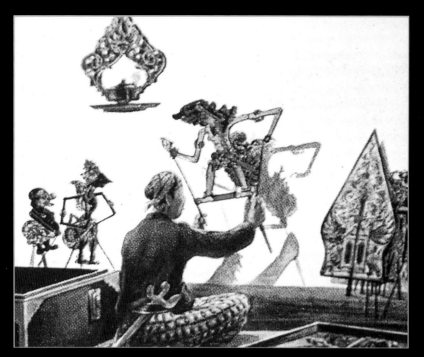

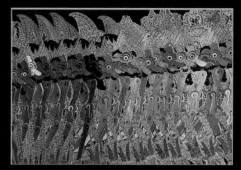

(Above) A row of wayang kulit *shadow puppets from Central Java representing monster characters. Although* wayang golek *performances have become increasingly rare,* wayang golek *puppets have become an important commodity on the tourist market. (Right) A* wayang cepak *puppet representing a female character. (Opposite, bottom) A* wayang golek *puppet representing a noble man.
(Below) Flat leather puppets are played against a cotton screen and their shadows are projected clearly to watchers on the other side. Traditionally this shadow side was where the women and children sat. In Bali the shadow theatre has remained popular despite the advent of television and the cinema.*

(Above) The dalang *is not only a master of puppet manipulation but also a scholar who is well-versed in Indian and local literature from which he adapts the stories of his performances. The* dalang *is a person with great spiritual power. In literature like the Panji tales and historical texts on the Yogyakarta sultans and sultanate, the king, prince or sultan is revered for his ability to perform as a* dalang.

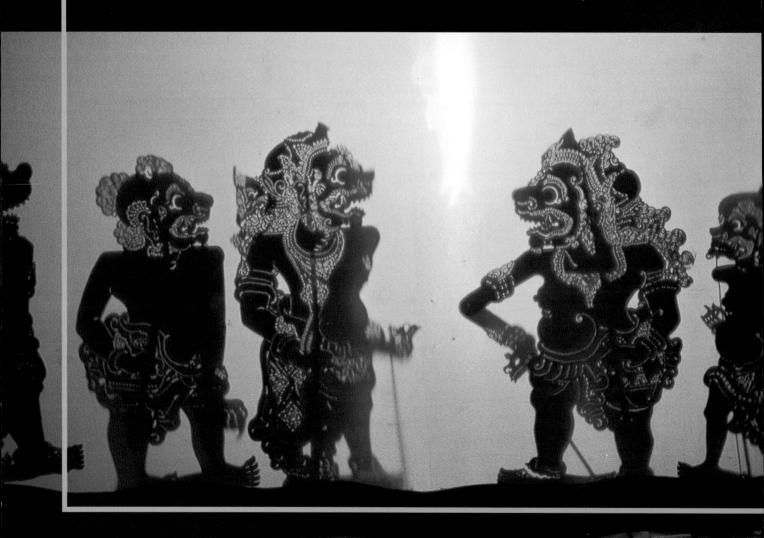

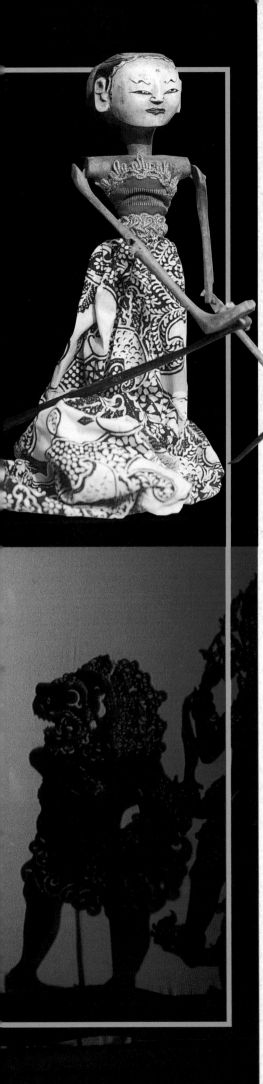

WAYANG THEATRE

Wayang is a difficult word to translate into English. It means both 'shadow' and 'image' or 'imagination'. The tendency has been to take the former connotation, and speak of the *wayang* theatre as being a 'shadow-puppet theatre'. This has led to the misconception that shadow is the medium of aesthetic expression throughout this class of performing arts. In actual fact, it is only so in the *wayang kulit* theatre with its two-dimensional leather puppets. The three-dimensional *wayang golek* (a variety of wooden puppets from Java and Sunda), for example, is not projected against a screen, and therefore shadows do not play any part in the performance.

The *wayang* represents the human, animal or ogre form and also refined, strong and clownish characters. Furthermore each dominant character can have varieties and the varieties are called *wanda*. *Wanda* is a particular rendering of a character to express a special mood and setting. Each single character can have four, five or even twelve versions representing a different mood and distinguished by a particular bent of head, bent of body, degree of slant to eyes and mouth, distance between eye and eyebrow, distance between eyes and mouth, and colours used.

The *wayang* performance constitutes a festival of local culture that encompasses elements of religion, social customs and traditions, art, mysticism, education and philosophy of life. These occur on and off the stage. The host, the *dalang* (puppeteer/manipulator/narrator) and his musicians, the audience and the food vendors all constitute elements of this unique cultural festival. Each presentation must fit into this particular ambience. No two *wayang* performances can ever be identical, even with the same *dalang* or the same story.

There are no fixed scripts; the story outline, called the *balungan lakon*, is filled by the *dalang* as he feels appropriate. The proficiency of the *dalang* is the determinant. He must be able to provide solutions to problems while keeping within the parameters of justness and the reality of life, because the audience will not only be comparing solutions provided by various *dalang*, but will probably discuss them with friends. The *dalang*'s freedom in giving content to the story outline is called *sanggit*.

Several forms of *wayang* theatre are described on the following pages, ranging from the ancient *wayang purwa* of Java and *wayang parwa* of Bali to others created in the post-Independence era as means of disseminating information on the struggle for independence.

Javanese Wayang Purwa

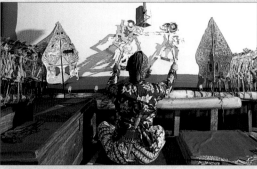

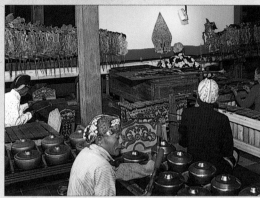

Wayang kulit purwa *is a very popular form of shadow-theatre in Java. Although it is very old, traditional and classical, it has been able to keep up with the passage of time, adapting to contemporary ideas and needs. It serves many functions: formerly a vehicle for ancestor worship (seen today in such rituals as* ruwatan, sadranan, bersih desa)*, it promotes religious preaching, education, dissemination of information or propaganda, and inculcation of moral standards. It is simultaneously a source of entertainment.*

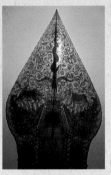

The stationary gunungan *signifies the beginning and end of each scene in the* wayang kulit *performance. It is also waved around by the* dalang *to signify natural forces at work.*

The dalang *easily manipulates the puppets to represent a fighting scene between Hanoman and a* raksasa. *(Below) The gamelan players of the shadow play theatre.*

The Puppets and Equipment

The *wayang kulit purwa* is a flat, two-dimensional figure made of buffalo hide intricately perforated and painted; it is furnished with a central supporting stick and manipulating sticks made of buffalo horn. The figures represent deities, humans, giants, animals and symbols of nature. A collection can contain a total of 150 to 300 of these leather shadow-puppet figures, which are kept in a chest.

The shadows are projected onto a screen (*kelir*). The *kelir* is white with a red or black frame and is stretched out both horizontally and vertically. A banana-tree bole (*gedebog*) lying flat along the bottom edge of the *kelir* is used to hold the figures: the soft trunk is easily penetrated by the puppets' sharp central rods of buffalo horn. An oil lamp (*blencong*) is hung above the *dalang* (puppeteer/ narrator/manipulator). Musical accompaniment is derived from a set of Javanese gamelan instruments while additional depth is provided by use of the *ke-prak* (slit wooden signal box sounded with a wooden mallet, *cempala*). Banana boles are also placed on the left and right sides of the screen to hold the array of *wayang* not being used for the performance. The *wayang* are arranged upright and almost overlapping one another. The array of *wayang* is called *simpingan* and it serves as additional decoration.

The Performance

The *wayang* performance is led by the *dalang* who acts as the storyteller, narrator and director of the play, as well as director of the gamelan orchestra. He is assisted by about 18 musicians and five male and female vocalists. The duration of the performance is about eight hours, from 9:00 p.m. to 5:00 a.m.

It is divided into three parts: *pathet nem*, *pathet sanga,* and *pathet manyura* which correspond to birth, growth and death, symbols of the chain of human life in traditional Javanese philosophy.

The stories are built around births, weddings, contests, revelations, ascensions, heroic death and war. They are rooted in the stories of the Arjunasasra, Ramayana and Mahabharata, traditional Javanese mythology, and fictional tales created by the *dalang* or narrator. Among the most popular are stories extracted from the Mahabharata cycle concerning the eternal rivalry between the Pandawa and Korawa families.

The most interesting aspect of a *wayang purwa* performance is the underlying message in each story. This can refer to actual community problems, make criticism of social conditions, and even encourage reform. Other significant elements are the narrator's skill in manipulating the *wayang* figures and the sharp sense of humour expressed by the *panakawan* (servants) in their role as faithful servants whose duty is to provide their masters with amusement as well as advice. The *panakawan* are unique to the Indonesian *wayang*; they are not found in the original Indian

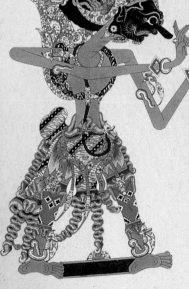

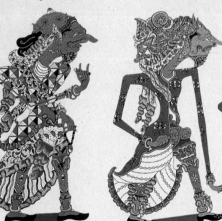

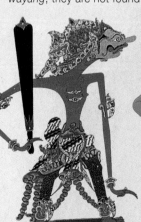

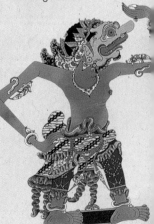

PARTS OF A *WAYANG KULIT* PUPPET

The flat leather puppets of Central Java are finely worked, every space filled with intricate detail. Perforations are made with small sharp stamps that are hammered into the buffalo hide. No motif or colour is perchance; but they follow age-old tradition to indicate mood and rank, and identify the character. Kresna (right) is first cousin to the Pandawa. Kresna is part deity, an incarnation of the Hindu god, Visnu.

1. *makuta* (crown)
2. *jamang* (diadem)
3. *garuda mungkur* (Garuda facing backwards)
4. *sumping* (ear ornament)
5. *praba* (backwing)
6. *saputangan* (ornamental collar)
7. *ulur-ulur* (long necklace)
8. *kelatbau* (arm band)
9. *gelang* (bracelet)
10. *sabuk* (waistsash)
11. *pending* (buckle)
12. *kunca* (tails of dress)
13. *kampuh* (royal cloth)
14. *uncal kencana* (gold pendants)
15. *lancingan* (trousers)
16. *kroncong* (bracelet on wrists and ankles)

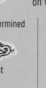
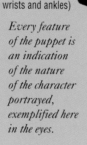

refined · patient · tranquil · determined · very determined

jealous · sly · looking for sympathy · clever · dishonest

forthright · anxious · frightening · blames others · wilful

Every feature of the puppet is an indication of the nature of the character portrayed, exemplified here in the eyes.

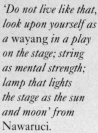

'*Do not live like that, look upon yourself as a wayang in a play on the stage; string as mental strength; lamp that lights the stage as the sun and moon*' from Nawaruci.

The shadow-puppet figures featured at the bottom of these pages are taken from the Mahabharata cycle of stories.

The colours are carefully applied to the newly-made puppet.

(Below, left to right) Jayadrata is a powerful ally of the Korawa. Durna is a brahmana and teacher to both the Pandawa and Korawa. Bisma is Astina's elder statesman and is well-loved by both the Pandawa and Korawa. Citraksi and Durmagati are two of the antagonists of the Pandawa. Pandu is the father of the five Pandawa brothers, namely, Yudistira, Arjuna, Nakula/Sadewa (identical twins) and the mighty Bima.

epics. A *wayang* performance also carries lessons on morals, ethics and philosophy.

"The trunks of banana trees that the puppets are inserted in are symbols of the world of man's spirit. Man's spirit is the puppeteer, symbol of truth and meaning. The screen's the unseen world above, man's characters the wayangs, and the lamp's rays the Almighty. The audience is the all-perceiving wise man." (quoted by dalang/writer, Sri Mulyono).

The Role of the *Wayang Purwa*

The audience at a *wayang purwa* performance is not required to give undivided attention to the narrative. People are free to sell things, eat or drink at the little stalls, talk with each other, and even take a nap. The play can be watched from both sides of the *kelir*, either behind the narrator or on the shadow side.

Wayang performances are held at many social and family events to ensure welfare and safety, for example at seven-month pregnancy rituals, when a baby is five days old, at circumcisions, weddings and on birthdays. They are also performed at traditional rites with a spiritual-religious context, like *ruwatan* (ritual to release a person from ill fortune), *nadaran* (to fulfil a vow made or a wish granted) and *bersih desa* (village purification). A *wayang* show is often performed in government circles or social institutions to convey a message or some information, for example at the celebration of Independence Day or the inauguration of a new building or bridge. On such official occasions, messages referring to the national development programme may very well be inserted. The *wayang* characters are so popular that their names are often used as names of people, schools, hotels, restaurants, streets, transportation vehicles and shops.

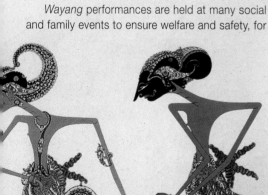

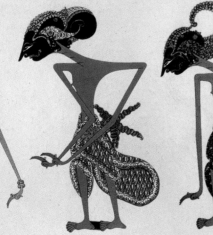

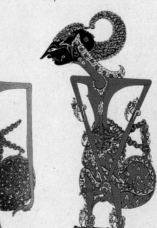

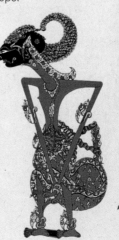

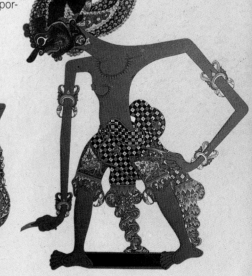

Balinese Wayang Kulit Parwa

Wayang *puppets in Bali are made of cowhide. A full set contains 100 to 135 characters. The shape and decoration of each puppet provide immediate clues to the character. Refined (alus) figures are generally small, have closed foot stance, almond eyes, slim profile and downward head posture. Coarse (keras) characters, on the contrary, are usually larger in size, have splayed foot stance, gross profile, round eyes and upward head posture.*

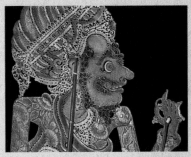

(Above) A rsi *who features in both the Indian epics and many local stories. Most heroic and other supporting characters speak in ancient Sanskrit-based Kawi, not always understood by the general audience. Dialogue is interpreted, paraphrased and commented upon at several levels of the contemporary vernacular by the buffoon attendants.*

(Below) The calonarang/barong *was also adapted for the* wayang *theatre.*

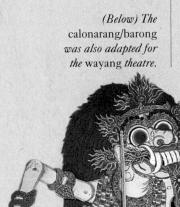

Wayang Parwa

Sources for the *wayang parwa* stories are the Hindu Mahabharata and Ramayana; local literature such as the *Panji* romances, *Cupak*, and *Calonarang*; and recently, the *Tantri Kamandaka*.

The Performance

A performance is usually an offering marking the completion of a ceremony or ritual such as a wedding, funeral or other major event for the individual or the community. It may last from two to five hours after sundown.

At the performance site, the *dalang* recites a *mantra*: 'The god of love is arrived! Ohmmm!' He then dines with the sponsor of the performance. When eating, the *dalang* must face east or north; if south, there will be interference by demonic spirits, and if west, he could become forgetful and confused during the play.

Before the action can begin, an invocation and explanatory narration are delivered. First, the *dalang* prepares his speaking voice for the extraordinary demands of the two-to-five-hour performance. Secondly, he requests permission from the gods for the performance and apologises for any errors he might make. Thirdly, he establishes the background for the story beginning with creation, then sets the basic circumstances of the night's particular play, in the Kawi language.

When preparations are complete and the lamp has been lit, the musicians commence with the overture, which signals the audience to be seated. After approximately 20 minutes of music, the *dalang* takes his place behind the screen, and invokes divine protection for himself and his troupe. He strikes the lid of his puppet chest three times, as he prays, calling the puppets to life.

The musicians play the *Pemungkah*. The puppet chest is opened and the lid placed beside the *dalang,* on his right. On each side, beyond lid and box is a *ketengkong* (assistant) who assists by filling and adjusting the oil lamp and helping the *dalang* keep his puppets in good order.

The performance opens with the *kayon* which the *dalang* holds behind his lamp, he presses his head forward against it, praying that the gods of the nine directions gather in his *kayon* to grant him their protection and power for a successful performance. The prologue begins when the *dalang* gives a signal with his *capala* (a mallet), and the musicians move to the next section of the *Pemungkah*.

The *dalang* now performs the *dance of the kayon* in which the figure flutters and spins between lamp and screen in time with the music. This represents the creation of the macro-cosmos from the void: every story begins with this backdrop of eternity. The *kayon* is then planted in the centre of the screen, indicating that creation is complete.

Next, the *dalang* takes each of the puppets from his chest and assigns it to its appropriate place on either the right (good characters) or left (evil characters) side of the screen. Puppets that will take part in the performance are stuck upright in the banana bole on either side of the *kayon* and placed against the screen in such a way that their features are only vaguely indicated by their shadows. This symbolises the indistinct nature of human character at the point of creation. Unused puppets are stacked in packs at the sides. In the centre is a special figure, Lord Acintya, who represents the ineffable single godhead presiding over the action of all the stories. The musicians move ahead to the next phase of *Pemungkah*. The four *penasar* (clown attendants) are placed on the lid of the box. Weapons and props are close at hand. The puppets to be used in the story are removed from the screen and placed to the sides. Before the story may begin, a shorter *kayon* dance is performed to represent the worldly struggle of humankind.

The *dalang* raps sharply with his *capala,* calling for a change in the music. The musicians know which piece to play when they see the *dalang* pick up the first puppet. The principal characters of the first scene are brought on rather formally, accompanied by the singing of the *dalang.* The highest ranking character enters first, followed by the less important characters and concluding always with the appropriate pair of *penasar,* depending on whether it is the 'good' or 'evil' party that is meeting.

When he has completed his opening routine, the *dalang* signals to his musicians to change to *Alas Harum* (The Perfumed Forest), a composition suitable for the entrance of a refined character. Finally, the performance begins.

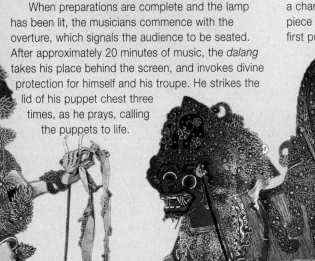

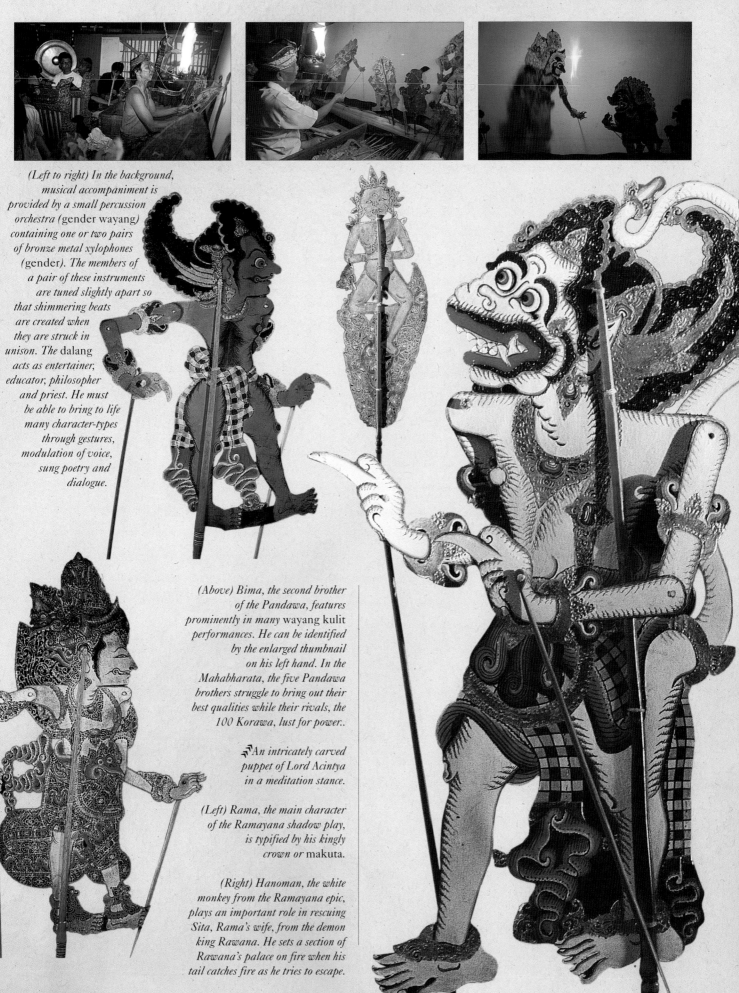

(Left to right) In the background, musical accompaniment is provided by a small percussion orchestra (gender wayang) containing one or two pairs of bronze metal xylophones (gender). The members of a pair of these instruments are tuned slightly apart so that shimmering beats are created when they are struck in unison. The dalang acts as entertainer, educator, philosopher and priest. He must be able to bring to life many character-types through gestures, modulation of voice, sung poetry and dialogue.

(Above) Bima, the second brother of the Pandawa, features prominently in many wayang kulit performances. He can be identified by the enlarged thumbnail on his left hand. In the Mahabharata, the five Pandawa brothers struggle to bring out their best qualities while their rivals, the 100 Korawa, lust for power..

An intricately carved puppet of Lord Acintya in a meditation stance.

(Left) Rama, the main character of the Ramayana shadow play, is typified by his kingly crown or makuta.

(Right) Hanoman, the white monkey from the Ramayana epic, plays an important role in rescuing Sita, Rama's wife, from the demon king Rawana. He sets a section of Rawana's palace on fire when his tail catches fire as he tries to escape.

The Wayang Cepak of Cirebon

The Cirebon cultural entity extends beyond Cirebon regency to include the regencies of Indramayu, part of Majalengka, Kuningan, Subang and Brebes, embracing a total population of some five million. This cultural unit is home to a special form of wayang *theatre known as* wayang cepak *or wayang papak. Both* cepak *and* papak *mean 'flat', 'equal' or 'closer'. The headdresses of these puppets are flat compared to the high, rounded forms of* wayang golek.

A panji puppet from the wayang cepak. *The term 'panji' is not used specifically to refer to the prince of the Panji tales but rather a hero character.*

EXTENT OF THE POPULARITY OF THE WAYANG CEPAK

Subang
Indramayu
Cirebon
Majalengka
Kuningan
Brebes

WEST JAVA

wayang cepak sites

Origin

Chronicles and oral history attribute the origins of the wayang cepak, and many other traditional art forms, to two of the wali sanga, Sunan Kudus and Sunan Kalijaga. The wali sanga are a group of nine Muslim proselytisers who propagated Islam in Java from the 15th to 16th centuries. It is traditionally believed that the puppetry tradition was established by the wali.

The spread of Islam in Java coincides more or less with the downfall of Majapahit, and concentrated along the north coast of the island, creating a unique pesisir culture. Islam created an unusual blend of syncretic culture composed of old and new elements. Religious texts (suluk) found in manuscripts, and oral performances reflect this phenomenon.

A Ritual Role

Along with a few other traditional art forms, the wayang cepak continues to play an important role in communal rituals. Even with diminished appearance in individual celebrations, its function in religious ritual still pertains. The annual ngunjung (ancestral)

rites held at village grave sites, for example, involve the performance of wayang cepak. Though the artistic and communicative aspects of wayang cepak as a form of entertainment are no longer popular with the general public, there is still a strong spiritual connection with farming and fishing communities. The three-day ceremony at the tomb of Sunan Gunung Jati in Cirebon — together with sidekah bumi (earth blessing) and nadran (fisherman's thanksgiving for a prayer fulfilled) held in November or December — can attract over 70, 000 participants.

Personae and Plots

On the basis of the costume, especially shirts and headcloths of the wayang cepak puppets, about 30 figures do resemble humans. The assumption that wayang puppets became stylised beyond resemblance to human beings is thought to pertain to Islamic tenets. Another 60 or so puppets, portraying kings wearing crowns, demons and princesses are, however, not dissimilar to wayang golek purwa puppets, except for the absence of the cupit urang ('shrimp pincer') headdress, which is so typical of the wayang purwa style.

The handsome, heroic and noble knight or prince (satria) in the wayang cepak, comparable to the Arjuna figure of the wayang purwa, is referred to as panji. There are about ten panji in one set. The primary hero is accompanied by one or two clown-attendants, panakawan. Lamsijan is the ever-present clown-attendant, somewhat reminiscent of Cepot of the Sundanese wayang golek. The other is Saragonja, who resembles Semar.

Unlike the wayang golek menak of Central Java which is restricted to the presentation of stories from the Menak cycle, the wayang cepak draws its repertoire from a great variety of sources: Panji, Damarwulan, Menak and the babad (local histories). The most commonly presented, at least since the

---

WAYANG CEPAK PUPPETS

'Wayang cepak' in general is used for wayang *forms in which the puppets have rather flat headdresses. The repertoire consists of Javanese history and Muslim stories.* Wayang cepak *puppets can be either of leather (shadow puppets) or of wood (wayang golek cepak). The* wayang golek cepak *puppets were probably derived from the* wayang kulit cepak *and therefore do not resemble the* wayang golek purwa *puppets.*

(Below) A group of wayang golek cepak *puppets representing* *female characters of a princess and two ladies-in-waiting.*

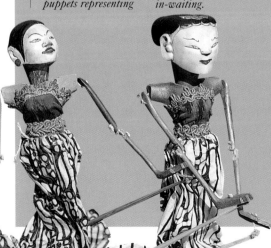

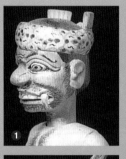
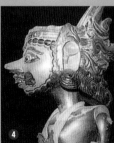
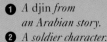
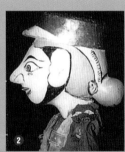
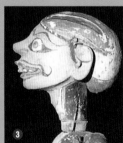

❶ *A djin from an Arabian story.*
❷ *A soldier character.*
❸ *A patih or minister.*
❹ *Menak Jingga from the Menak stories*

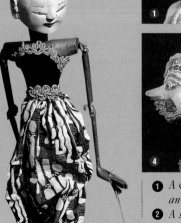

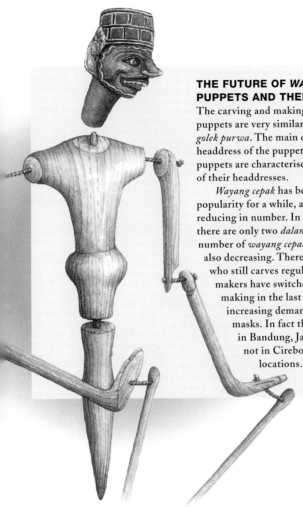

THE FUTURE OF *WAYANG CEPAK* PUPPETS AND THEIR *DALANG*

The carving and making of *wayang cepak* puppets are very similar to that of the *wayang golek purwa*. The main difference lies in the headdress of the puppet. *Wayang cepak* puppets are characterised by the flatness of their headdresses.

Wayang cepak has been declining in popularity for a while, and *dalang* are rapidly reducing in number. In the Indramayu regency, there are only two *dalang* still active. The number of *wayang cepak* puppet-makers is also decreasing. There is now only one maker who still carves regularly. Most of the other makers have switched to *kedok* (mask)-making in the last two decades. There are increasing demands and markets for masks. In fact these 'markets' are based in Bandung, Jakarta and abroad, and not in Cirebon or other traditional locations.

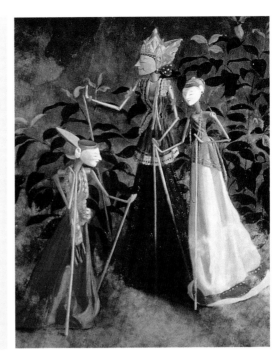

A painting of a trio of wayang golek cepak *puppets by Lodewijk Karel Bruckman.*

though, is that no matter what story is presented, the structure (sequences of the scenes), the nature of the play (good against bad), and character portrayal (*sakti* or supernatural/magical) are similar to those of *wayang* in general.

Musical Accompaniment

The *wayang cepak* performance is accompanied by gamelan music, tuned to either the *prawa* (five-toned) or *pelog* (seven-toned) scale. There are only a few pieces of music unique to *wayang cepak*. The most notable one is the accompaniment to the fight scene, named accordingly, *Perang Golek* ('Wooden Puppet Fight'). Musical presentation is also very dominant. People may request for favourite songs to be sung by the singer, *sinden*, with some tips, and these songs may vary from traditional Cirebon pieces, to Sundanese *jaipongan* (today's popular song-and-dance genre), to *dangdut* (popular diatonic songs).

early 20th century, is the *babad* concerning the Islamisation of the Hinduised kingdoms of Cirebon and vicinity by the *wali sanga*, particularly Sunan Gunung Jati, founder of the kingdom of Cirebon, and Sunan Kalijaga, the *wali* mostly credited with the creation of many Javanese art forms. Although related to history, the stories have been adopted from orally transmitted sources, and then redefined or recreated individually. The same story therefore varies from *dalang* to *dalang*. This reference to oral sources (to some degree esoteric), and to individual (meditative) interpretation, is called *sejarah peteng* (dark history), which generally differs from the royal *babad*, for instance. For this reason, the *wayang cepak* is almost never performed in the courts of Cirebon. One of the most controversial stories is that of Sekh Siti Jenar, because of the message implied by many of the *dalang* that Siti Jenar is more on the 'right side' than the other *walis*.

Although acknowledging the nobility as a source of power upon which the common folk depend, the *wayang cepak* stories relate more to the village world than do the *wayang purwa* stories which primarily concern conflicts between kings and kingdoms. Stories about the knight who must find a magical treatment for rice pests, or to open an irrigation dam blocked by evil characters, are commonly performed for village ceremonies. No differentiation is made in the ethnic origins of this noble power, at least not in the story itself. The kings of Bagdad (Iraq), Majapahit (East Java), Mataram (Central Java), Sunda-Pajajaran (West Java) and Cirebon itself are viewed as 'their own' and able to give protection or blessings to the common people. More important,

WAYANG CEPAK PUPPETS WITH LEGS

There was a form of 19th-century *wayang cepak* from Central Java whose puppets were portrayed with feet. For the performance, a wooden plank with holes was used, instead of the traditional banana bole or trunk. Many of these puppets have red faces, but by contrast with the *wayang golek purwa* puppets, none have fangs. Some of the paraphernalia are different: table, chair and a horse with a hole in its back.

(Below, left to right) A puppet representing a prince. A king on his horse; the crown is similar to that of *wayang golek purwa* puppets but is less ornate. A royal character on his throne, with a table in front of him. Tables and chairs are not found with *wayang golek purwa*.

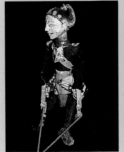

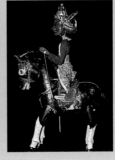

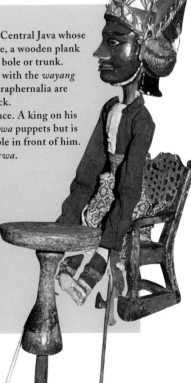

Wayang Golek and Wayang Krucil

*T*he wayang golek *and* wayang krucil *are made of wood. The* wayang golek *is found in Central and East Java, with performances in the Javanese language, and in West Java, using the Sundanese language. The* wayang krucil *is native to Central Java; performances are in Javanese.*

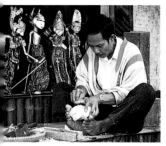

(Top right) An oil painting of wayang golek *puppets by Jan Sluyters.* Wayang golek *puppets have always been a source of inspiration for Indonesian and foreign artists alike.*

Wayang golek *puppets have become such popular tourist goods that demands for them has kept many carvers such as this man in the profession.*

(Below) Wayang klithik *lithographs taken from H.H. Juynboll's book on* Wayang kelitik oder kerutjil. *Characters depicted here are taken from the* Damarwulan *and* Babad Majapahit *stories.*

Wayang Golek

The *wayang golek* are three-dimensional puppets. The word *golek* literally means 'puppet', 'a small statue', or 'searching' (for the meaning of the story). Head, body and limbs are carved from wood: the *tuding* (manipulating rods) are generally made of bamboo, as is the central stick (*sogo*). The *sogo* passes through the body to the head and functions as a handhold. The puppets are clothed in a very long skirt (*kain*) bound at the waist with a sash into which may be slipped a *keris* (dagger), and a collar or breast-covering, and in some cases a jacket.

According to the *Serat Centhini* (early 19th century) and *Serat Sastramiruda* (early 20th century), the Javanese *wayang golek* was introduced in 1506 anno Java (AD 1584). The Sundanese *wayang golek purwa* became known in Priangan early in the 19th century.

Source of the Stories

Wayang golek can be classified into several types based on the stories performed:

- *wayang golek purwa*, which takes its stories from the Mahabharata and Ramayana, is found in West Java, and uses the Sundanese language;
- *wayang golek menak*, which presents stories from the Islamic-influenced *Serat Menak* group of literature, is found in Central and East Java, and uses the Javanese language;
- *wayang golek babad*, which portrays *babad* (traditional historical account) such as *Babad Majapahit* from Central Java and the *Babad Pajajaran* in West Java; now very rare;
- *wayang potehi*, with Chinese-based stories and

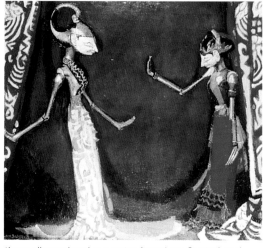

three-dimensional puppets; found on Central and East Java's north coast; performances are rare today.

Presentation

A *wayang golek* performance is generally presented to accompany ceremonies related to the life cycle, but also on national holidays like New Year and Independence Day. Shows begin at night (9:00 p.m. to 5:00 a.m) or in the daytime, depending on their purpose. They are presented by a *dalang* (puppeteer-narrator) and accompanied by a gamelan orchestr a with its musicians and vocalists. Also required are a stage, the puppets, *kotak* (storage box), *gedebog* (banana bole), *blencong* (oil lamp), *cempala* (small mallet) and *kepyak* (rattle made of metal plates strung together).

The *dalang* must be able to carry dialogues and move each *wayang* in a manner complementary to its character. In a performance, he must bring to life up to 30 characters, sing in the required style (*suluk*), conduct the music and entertain. The skills needed for the work are usually passed orally from one generation to the next.

A wayang krucil *puppet of* Bhatara Guru *(otherwise known as the Hindu god Siva). The* wayang krucil *is very rarely performed today.*

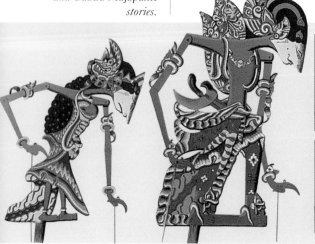

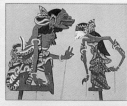

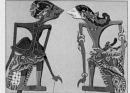

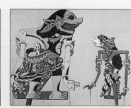

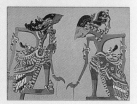

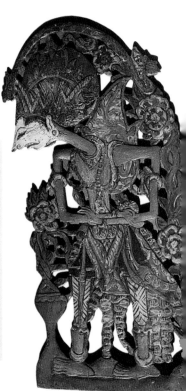

THREE TYPES OF *WAYANG GOLEK* PUPPETS' HEADDRESSES

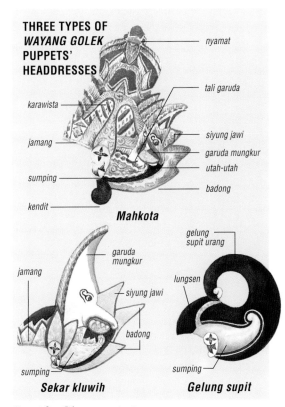

nyamat

tali garuda

karawista

siyung jawi

jamang

garuda mungkur

utah-utah

sumping

badong

kendit

Mahkota

gelung supit urang

garuda mungkur

jamang

lungsen

siyung jawi

badong

sumping

sumping

Sekar kluwih

Gelung supit

This story combining the Mahabharata and Panji cycles was obtained orally by artist Tyra de Kleen in 1947. Arayana (Narayana?) decides to travel to Daha to participate in a contest for the hand of the princess. Arayana seeks permission from his father. But his father refuses which compels him to run away. Meanwhile in Astina, Arjuna has also decided to join the contest. He is seen in conference with his clown servants, Semar, Trepot and Petruk. When they arrive at Daha, the contest has already begun between Arya Gandamani, the Chief Minister of Daha, and Arya Dursana.

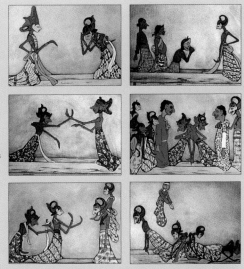

Sumandra (Sumbadra?), sister of Arayana, who is perched on the shoulders of elder brother, Alladarat (Jaladara?), catches the eyes of Arjuna who is on Bima's shoulders. Arjuna tries to catch the attention of Sumandra but incurs the wrath of Arayana instead. Arayana challenges Arjuna to a fight. It soon develops into a battle in which Arayana, Arjuna, Bima and Alladarat will all be killed. However a god is sent down and he revives all of them. In the end, Arjuna wins the love of Sumandra for his persistence.

Specific Characteristics

There are several characteristics specific to the *wayang golek*. The puppet's head can be moved to right and left and the body, up and down as well as to right and left. The arms can be moved freely to imitate a person dancing, or even perform martial arts movements.

Recently, *wayang golek* performers have become quite innovative in their presentations, to make them more realistic and interesting to the modern public, such as the actual cutting-off of heads when required in battle. This tendency is particularly true of the West Javanese genre.

Wayang Krucil

Wayang krucil (also called *wayang klithik*) is a flat, two-dimensional figure made of carved and painted wood with leather arms; only the arms are movable. Occasionally, the head can be more round than flat. According to the *Serat Sastramiruda*, the first was made by Ratu Pekik in Surabaya in the year 1571 Saka (AD 1648). Stories or themes are taken from the *Serat Damarwulan* depicting the Majapahit legend, the most popular segment being the fall of King Menakjingga (*wayang klithik*), and the Mahabharata (*wayang krucil*).

Used in a performance are the *kotak* (wooden storage box), *cempala* (to knock the storage box), and a limited, *slendro*-tuned gamelan, but no screen

(*kelir*). Instead of a banana bole (*gedebog*), the puppets are inserted into a length of bamboo or wood with holes (*slanggan*). Each scene is accompanied by *tembang macapat* (*macapat* songs) sung by the *dalang*. Performances usually take place during the day between 10:00 a.m. to 4:00 p.m., to accompany important events such as *kaulan* (thanking God for a wish fulfilled), weddings and circumcisions. *Wayang krucil* performances are very rare today.

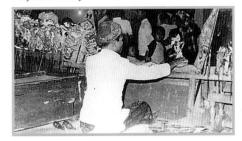

THE ARRANGEMENT OF MUSICAL INSTRUMENTS IN THE *WAYANG GOLEK* GAMELAN
(After Buurman, 1987)

kendhang

bonang

saron   saron

gong

pesinden

rebab

kempul

gambang

dalang

puppet chest

stage

puppets for the right hand   puppets for the left hand

(Right, top) As wayang krucil *puppets do not have intricate and perforated details on their bodies, performances are conducted without a screen. Stories are taken from the Damarwulan cycle which portrays the exploits of the Javanese hero, Damarwulan. (Right) A 1920s image of a* wayang golek *performance in a traditional village in Central Java.*

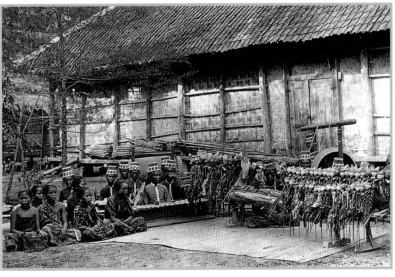

New Forms of Wayang

The wayang *theatre is a continuously developing form of entertainment and education. The leather-puppet genre of the* wayang *theatre is particularly popular and flexible, inspiring the creation of a number of new forms in the 20th century. Six of these have been particularly well-received: the* wayang suluh, wayang revolusi, wayang pancasila, wayang kancil, wayang sadat *and* wayang wahyu. *What is interesting about these is that they are all used as a medium of instruction.*

»»The wayang suluh *gunungan features the Garuda Pancasila in the centre of the leaf-like figure. Sometimes at the bottom, a map of the Indonesian Archipelago may be represented.*

Wayang Suluh

The *wayang suluh* came into being after Indonesia's proclamation of independence in 1945. The first performance took place at the Balai Rakyat (Public Hall) in Madiun city on 1 December 1947, which was attended by representatives of the government's information service. By 1950, the new genre was being used by the Department of Information to disseminate information emanating from the government at that time, since not only were radios few and far between, and television non-existent, but a great many of the people were still illiterate. With time, this form of the *wayang* art developed into a folk theatre, but only in Central and East Java, with East Java dominating.

The Puppets

The *wayang suluh* figures are made from cow- or buffalo hide, and the bodies of the personalities presented in profile. There are not as many personalities in the repertoire as in the more ancient *wayang purwa*, and the figures are shorter in height. The figures are modern men and women wearing everyday clothes, sometimes local dress and sometimes Western dress, depending on the character portrayed. Like the older *wayang*

WAYANG PANCASILA

One of several new forms of *wayang kulit* created in the post-Independence era is the *wayang pancasila*. It was conceived by Mr Harsono Hadisoeseno, a puppeteer and leader of a government information unit. In the *wayang pancasila*, the five Pandawa brothers of the Mahabharata became symbols for the five principles of the modern Indonesian state.

These five figures at the bottom of the page represent characters from the wayang suluh. *The subject of this performance is the Asia-Africa Conference in Bandung in 1955. The characters (from left to right) are the government leaders of Sri Lanka, Pakistan, Egypt, Burma, and India respectively.*

forms, the *wayang suluh* performance is accompanied by gamelan music but now playing modernised compositions.

Stories and Themes

In line with their original purpose, *wayang suluh* performances are usually built around events that took place during the Indonesian nationalist movement, but the repertoire and the variety in personalities were expanded to suit new uses, such as entertainment for guests at a wedding or a circumcision celebration or annual independence day celebrations. Since then themes have been incorporated that are derived from the Mataram Chronicles, the Diponegoro War (1825-1830), the heroism of Suropati fighting against the Dutch (late 17th to early 18th centuries), and others. Stories are presented in any language or vernacular necessary to reach the common people.

Wayang Wahyu

The *wayang wahyu* was created in 1957 by Brother Temotheus Mardji Wignjasoebrata to teach the Roman Catholic faith through an already-popular medium, the shadow-puppet theatre. Taking his stories from the Old and New Testaments, he designed a total of 225 characters which in performance are lined up to the right and left of the *dalang*. Those on the right side represent the good characters with Samson at the beginning. On the left side are the darker characters, beginning with Goliath. In the middle is Jesus Christ, who is always placed slightly higher than the rest. The *gunungan* bears the traditional shape, but depicts the universe according to Catholic iconography: the crucified Christ rises from the dome of St. Peter's with the symbol of the Holy Ghost hovering above Christ. Music is provided by the gamelan but is interlaced with strains of diatonic church music.

New Creation — Wayang Sandosa

The newest creation in contemporary *wayang* performances is the *wayang sandosa*, which makes use of special effects, Bahasa Indonesia (rather than Javanese), and two screens flanking a stage. Stories are generally conventional but given new interpretations. While the screens are used in the usual way to project shadows from puppets, the stage allows dancing and singing to be used as additional acting media. The *wayang sandosa* which came into being in the 1980s at the College of Indonesian Art (STSI) in Surakarta has understandably been received with mixed feelings by the *wayang* community.

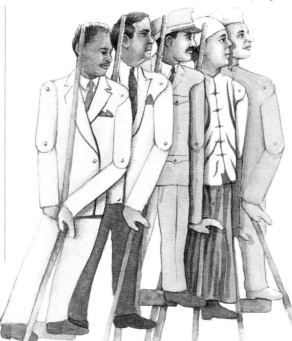

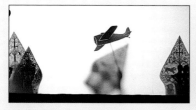

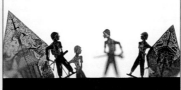

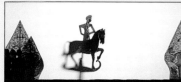

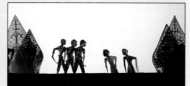

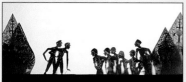

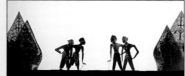

WAYANG KANCIL

Indonesia has a long-established tradition of animal stories. Those of *kancil*, the clever little mouse-deer, are particularly popular. Couched in easily understood terms, the entertaining *kancil* tales educate listeners, pass on moral teaching, and even make social criticism through animals that have the gift of speech. Through wit and cunning, little *kancil* always attains his goal, frequently against much larger adversaries such as the crocodile and the tiger, and with a great deal of penetrating logic in its methods.

The *wayang kancil* was created around 1924 or 1925, reputedly by Bo Lim, an Indonesian-born Chinese from Surakarta. In 1943, R.M. Sayid enlarged the puppet collection to about 200 figures including new figures, like nurses and village administrators, to expand its use as a medium of education amongst an as yet largely illiterate populace.

Although the *wayang kancil* is no longer presented, *kancil* stories have remained popular in children's storybooks. In 1983 a version of the *wayang kancil* was developed in the Universiti Sains Malaysia in Penang, Malaysia.

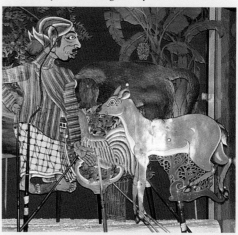

WAYANG REVOLUSI

During the years of the Revolution (1945-1949), the Indonesian struggling nationalist government sought various ways of rallying the support of the people. As conventional means of disseminating information such as the radio and the newspapers were in the hands of the Dutch, the nationalist government turned to using the *wayang* theatre for propagating their cause.

Puppets in the *wayang revolusi* represented various contemporary personalities such as Soekarno (Former President of Indonesia), Nehru (Former Prime Minister of India), revolutionary soldiers, the Dutch and the peasantry. The many figures are cut and painted realistically to represent modern people. Stories in the *wayang revolusi* were taken from real-life events such as the bombing of Hiroshima, Japan, and the skirmishes and outbreaks of fighting between the Dutch and the student guerillas or peasants. With the end of the revolutionary years, the *wayang revolusi* soon ceased to be popular.

WAYANG SADAT

In mid-1985, Suryadi Warnosuharjo, a mathematics teacher at the Muhammidiyah Teachers' College in Klaten, Central Java, realised his dream of a specifically Muslim *wayang* theatre, which he named *wayang sadat*. Since his high school days, Suryadi had spent his spare time learning to be a *dalang*, pouring over books on the *dalang*'s art, the historical stories of the early Muslim kingdoms of Java, and the biographies of the saintly propagators of Islam on Java, and getting practical experience as a *dalang*. The result was 20 stories and 40 puppet figures (of a planned eventual 100).

The word *sadat* derives from *syahadatain* (the two sentences of commitment to Islam), but it is also seen to be an acronym for <u>sa</u>rana <u>da</u>kwah dan <u>t</u>abligh, which translates to something like 'means of calling together and sermonising'. In using the popular Javanese puppet theatre for spreading the faith, Suryadi was emulating a method used in the 15th and 16th centuries to popularise the new faith in Java.

The entire performance of the *wayang sadat* is thick with Islamic nuances. It opens with the *bedug*, the large resonant drum used to call believers to prayer. This is followed by the greeting, *assalamu' alaikum*, then the strains of the Middle Eastern-derived rebecca (*rebab*) and the Javanese gamelan. The music is fundamentally Javanese, but it is interspersed with Muslim-oriented music of the tambourine-based *qasidah* type. The puppets do not resemble the classic *wayang purwa*, but are much more finely worked than the paperdoll-like *wayang suluh*. Musicians and *dalang*, all men, wear white turbans and jackets, while the female singers wear Javanese dress with a veil covering their hair and only face, hands and feet are exposed. The *wayang sadat* has been performed less than a dozen times to date.

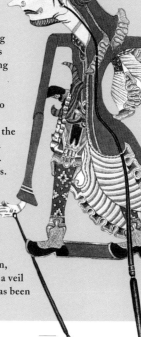

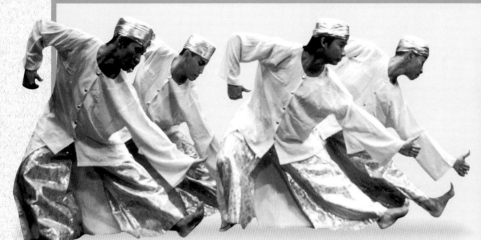
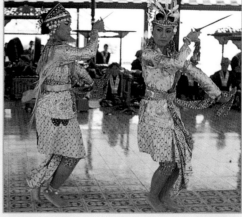
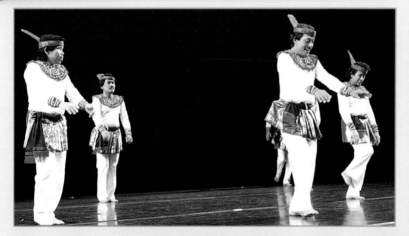
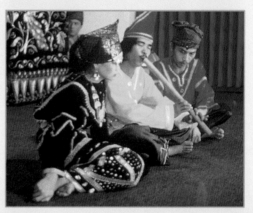
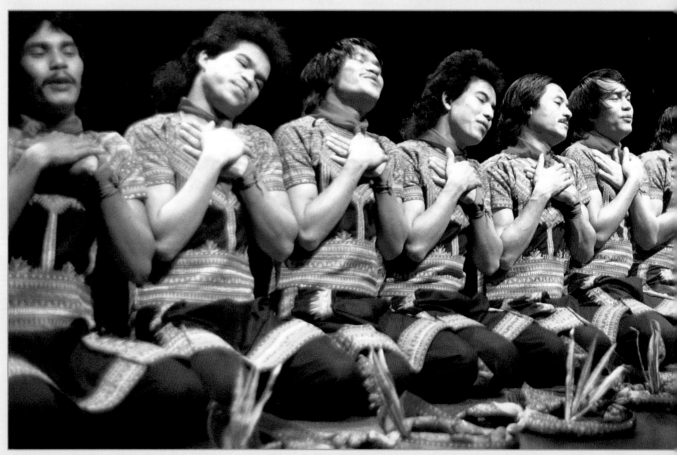

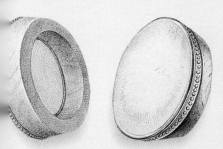

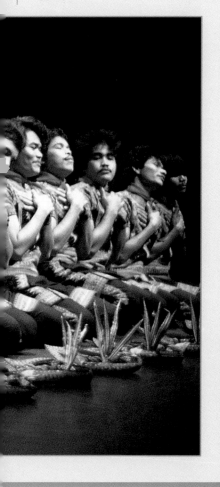

ISLAMIC PERFORMANCES

The term 'Islamic Performances' designates performing arts associated with Islam in a historical and socio-cultural sense. The word 'Islamic' is preferred because these art forms are not at all tightly integrated into the structure of the teachings and rules of the religion itself, but constitute peripheral phenomena in Islam as a religion. Nevertheless, some of the older forms did play an instrumental role in the spreading of the faith amongst the populace. Art is not part and parcel of the religious teachings of Islam. The only form of 'art' referred to in the Hadiths, the recorded sayings and doings of the Prophet, is the recitation of the Qur'an, of which a variety of modes were found acceptable to early Muslim religious leaders.

Three kinds of Islamic association can be identified in Indonesia's performing arts. First are art forms established before the introduction of Islam, that were subsequently transformed by the intervention of Muslim messages. The Menak story cycle in the *wayang golek menak* and the mid-20th century *beksa golek menak* tells of Islamic heroes and carries Islamic messages, while dramaturgy and basic characterisation of roles are based on the ancient Javanese *wayang purwa*.

A second form is the newly introduced art form which arrived in Indonesia already laden with Islamic messages. One manifestation of this is performances in which dancers stand in rows while singing and reciting texts and making rhythmic body movements. Most of the texts are Arabic laudations of the Prophet Muhammad; occasionally they are coloured with verses in the local language. This kind of presentation together with certain musical instruments used in accompaniment is believed to have come from Persia.

Finally, there are contemporary works which are not tightly bound to any particular tradition, but bear an obviously Islamic imprint.

Islamic-ness in Indonesia's performing arts is detectible through texts, visualisation and musical instrumentation. Texts may be totally Arabic, taken from religious scriptures, or in the local language with or without the insertion of Arabic religious terms but with a clearly Islamic message. Visualisation may include Arabic calligraphical traits, *arabesque* floral motifs and costumes. Musical instrumentation features the *gambus* (lute) and *rebana* (frame-drum) as an Islamic trait. The *rebana* have tubular bodies made of wood or metal, a membrane covering only one end, and sometimes metal discs attached around the perimeter of the drum which produce a shimmering sound when shaken.

Salawat and Santiswaran

*T*he diffusion of Islam throughout the Indonesian Archipelago also meant the spread of Islamic music, including forms which had already become rooted in the local traditions of propagation centres. Even today, such centres continue to provide fertile grounds for the growth of this kind of music.

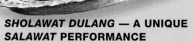

Islamic Music

This genre of music consists of songs vocalised by a soloist and a choir in alternation, to the accompaniment of frame-drums played in unequal patterns. These unequal patterns, when combined, intermingle to produce a single complex musical arrangement. Additional local musical instruments may also be used, though not always from the frame-drum family. The lyrics are a mixture of the vernacular and Arabic adjusted to local pronunciation systems. The text is divided into two parts. The first is in the vernacular with variable content; the second part is in Arabic and contains praises, and the teachings and stories of the prophets. In some cases, only Arabic is used and in others, only the local language. Performers are generally men.

Salawatan. The singers rise as they reach the srokal, *the part of the text that relates Muhammad's birth, Central Java.*

Salawat

The distinctive characteristic of *salawat* is the dominant use of the frame-drum, which in Javanese is known as *trebang* or *terbang* and the music *trebangan* or *terbangan*. The second characteristic is the presence of *salawat* or *sholawat*, prayers presented in the Arabic language in song form. A third characteristic is the melodic arrangement.

The melodic arrangement of the *salawat* has not been studied to determine exactly what it is that gives it its Islamic nuances. To the traditional 'ear', however, *salawat* music has a distinctly Islamic nuance. It is true that the frame-drum is the principal instrument in this kind of music, but this does not mean that there must always be such accompaniment. The lack of this instrument in no way impedes the local genius in producing the sounds needed.

A unique form of *salawat* music has evolved on Lombok island, amongst the Muslim Sasak people. It is related that in a

Islamic religious chant with round dance by boys or young men. Drawing from Yogyakarta plate album.

»Frame-drum played in the salawat *in Cirebon, West Java.*

(Below) Cakepung *performance in Lombok.*

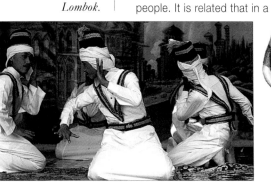

SHOLAWAT DULANG — A UNIQUE SALAWAT PERFORMANCE

A form of *salawat* music has evolved in Padang Panjang, West Sumatra, a centre of Minangkabau culture that claims to be Mecca's Front Porch. The *sholawat dulang*, as it is known locally, is accompanied by beating the *dulang*, a round footed tray of brass on which food is generally served to guests. It is said that once upon a time, a thanksgiving ceremony was supposed to have been highlighted with frame-drum music, but the players did not show up. So, two *santris* (students of religion) who dearly wanted to sing a *sholawat*, rushed forward, snatching two trays of food as they went. Removing the food from the trays, they sat themselves in front of the guests and sang to a rhythm beaten out on the *dulang* trays. The result was quite successful, so the *santris* continued singing until dawn.

celebration of a religious nature, the men paid to play the frame-drums failed to turn up. The day grew darker and darker. After a brief discussion, seven *sholawat* artists came forward; they knelt on the floor in a half-circle and suddenly was heard the alternating beat of three frame-drums followed by the sounds of the *kendhang* (double-headed drum) and the *kempluk* (a small gong beaten regularly to strengthen rhythm), and then the *sholawat*. Apparently, three of the *santris* had imitated the sound of three kinds of frame-drum orally, a fourth had replicated the *kendhang* beat, and a fifth the *kempluk*. *Sholawat* singing is generally vigorous and performed in chorus by many people, so in the Sasak case, the 'musicians' had to stop making music in order to join the singing. Thus, the 'music' alternated with the vocalisation.

Another feature of the Sasak version of the *sholawat* is that the hands were left free for movement. There is a prohibition on dancing when presenting the teachings and stories of the prophets; in addition, one may not stand, but must sit respectfully on the ground. However, the spirit of the folk dances in the area ranging from Banyuwangi in East Java through Bali to western Lombok depends upon hip movements. The Lombok solution was to sit in a kneeling position which allowed the required hip movements while mouthing the music and singing. In Lombok, this form of entertainment has become known as *cakepung* — the same name as the *cakepung* from Bali which is

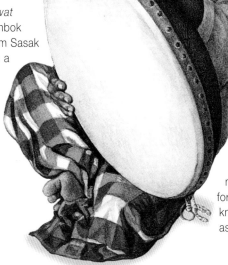

64

performed by as many as 10 to 20 male dancers.

Along the coasts of Indonesia, frame-drum music flourished. Today, each region continues to retain its own style. On the north coast, the frame-drum music of Banten in West Java differs from that of Tegal in Central Java, which in turn differs from that in Situbondo in East Java. In inland regions, the local genius has provided a specifically local flavour, but the Islamic nuance remains strong. In Central Java, the local cultural influence is quite forceful; the resultant cultural product is popularly nicknamed *Islam Jawa*. One manifestation of this is the *santiswaran*.

Santiswaran

Santiswaran may be defined as a Javanese cultural product inspired by Islam. The 19th-century *Serat Centhini*, a Javanese encyclopaedic treatise, contains an illustration known as *gendhing trebangan* (below right). The old term for this kind of music, *gendhing trebangan* or *terbangan* is derived from the dominant instrument which is the frame-drum.

The actual time when *santiswaran* began to develop is not known. The first specific record of the *santiswaran* is perhaps cited in the *Serat Centhini* which describes the Javanese post-Majapahit period (16th century) and after. The *Serat Centhini* contains all kinds of information on the Javanese culture of that period, including a description of the *santiswaran*.

Santiswaran melodies follow the five-toned *slendro* musical scale of Javanese music. The verses carry the teachings of Islam and information on Javanese culture, including examples of Javanese literary forms, interpolated here and there with *sholawat* in Arabic adapted to the local tongue. The *santiswaran* is accompanied by three pairs of big, medium and small frame-drums, a pair of

kemanak (hollow bars struck with a padded mallet) and a *kendhang ciblon* (medium-sized double-headed drum).

The music commences with an opening song rendered in solo with free rhythm. Near the end of the song, the rhythm becomes metrical. The song is *tembang gede* or *tembang tengahan* which are classical forms of Javanese verse.

The main song was presented in metrical rhythm by a totally male chorus in the past but this has changed in recent times. Accompaniment is provided by the *terbang*, *kendhang* and *kemanak*. The melody consists of several couplets, sometimes more than ten. Each couplet is followed by a *sholawat*.

The *sholawat* is likewise sung in chorus, or one voice after another. The atmosphere of the *sholawat* is much more cheerful than that of the main song. It is often interrupted with *senggakan* which are amusing verses composed of two lines of eight syllables each.

The *santiswaran* was developed by artists of the Surakarta palace in Central Java during the reigns of Pakubuwana IV (1788-1820) and Pakubuwana V (1820-1823). Under Pakubuwana VI (1823-1830), the kingdom was too occupied with fighting against the Dutch colonialists to think of cultural endeavours. Hencefore it was not until the accession of Pakubuwana X in 1893 that the palace continued again to develop its various cultural traditions and arts and at this time the *santiswaran* was re-established.

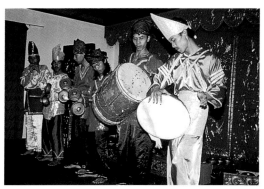

> " .....Tarebang ageng jumengglung, dereng minggah kang irama, dhung prang prong brung, dhung dhah dhung dheng, tong tung tung brang ..... "
>
> (Serat Centhini IV, 279:4-5)

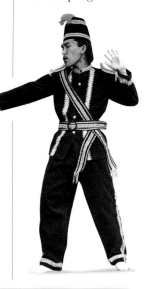

A salawat performance in Bukittinggi, West Sumatra.

Besides the cakepung, other forms of Islamic performances are also held on the island of Lombok such as the one below. It is held in conjunction with the cakepung.

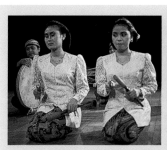
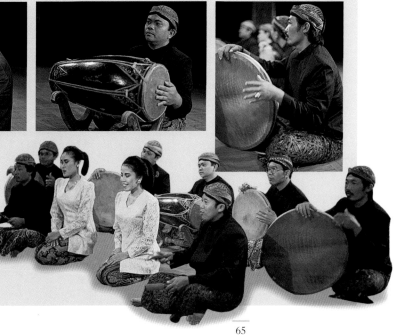

SANTISWARAN MUSICIANS

A *santiswaran* presentation is accompanied by a two-headed drum (*kendhang*), the frame-drum (*terbang*), the *kemanak*, and a vocalist (*sinden*). The musical ensemble is mainly Javanese, except the *terbang*, and tuned to the five-toned Javanese scale, but the sung verses contain Islamic teachings and prayers, as well as Javanese themes. The *santiswaran* musical accompaniment is totally percussive.

A modern phenomenon in Indonesian Islamic performances is the participation of women. In fact, in some cases, women performers have totally supplanted male performers. These two women (above) double up up as vocalists (*sinden*).

Frame-Drum Ensembles

In Indonesia, the frame-drum is closely associated with Islam. All over the country one encounters ensembles of several or many frame-drums which are played for Muslim weddings and circumcisions, both in parades and processions preceding the ceremony and as entertainment afterwards, and for devotional meetings.

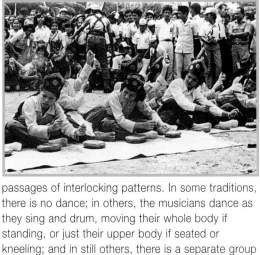

»»*Many of the folk performances throughout Indonesia are held by torchlight at night, such as this* indang *performance in West Sumatra.*

Defining Frame-Drums

In a frame-drum, by definition, the diameter of the head is greater than the depth of the body. Frame-drums may or may not have jingles attached (tambourine), and they may have one or two heads (membranes), although in Indonesia the single-headed variety is more common. The single-headed drum is often called *rebana;* some other names are *terbang, rapa'i, rapano* and *gendang.*

Frame-drum music is believed originally to have been used in the dissemination of Islam. It is, even today, a combination of art and religious teaching, however the Arabic verses have become largely unintelligible through the centuries and the assimilation of local languages.

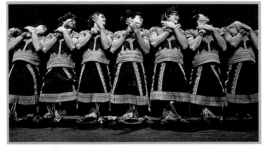

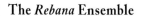

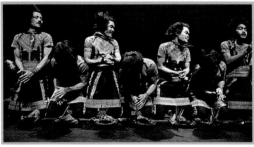

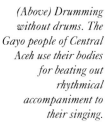

(Above) Drumming without drums. The Gayo people of Central Aceh use their bodies for beating out rhythmical accompaniment to their singing.

The *Rebana* Ensemble

The number of single-headed frame-drums in an ensemble ranges from two or three to 20 or 30, and even more for a spectacular occasion. Typically, some of the frame-drums are larger than others, and thus lower in pitch, and different musical functions are assigned to various drums. The lowest-pitched drums may function, for example, as gongs, marking strong beats of repeating patterns. It is very common in these ensembles for the drummers to divide into several groups playing interlocking patterns of considerable complexity and variation.

The drummers, who are usually male, generally sing as they drum, more or less in unison, songs with Muslim content: praises of Allah and Muhammad, or statements of Islamic rules and principles. One common text is the Arabic poem known as *Barzanji,* after its author; many texts are in Indonesian or in regional languages. While the singing is going on, the *rebana* will typically play a repeating pattern quietly. In pauses, the drums will state their pattern vigorously or burst into impressive

passages of interlocking patterns. In some traditions, there is no dance; in others, the musicians dance as they sing and drum, moving their whole body if standing, or just their upper body if seated or kneeling; and in still others, there is a separate group of dancers. *Dabus* in Aceh, West Java and Maluku, *indang* in West Sumatra, *rebana biang* in Jakarta, and *selawatan* throughout Java are typical genres featuring ensembles of *rebana.*

Variations

Many variations and expansions of this nuclear combination of frame-drums and Islamic content or context have developed. Melody instruments — guitars and electronic keyboards, for example — are added, and a female chorus substituted, to make a popular form known as *qasidah,* or *nasyid.* The *gambus* ensemble uses a plucked lute, the *gambus,* which can be an Arab-style *ud* or an indigenous Indonesian lute, and three to five small two-headed frame-drums, *marwas* or *marwis,* to accompany singing by the lute-player. The drums play in the style described above for *rebana.*

In Banyuwangi, at the eastern end of

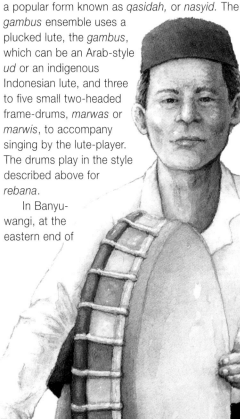

»»*This man demonstrates the technique of playing the* rebana biang.

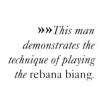

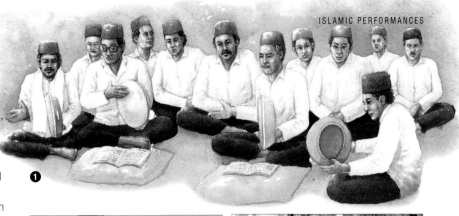

Java, the *kuntulan* ensemble augments a group of some ten *rebana* with European military drums, some instruments typical of a local dance tradition (*gandrung Banyuwangi*) and, apparently, anything else that comes to hand — Balinese *reyong,* singers, dancer and Casio keyboards are among the possibilities. The frame-drums, together with the military drums, tend to play in alternation with the other instruments, rather than simultaneously; this musical opposition reflects *kuntulan*'s history as a genre that originated in religious performance, *hadrah,* and then over time, acquired secular elements.

In Muslim areas of Lombok, there is a *rebana* ensemble that is also a 'drum chime', that is a set of precisely tuned drums which use, in this case, a five-tone scale. At least one of these ensembles plays music borrowed from the Balinese processional gamelan, *bebonangan*: each drummer drops in his pitch whenever it comes around in the melody. Here, there appears to be no Islamic content to the performance, but other Lombok *rebana* ensembles are reported to perform more typically Muslim music.

Frame-drum music is very popular amongst the Betawi of Jakarta. The *rebana burdah*, which is believed to be the oldest form, consists of four frame-drums, conforming to a Muslim's 'four' obligations: to God, to nature, to the community, and to the self. The songs are rendered traditionally in Arabic, which has become garbled with time and is now largely unintelligible, but today quite often in the vernacular.

The Islamic nature of frame-drum music is reinforced by the costumes worn by the musicians and vocalists. These are invariably long trousers, shirt and a Muslim cap or turban for men, and perhaps a scarf around the neck; and trousers, a long tunic, and a veil worn over a head-hugging cap for women.

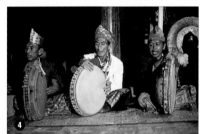
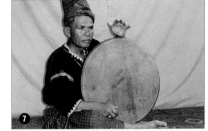
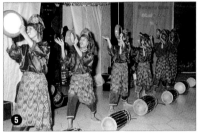
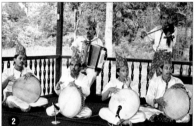
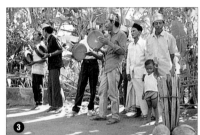
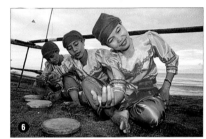

Drumming without Drums

In Aceh, there are two instances of what could be considered frame-drum ensembles without the frame-drums. The *seudati* genre of the Acehnese is derived from Sufi ecstatic rites; it involves male singers who dance and make percussive sounds, but their instruments are their own bodies, as they clap their hands, slap their chests and sides, and snap their fingers. Among the Gayo, who live in southern Aceh, *didong* is performed at Muslim celebrations, although its songs do not necessarily have Muslim content. Some of the singers, traditionally always male and always seated, clap while others produce surprisingly loud sounds by slapping small square fabric pillows.

❶ *The entire entourage of the* rebana burdah.
❷ *A* zapin *performance using frame-drums.*
❸ *A frame-drum ensemble in Sumbawa.*
❹ *A* rebana *performance near*

Sumbawa Besar.
❺ *A combined frame-drum performance,* Sulawesi.
❻ *An* indang *dance, West Sumatra.*
❼ *A Minangkabau frame-drum player from West Sumatra.*

TERBANG GUDRUG OF CIRANGKONG, TASIKMALAYA

The *terbang gudrug* of the Cirangkong area of South Tasikmalaya, West Java, is a set of frame-drums which are played by three to five drummers. The players are taken from the male community. Usually, two players take turns to play a drum because the performance continues until late at night.

The form of the *terbang* is unique and distinctly different from the usual frame-drums found in other areas. The structure of the drum is superior, strong and antique. Each drum measures about 70 centimetres in diameter. The membrane is made from two-year-old buffalo hide and small holes surround the edges of the membrane for interlacing strings. The body is surrounded by 66 symmetrically placed wooden pegs.

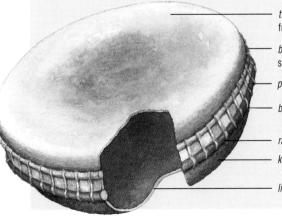

tutup (membrane made from buffalo hide)

beubet nyere (little holes surrounding the membrane)

paseuk (pegs made from new wood)

bengker (rattan coil)

rarawat (string)

kuluwung (body)

liang or lubang (hole)

Zapin

The zapin dance is common to almost all of coastal Indonesia, and especially areas where Islam is the dominant influence. Deli on the eastern littoral of North Sumatra, the Riau islands, Jambi, South Sumatra, Bengkulu, and Lampung; Jakarta, Pekalongan, Garut, Tuban, Gresik, Bondowoso and Yogyakarta in the Javanese coastlands; Madura, Nusa Tenggara, all of the Kalimantan and Sulawesi coastal districts, Ternate, Seram and several other Malukan islands, each has its own version of the zapin dance. Aceh and West Sumatra are the exception, despite the predominance of Islam and the presence of the right traditional musical instruments and rhythms for accompaniment.

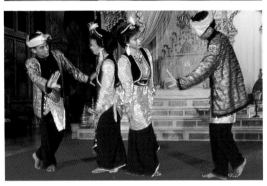

(Top right) This zapin 'Mak Inang' was performed by Sanggar Tari Dahlia in Medan, Sumatra. (Bottom) A performance of the zapin 'Kasih dan Budi'.

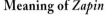

(Above) A stage backdrop for a zapin performance at TIM Art Centre in 1984.

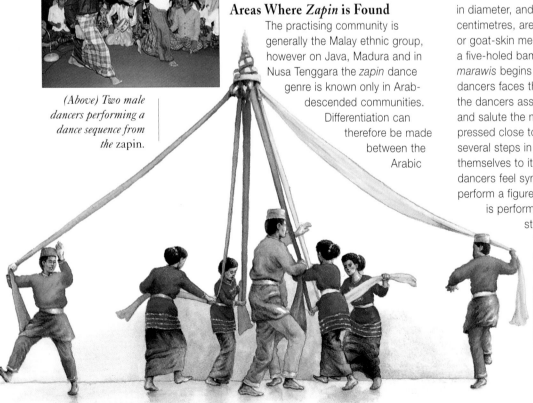

(Above) Two male dancers performing a dance sequence from the zapin.

Meaning of *Zapin*

Zapin, the word, has a variety of interpretations, all derived from Arabic. In the Arab-descended community of Bondowoso (East Java), it is variously attributed to the word *zafin* (step or to take a step), *zaf* (which is a plucked 12-stringed musical instrument for dance accompaniment) and *al-zafn* (to take a step or to raise one foot). *Zapin* dance movement emphasises footwork. Hand and arm gestures act as a balance and have a form of their own, like paddling a canoe, swinging freely, taking hold of the shirt front with one hand, the other behind the body, palms loosely open or clenched with a protruding index finger elegantly curved.

Amongst the Malay peoples of Indonesia, the word *zapin* has various equivalents. In Deli and Riau, *zapin* prevails, in Jambi it becomes *dana sarah*, and in Lampung *bedana*. On Java and Madura, the dance is known as *zafin*, on Kalimantan, Sulawesi and Maluku *jepin* or *jepen*, and in Nusa Tenggara *dani-dana*.

Areas Where *Zapin* is Found

The practising community is generally the Malay ethnic group, however on Java, Madura and in Nusa Tenggara the *zapin* dance genre is known only in Arab-descended communities. Differentiation can therefore be made between the Arabic

zapin and the Malay *zapin*. The Arabic *zapin* is so institutionalised with respect to style and accompanying music that it can be performed by any dancers anywhere. The Malay *zapin* is greatly varied. On Sumatra, for example, we have the *zapin Deli*, *zapin Siak*, *zapin Pulau Penyengat*, *zapin Tembilahan*, and *zapin Palembang*. All may be linked by dance pattern and musical accompaniment, but they differ extensively with respect to style.

Arab *Zapin*

The Arabic *zapin* (*zafin hajjir marawis*) is derived from the double-headed *marwas* or *hajjir* drums which provide the accompanying rhythm. Both ends of the *marwas* drums, which are 15-20 centimetres in diameter, and the larger *hajjir* drums, 30-40 centimetres, are covered with tightly stretched calf- or goat-skin membranes. The melody is carried by a five-holed bamboo flute, *madruf*. The *zafin hajjir marawis* begins with the *julus*, in which a pair of male dancers faces the musicians. As the music begins, the dancers assume a standing position, *qiyam*, and salute the musicians with raised hands, palms pressed close together. They move back and forth several steps in time to the music as they adjust themselves to its rhythm and tempo. When the dancers feel synchronised with the music, they perform a figure-eight movement. This basic step is performed at the completion of each dance step or movement. This is then followed by the *tahtoh* which is to move forward, shift one foot to the back, then turn in place and sit on

The modern zapin are presented in theatres, open fields and schools in diverse styles and forms. By devising new modes of expression, the genre is expanded into a creative 'work', while on the village level the zapin continues to fulfil its traditional role.

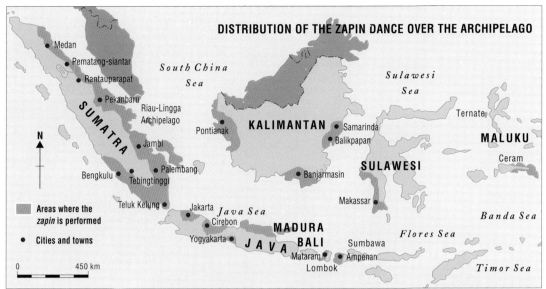

DISTRIBUTION OF THE ZAPIN DANCE OVER THE ARCHIPELAGO

The zafin gambus *is accompanied by the* gambus *(6-stringed lute), violin, double-headed* marwas *drum,* madruf *flute and singing. Vocal accompaniment appears in the form of quatrain-versed* pantun *and* syair. *This is delivered in the Arabic language for the Arabic* zapin *and Malay and Arabic for the Malay* zapin. *Both contain advice, a story, romance and humour which are closely linked to Islamic poetry.*

onc folded leg. The figure-eight is followed by a voluntary step, then repeated. The *tahtim,* which is identical to the *tahtoh,* is executed after each dance step. The dance concludes with the closing *tahtoh.*

TAKSIM SECTION	*MAIN* SECTION	*WAINAB* SECTION
Zapin Music: *gambus* solo and introduction	**Zapin Music:** A B C } (ABC sung-verse unit) Three-bar loud *kopak* pattern A B C } (ABC sung-verse unit) Three-bar loud *marwas* pattern (The two ABC units alternate a number of times).	**Zapin Music:** An extended form of the three-bar loud drumming pattern and a cadence.
Zapin Dance: *sembah* or *salam* salutational dance phase	**Zapin Dance:** dance motives clustered within each repeated ABC musical unit.	**Zapin Dance:** Variation of skips, turns, low *plié,* and standing and squatting positions.

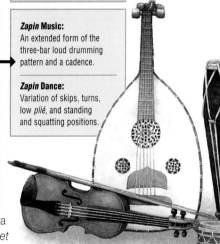

The Malay Form

The Malay *zapin* has a great many regional styles and steps. The pattern of the dance is similar to that of the Arabic *zapin.* It opens with the salute (*salam*) executed while standing, or sitting (*duduk sembah*), followed by the *langkah buka* (opening movement), *langkah tari* (dance step), *tahtim, langkah tari,* and closing *tahtoh* or *sembah penutup* (closing salute). The actual number of dance steps used in each *zapin* depends on the dancers.

The Malay *zapin* differs with the Arabic *zapin* in that the dancers face the audience and not the musicians. The opening step is simple, merely stepping forward, rising on the toes with feet together on every fourth count, pressing or brushing heels on ground, or raising one foot, turning 180° to return to the original position with the same step, and making another 180° turn so as to end up facing the audience. Musical accompaniment is provided by the same instruments as the *zafin gambus.*

Some Malay *zapin* make use of dance accessories, in which case the dance adopts the name of the accessory. This technique is particularly popular in West Kalimantan where we find the *jepin tembung* (pole), *jepin kerangkang* (fishing net), *jepin payung* (umbrella), and *jepin selendang* (stole/shawl).

Occasions for Performances

The *zapin* dance is generally presented on specific occasions such as ritual gatherings, circumcisions, ritual bathing ceremonies and commemorations of Islamic holy days. Initially the performers were all men who danced in pairs and dressed in *sarung* (cylndrical skirt-cloth), shirts and black *kopiah* hats,

or the *teluk belanga* (pajama suit) with *sesamping songket* (gold-brocaded sarong over-skirt) and *lacak* or *destar* headcloth. The Arabic *zapin* is still performed by an all-male company, but the Malay *zapin* is now performed as well by an all-female or mixed troupe. Female dancers wear the *songket* sarong, *baju kurung* (pullover blouse) or *kebaya panjang* (cardigan blouse), and a *selendang* (stole). The stole may be worn to cover the hair, draped diagonally across the chest, or wound around the waist. When the hair is not covered, it is wound in a *sanggul* knot and ornamented with *sunting* (decorative hairpins) or flowers.

The *Zapin* in Present Day

The origin of the *zapin* dance is contemporaneous with the arrival of Arab, Persian and Indian traders in the 13th century. It has become a cultural heritage, a root from which have sprouted new forms of Indonesian dance, a process greatly facilitated by the wealth of existing *zapin* forms and its demand for both spontaneous and pre-conceived improvisation.

(Below) The zapin *dancers perform a figure-eight movement taking a diagonal step forward to the left, a jump to the right, a 180° turn, a diagonal step to the right, a jump to the left, and another 180° turn, arriving back at the starting point.*

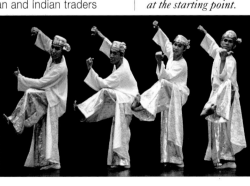

Seudati

Seudati *is a traditional folk dance from Indonesia's most northern province, the Special Territory of Aceh on Sumatra island. It is said that the word* seudati *derives most likely from the Arabic 'syahadatain', or 'meusaman' to some. The dance itself is generally believed by the Acehnese to have originated in Aceh contemporarily with the spread of Islam. It was used to teach the new religion to the people in an entertaining way.*

Historical Development

During the process of development, *seudati* evolved into a forum of competition between troupes. The *seudati Tunang,* as the competition is called, is usually held for thanksgiving purposes, such as after a successful harvest, beginning just after evening prayers and ending at dawn the next morning. According to Nurdin Daud, Acehnese dance expert from the Jakarta Institute of the Arts, one should look for the roots of the *seudati* in the folk theatre of the pre-Islamic period. One of these is the *aneuk dhiek* folk play, now near extinction, in which boys, sporting earrings, a generally female adornment, sing and dance to entertain the public at large.

THE SPECIAL TERRITORY OF ACEH

Banda Aceh
Indrapuri

Areas where *seudati* is popular

Pasir Panjang
Medan

SUMATRA

Elements of the Performance

As a dance performance, the *seudati* contains certain literary elements and sound accompaniment produced physically by the dancers themselves by snapping the fingers, clapping the hands or slapping them against the breasts (by male dancers) and thighs (by female dancers), and stamping the feet on the ground.

The songs of the *seudati* are taken from holy books or developed creatively by the *aneuk syahi,* the two poet-singers. The development of the *seudati tunang* has given prominence to the captain of the troupe who is called the *syeh.*

Movements of the Performance

The movements of the *seudati* have been inspired by the natural environment: branches blown by the wind, the ferocity of an eagle, a rooster's courage. The naming of the choreographic patterns in traditional terminology conforms to the 'nature' theme: *puta taloe* in which the dancers move in criss-crossing

(Below) The saman la hoyan *constitutes one of the basic standard movements in the* seudati *genre.*

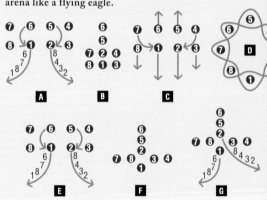

Bak saman. Before the *seudati* begins, the performers gather in a circle around the *syeh* to tune their voices to his. It is also seen by some as an adaptation of the *azan,* the Muslim call to prayer.

DANCE STEPS IN THE SEUDATI

A and **B** *Kapai teureubang* movements in which the dancers move around like an aeroplane. The idea of the aeroplane was adopted in the 1930s when the Acehnese first became aware of their existence.
C and **D** *Puta taloe* which means twisting the rope (or traversing rivers), in which the dancers move in criss-crossing patterns.
E, **F** and **G** *Kleung pho* in which the dancers move freely and ferociously around the dance arena like a flying eagle.

patterns; *bintang beuleun,* literally stars and moon (the dancers form a pattern resembling the crescent moon while the *syeh* and his assistant, the primadonnas, move around like stars); *kapai teureubang,* aeroplane (the dancers move around like an aeroplane). The inspiration for the *kapai teureubang* was received when the Acehnese first became aware of the aeroplane, around 1930. Previously the formation had been known as *kleung pho,* or flying eagle. The choreographic patterns of the *seudati* are unique in their strong feeling for space and a dynamism that stands out in comparison to the other ethnic dances of Indonesia.

The *seudati* consists of six parts, known as *saleum, likok, saman, kisah, nasib,* and *lanie,* performed by eight dancers and two *aneuk syahi.*

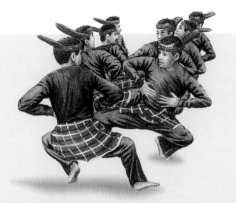

Saman la hoyan. Dividing the *seudati* into three main parts, this movement comes in the middle. It constitutes merely rhythmic movements accompanying the singing of words no longer understood.

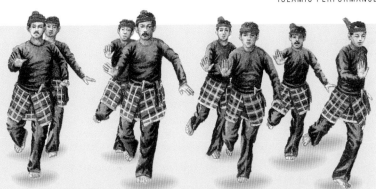

Kisah. The *syeh* begins the telling of a story (*kisah*), which is taken over by the *aneuk syahi*, while the dancers perform rhythmic movements that have no relationship to the story.

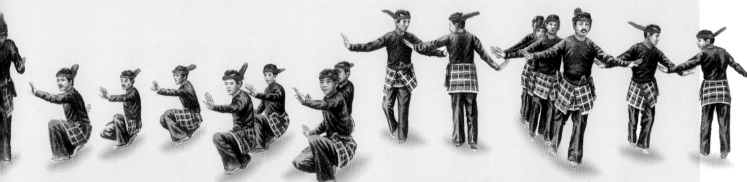

Likok. *Likok* merely means 'winding, twisting' (like a road). It follows the *kisah* and therefore tells the audience that the story is finished.

Likok *Kapai teureubang.* The dancers construct a variety of compositions like the *kapai tereubang* (flying aeroplane).

Likok *Meleut manok.* Otherwise known as fighting cocks. The dance has been inspired by a rooster's courage. The various parts of the *seudati* dance adopt ideas from the natural environment itself.

Order of movements depicted in these illustrations:

> bak saman
> saman la hoyan
> kisah
> likok
> likok kapai teureubang
> likok meleut manok

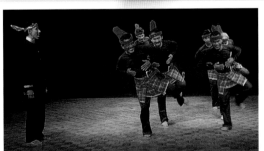

It opens with the *saleum* (greeting) followed by certain movements and patterns known as *likok*. The third segment, *saman*, is a dance and song led by the *syeh*. The *kisah* is the story to be conveyed; it consists of poems of an educational and religious nature. *Nasib* is the term for the creative expression of the *aneuk syahi* (poet-singer) which may take the form of social criticism or a game in which poetic sayings are thrown at competitors as the bases for their ripostes. The final segment of the *seudati* is the *lanie*, a dance with no other motive than pure entertainment that is performed through movement and songs depicting such events as rice-stamping (*top padi*), to free the grains from the chaff, chasing birds (*paroh tulo*), working in the ricefields (*tron u blang*) and other popular and up-to-date themes and songs.

Today the *seudati* is performed in a more flexible manner, to accommodate newly created works arising from contemporary aspirations and needs. It has also become an important teaching tool in Indonesia's dance schools.

(Left) The syeh *(on the left) sings the poetry, and often composes it himself as he is singing, while the dancers slap out the rhythms on their bodies and by stamping their feet, and sing the chorus. The verses are not always poetry, but may contain comments on everyday life and advice.*

Beksa Golek Menak

The beksa golek menak dance was created by Sultan Hamengkubuwana IX of Yogyakarta in 1941. It differs from all the other dances of the palace in dance technique, costumes and story performed. Technique and costumes are based on the movements and clothing of the three-dimensional wooden puppets of the wayang golek performance.

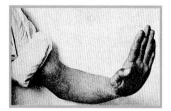

(Above) The ngruji *position with the fingers pressed together tightly and the thumb slightly bent.*

»»Rengganis in her lovely feathered headdress and the golden-clad princess, Widaninggar, in the beksa golek menak *of Yogyakarta.*

(Below) An example of a page from a Serat Menak, *an Islamic Javanese genre of literary works.*

Movement and Development

While the other dances of Yogyakarta generally imitate the lateral movements of the flat leather shadow puppets of the *wayang kulit* theatre, the actions of the *beksa golek menak* can be in any direction. Dance movements are rather stiff, with the hands maintaining the *ngruji* position, in which the fingers are pressed tightly together and straight while the thumb is slightly bent. To enact breathing, the dancer lifts and relaxes his shoulders, as do the rigid wooden *golek* puppets. The source of the stories presented is always the *Serat Menak,* an Islamic Javanese genre of literary works depicting the Prophet Muhammad's predecessors and the situation in the Arab countries before his birth.

The dance was first performed as a duet representing the struggle between a protagonist who believes in the Almighty God and his antagonist who does not. After 1945, the Yogyakarta palace was no longer the centre of political activities and its cultural events became limited to important ceremonies. As a result of this, the *beksa golek menak* evolved outside the palace, without close reference to its origins. Even a *golek menak* dance-drama was developed. The *golek menak* has been a favourite of Yogyakarta's dance community since the 1960s and is also popular with the wider Javanese audience.

Further Refinement

In 1986, the Sultan asked R. M. Soedarsono to coordinate a review of the *beksa golek menak* by artists and literary writers from Yogyakarta. Dance experts from the Yogyakarta palace who had performed in the original dance in 1941 and younger dancers held several workshops with martial arts experts from Minangkabau (West Sumatra) and *wayang golek* puppeteer-narrators in Jakarta, all watched closely by the Sultan. After several trials, the Sultan was satisfied and the gala premiere was planned for Yogyakarta in March 1989. Unfortunately Sultan Hamengkubuwana IX passed away on 3 October 1988 in the United States, but the perfected *beksa golek menak* was performed in the Kepatihan Hall as planned, presenting the story of *Kelaswara Palakrama* (The Wedding of Dewi Kelaswara). This version of the

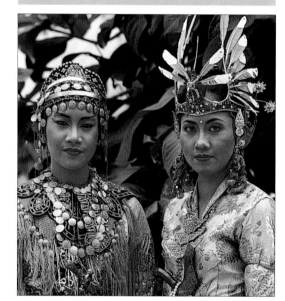

dance was subsequently included in the performing arts programme of the Festival of Indonesia in the USA 1990–1991.

Presentation

A performance of the *golek menak* dance-drama involves detailed preparation, because the dancing technique, costumes and musical accompaniment need special attention. Although characters like Jayengrana, Umarmaya, Kelaswara and Adaninggar (the Chinese princess) are not as numerous as those in the *wayang wong* dance-drama with its 21 character types, special skills are needed for presenting the various characters of the *golek menak*. Although the dancing technique of the golek menak is uniquely different from that of the *wayang wong*, the characterisation concept has great influence on both art forms. The female dancer performs with her arms and legs always slightly apart. The refined male character dances with legs apart, knees almost always bent, and feet lifted

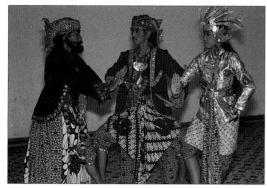

slightly, while the arms are somewhat open. For strong male characters, the legs are wide apart, arms apart and raised to the horizontal position; the legs can likewise be raised to a horizontal position.

While male *wayang wong* dancers are all bare-chested, except for the characters of the gods, giants, and apes; all *golek menak* dancers wear long-sleeved shirts like the *wayang golek* puppets. Some movements require a special talent: the stiff gestures imitating those of the *wayang golek* puppets must be presented smoothly, using only the *ngruji* position of the fingers; the special actions of the Chinese princess with index and middle fingers straight and stiff and much use of martial arts elements; and battle movements that must be based on the martial arts.

(Above) The beksa golek menak *performance in the Yogyakarta kraton.*
(Below) The Chinese princess-cum-military general, Widaninggar,

and Rengganis are engaged in a battle.
(Bottom) Rengganis enlists the help of Garuda to carry her to her father's hermitage on Mount Argapura.

As a result of the complex demands of movement, costumes and music, the *golek menak* dance is today only presented as a duet depicting the fight between characters in the Menak story cycle. Most popular is the fight between two princesses, Kelaswara and Adaninggar, or between Rengganis and Widaninggar. A special feature shows both or one of the battling princesses riding a *garuda*-bird. Another well-liked plot is the fight between two knights, Umarmaya and Raja Jayengpati. This latter dance is full of humour, because the Umarmaya of the Menak stories is well-known as a knight who often does funny things.

Relationship to the *Wayang Wong*

Although the *golek menak* dance is a new creation with a different concept of presentation, its characterisation is clearly based on the *wayang wong*. Not surprisingly, the characters in the *Serat Menak* are often identified with those in the Mahabharata.

The leading character in the *golek menak* is Jayengrana, which means 'One Who Always Wins the War'. He is a gentle knight, patient and modest, like Arjuna. Although he does not project an image of strength, he is always victorious. He is constantly being fought over by beautiful girls all over the world because of his good looks.

MENAK CHARACTERS AND THEIR EQUIVALENTS	
Menak Stories	**Mahabharata**
Jayengrana	Arjuna
Dewi Muninggar	Sembadra
Kelaswara	Srikandi
Sirtupelaeli	Larasati
Adaninggar	Banowati
Maktal	Kresna
Lamdahur	Bima
Nuserwan	Suyudana
Patih Bestak	Durna

A scene from the Menak Cina *directed by Sardono W. Kusumo in 1976 with Basuki Kuswaraga as dance-master.*

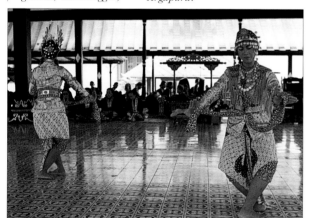

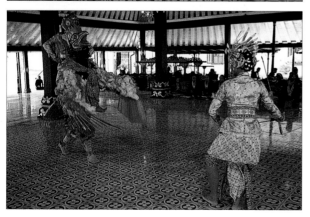

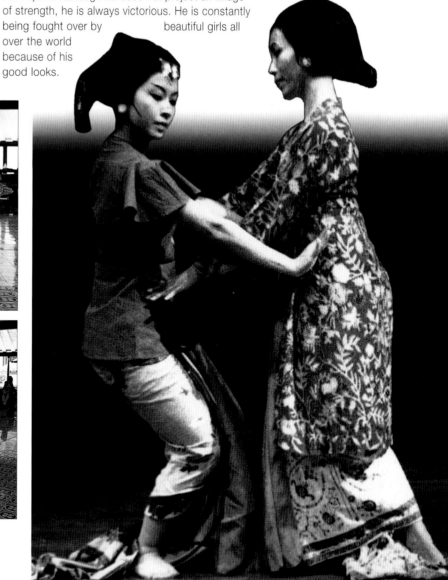

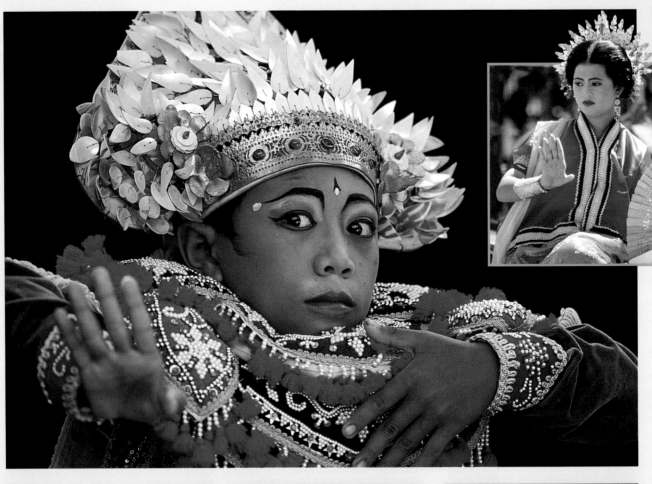
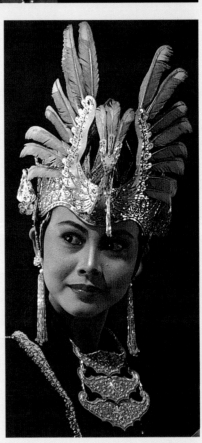
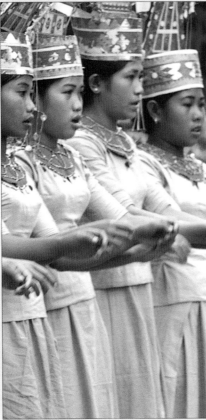
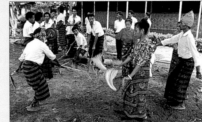
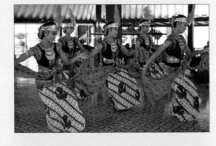
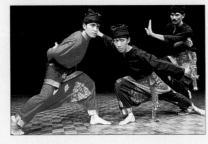

NON-REPRESENTATIONAL DANCE

(Left) The baris tunggal *(solo baris dance) has evolved out of the ancient ritualistic* baris gede *and is often performed by young boys.*

(Inset) The pakarena, *once a court dance of Makasar-Gowa, is presented as part of wedding ceremonies.*

(Below, extreme left) The Torajan dancers take such small steps that they appear not to be moving.

(Below centre, top) Traditional dance from Maumere, Flores. (Middle) The bedhaya *is a Central Javanese court dance believed to have been created by Sultan Agung himself in the early 17th century. (Bottom) Martial arts movements form the basis of the* randai barali'eh *of West Sumatra.*

(Below right) The costume and headdress of Javanese court dancers can be very elaborate.

(Below) The baris tumbak *dancer from Bali (Covarrubias, 1937).*

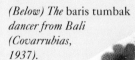

Indonesia has many non-representational dances that are performed for sheer delight in movement. A number have been known for centuries amongst the common people; others have developed within the confines of royal courts. More have been created since independence for public entertainment, based on the movements of ritual dances.

Dances which are rooted in ritual include the *pendet* and *gabor* in Bali and the *jathilan* in Central Java. Guests in Bali are welcomed with the *pendet* and *gabor* dances which were originally performed in the inner courtyard of Balinese temples to amuse deities during a temple's anniversary celebration (*odalan*). They were adapted in the 1950s for secular use. The *jathilan* was traditionally performed by a group of itinerant artists in Central Java who collected a fee from the audience who gathered voluntarily. The dancers hold a hobbyhorse made from bamboo matting between their legs.

Several dances are adapted for the theatre such as the *baris tunggal* of Bali and the *kanjet pepatai* of East Kalimantan. The *baris tunggal* is a solo dance performed by a young male dancer. Its movements derive from the older and ritualistic *baris gede*. The beauty of non-representational dances is epitomised in the royal courts. This is exemplified by the Javanese *bedhaya* and *serimpi*. The Balinese *legong* does have a narrative theme, but neither story nor dramatic plot is stressed in the performance. The aim is to execute phrases and series of movements with maximum skill, beauty and feeling.

Choreographed displays of martial arts skill were as much a part of the palace environment as they were of the populace at large. In West Sumatra, the *alang suntiang panghulu* emulates the agility and prowess in defending oneself, while the *alau ambek* takes the form of a martial arts contest with musical accompaniment.

The *gambyong, ketuk tilu* and *tayuban* originated in the rural communities of Java and subsequently developed into more refined forms.

True social dances are performed by young male-female couples. The best-known of these is the *serampang dua belas* of North Sumatra, popularised nationally in the 1950s and 1960s by President Soekarno as the Indonesian's answer to Western style of social dancing.

Central Javanese Dances

*T*he dances of Central Java can be crudely divided into two types, court dances and village dances. Court dances like the bedhaya and serimpi were developed by past kings and enjoy royal patronage even today. The jathilan is performed either in ritual such as village cleansing or as entertainment. The gambyong is a village dance which has been adapted and refined within one of the courts.

Bedhaya *dancer.*

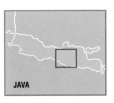

JAVA

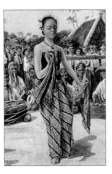

The gambyong *evolved out of a street dance.*

The bedhaya *dancers in Surakarta have always been women but in Yogyakarta they used to be boys clad in women's attire. Besides being dancers, the* bedhaya *also formed part of the ruler's ceremonial retinue.*

Gambyong

Gambyong is found in many parts of Central Java, the Special Territory of Yogyakarta and East Java. It is performed by female dancers. A variation of the *gambyong* was once found in West Java under other names; however it is now extinct.

Oral tradition places the beginnings of the *gambyong* in the reign of Sri Sunan Pakubuwana IX (ruled 1881-1893) of the sultanate of Surakarta, but written records show earlier development, during the reign of Sri Sunan Pakubuwana IV (ruled 1788-1820). *Gambyong* was included in *Serat Centhini* and *Serat Cabolang*, two authoritative sources on Indonesian performing arts written during the 19th century.

The erotic movements of the *gambyong* are accompanied by a gamelan orchestra and vocals in either *slendro* or *pelog* tone.

A *gambyong* dance is performed by one or more dancers on such occasions as a wedding party or to welcome guests, or as a prologue to the *wayang wong* theatre by such groups as the Ngesti Pandawa in Semarang and Sri Wedari in Surakarta. Even *ketoprak* folk theatre groups, like the ketoprak Siswo Budoyo in Tulungagung and the Sapta Mandala in Yogyakarta, may include the *gambyong* in their opening performances.

Costume and Makeup

The *gambyong* dancer wears a long skirt-cloth (*kain*) with pleats down the front, a breast-cloth (*kemben*), a stole (*selendang*) over her right shoulder, long hair knotted in a chignon (*ukel, gelung*) and ornamented with a small semi-circular comb (*cundhuk jungkat*), floral hairpins set on wobbly

THE *SERIMPI* DANCES

The *serimpi* is a classical Javanese dance which originated centuries ago in the courts. The dance continued to be performed and cultivated up to the present day. It is usually performed by four female dancers. There are vario forms of the *serimpi*, each carefully composed and choreographed during the reigns of various different rulers of Surakarta and Yogyakarta. The oldest form of the *serimp* according to a written source, was created by Pakubuwana \ in the Javanese year 1748. The *serimpi ludiramadu* derives from the tale of Sri Pakubuwana V who was of Madurese descent.

A recent form of *serimpi* is the *serimpi pandelori*. A composition by the teachers from the Yogyakarta dance association, Among Beksa, *serimpi pandelori* consists of eight dancers and takes its theme from the Menak stories.

springs (*cundhuk mentul*) and small decorative hairpins (*penetep*), and disc-shaped earpins (*suweng*), necklace and bracelets. Long garlands of jasmine flowers are sometimes draped around the neck, the ends fastened in the back at the waist. Make-up is natural.

Jathilan

Jathilan is a Javanese dance traditionally performed by male dancers. However, in several regions, such as Wonosobo (Central Java), and Gunung Kidul and Kulon Progo (Special Territory of Yogyakarta), the dancers are women dressed as men. The dance is known by various names — *kuda lumping* and *kuda kepang* (West Java), *jaran kepang, incling* or *ebeg* (Central Java and the Special Territory of Yogyakarta), and *jaran kepang* (East Java).

The *jathilan* dance is presented by two or more dancers in pairs, who execute war-like movements. In some regions, it is still perceived as a sacred dance to be performed in conjunction with *bersih desa* (village cleansing) or *memetri desa* (village commemoration) rituals. Otherwise, the *jathilan* has evolved into a secular *barangan* form of entertainment presented by travelling performers.

Musical Instruments and Story

The gamelan orchestra consists of three to five *bende* (small gongs), one to two *kendhang* (double-headed

THE *BEDHAYA*

The *bedhaya* dance is generally believed to have been created by Sultan Agung of Mataram during the first part of the 17th century. It belongs to the category of sacred heirlooms of the Central Javanese courts and until very recently, was performed solely in the palace on very special occasions. Danced by nine of the land's finest and most beautiful dancers, the *bedhaya* is replete with symbolism; it is also the epitome of refinement. Movements are exceptionally slow, creating an atmosphere of tranquility, well-being and solemnity.

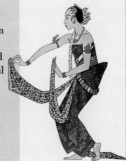
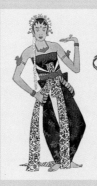
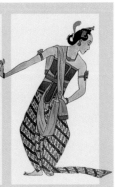

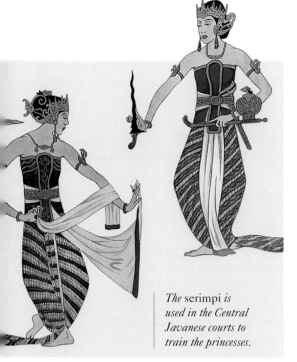

The serimpi *is used in the Central Javanese courts to train the princesses.*

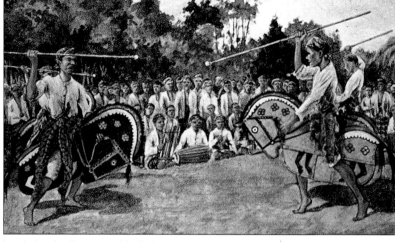

drums), three to five *angklung* (bamboo idiophones), and occasionally a *terbang* (frame-drum) and a *selompret* (trumpet). The gamelan and vocal accompaniments follow the five-toned *slendro* musical system.

Some of the regional versions of the *jathilan* present a story from the Panji cycle. These portray heroic battle-dances and include two comical figures, *Pentul* and *Tembem*, and sometimes a *barongan* figure (large mythical animal) which dances with exaggerated movements.

Pentul and Tembem wear knee-length pants, a batik skirt-cloth, *setagen, epek timang, ikel, sampur* and *rompi* (vest), and a mask. Pentul wears a white mask; and Tembem's is black. The *barongan* character wears a large mask that fits over his head in the shape of a lion's head or a giant's face. His body is concealed under a cloak attached to the mask.

(Above) Two horsemen brandishing lances in battle in the Javanese jathilan. *The plaited bamboo hobbyhorse is a popular dance and theatrical accessory.*

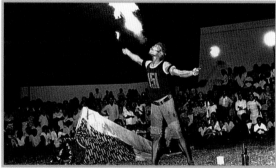

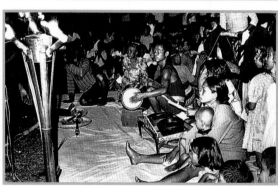

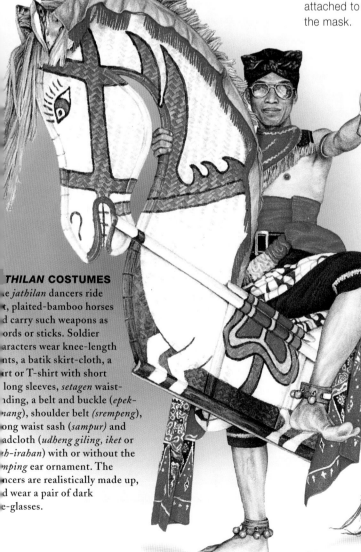

THILAN COSTUMES

e *jathilan* dancers ride , plaited-bamboo horses d carry such weapons as ords or sticks. Soldier aracters wear knee-length nts, a batik skirt-cloth, a rt or T-shirt with short long sleeves, *setagen* waist- nding, a belt and buckle (*epek-nang*), shoulder belt (*srempeng*), ong waist sash (*sampur)* and adcloth (*udheng giling, iket* or h-*irahan*) with or without the mping ear ornament. The ncers are realistically made up, d wear a pair of dark e-glasses.

(Top) Flame–throwing is one demonstration of magic shown at village fairs as part of the kuda kepang *performances.*

(Above) The orchestra accompanying the kuda kepang *is simple and portable. A basic set consists of* kethuk *and* kenong *kettle-gongs, hanging gongs and a* kendhang.

(Left) Jathilan *troupes are frequently invited to perform on special celebrations by the local administration, as they are very popular with the general public and the performances do not require long periods of preparation.*

77

Dances of Bali

Dances in Bali do not always have a storyline or plot. The main goal of the performer is to execute every movement phase and sequence in the dance with full expression. The beauty lies primarily in the visual and the kinaesthetic impact of abstract and stylistic movements. Among the best examples of the non-representational dances are the pendet, gabor, baris, sanghyang and legong.

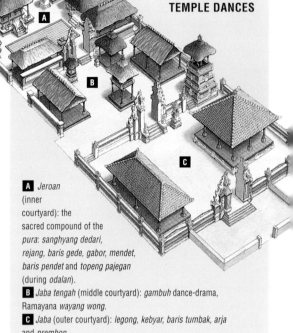

LOCATION OF TEMPLE DANCES

A *Jeroan* (inner courtyard): the sacred compound of the *pura*: *sanghyang dedari, rejang, baris gede, gabor, mendet, baris pendet* and *topeng pajegan* (during *odalan*).

B *Jaba tengah* (middle courtyard): *gambuh* dance-drama, Ramayana *wayang wong*.

C *Jaba* (outer courtyard): *legong, kebyar, baris tumbak, arja* and *prembon*.

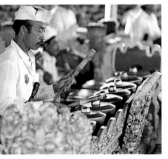

The gamelan gede *is an important set of musical instruments which is used in various dance and drama performances.*

»*In the story of Prabu Lasem, a raven warns the king of Lasem of impending death as he sets out for the battlefield. The king has taken the princess of Daha to his palace with the intention of marrying her, but she is unwilling. Her brother, the king of Daha, has instigated the battle to free his sister.*

Sacred and Secular Dances

These dances continue to have important functions in the socio-religious activities of the Balinese. While the *pendet, gabor, baris* and *sanghyang* are essential for Hindu-Balinese religious practices, and are classified as sacred (*wali*) or ceremonial (*bebali*), the *legong* is featured for non-religious events. Since the early 1950s, with the development of tourism on the island, the first four dances have also been featured on secular occasions, with some modifications.

Sacred and secular dances are presented at different times and places. Religious dances are normally performed in the temple's inner court (*jeroan*) or middle courtyard (*jaba tengah*), at the same time as the temple priest conducts the ritual or after the prayer. In contrast, the performance of secular dances normally takes place outside the temple (*jaba sisi*) at any site and time.

Using different musical compositions and melodic lines, these dances are accompanied by a *pelog* gamelan, the *gamelan gong kebyar*. If it is not available, the *slendro gamelan angklung* is used. The *gamelan gong gede* may also be used for the *baris*. The *sanghyang* is the only form using mainly vocal music by a male and female chorus.

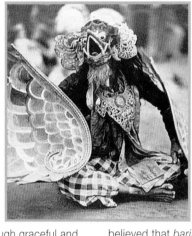

Pendet and Gabor

Pendet and *gabor* are welcome dances, expressions of joy, happiness and gratitude made through graceful and refined movements. Depending on the choreography, they may be performed by a pair or a group of female dancers of any age. In the past, they were temple dances to greet or please the gods and deities residing in the temple for the duration of the temple's anniversary festival (*odalan*). Today, they are staged purely as artistic entertainment.

The choreography of both includes three main parts: a brief introduction (*papeson*) with fast music, a slow-moving body (*pangadeng*), and a fast-ending (*panyuwud*). The traditional *pendet* and *gabor* may be performed by 10 to 30 dancers,

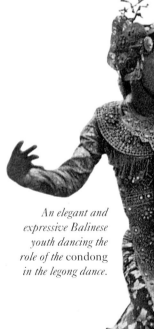

An elegant and expressive Balinese youth dancing the role of the condong *in the legong dance.*

in pairs or in groups of four to six, while each dancer carries offerings which are later placed on the altar in front or at the foot of a temple shrine. The secular versions can be performed by four or six dancers, each carrying a bowl of colourful flowers which they scatter over the audience to symbolise a warm welcome.

Baris

Baris is a type of heroic dance depicting great warrior(s). Performed by male dancers of any age, it expresses bravery and dignity through muscular, percussive and explosive movements. The name derives from *bebarisan* (a line or file formation) and appears in the *Kidung Sunda*, a semi-historical East Javanese poem of AD 1550. It is believed that *baris* was once a type of soldier used by the Balinese kings to protect their kingdoms.

Two kinds of *baris* are currently preserved by the Balinese. The *baris tunggal* is a dynamic solo piece characterised by quick and abrupt motions with lively facial expression. The *baris gede*, a ceremonial (*babali*) art form, is usually presented in a double-line formation with rather static but dignified movements. Both are accompanied by the same type of eight-beat gamelan music known as *gilak*.

Baris costumes are characterised by a cone-like headdress full of glittering leaves made of white metal or shells. They wear multiple-layers of decorative cloth bands (*awiran*) hanging from the breast to cover the body like an armour. Each dancer wears a differently coloured jacket and a dagger (*keris*).

Unlike the secular *baris* which can be seen almost everywhere, the ceremonial *baris gede* is only

NON-REPRESENTATIONAL DANCES

Dances	Occasions	Number of Dancers	Basic Progression in Dances
Pendet and **Gabor**	Welcome dances performed during the temple's anniversary festival or for guests.	No particular number but usually performed in pairs.	Brief introduction (*papeson*) with fast music, a slow-moving body (*pangadeng*), and a fast ending (*panyuwud*)
Baris	*Baris gede* (*babali*) sacred dance performed during temple's *odalan* and cremations. *Baris tunggal* (*balih-balihan*) secular dance presented for entertainment.	*Baris gede* dance consists of 12 to 40 dancers carrying weapons. *Baris tunggal* is a solo dance.	Dancers come into the *jeroan*, marching in unison, accompanied by the *gamelan gong gede*. When the formation is complete, all shout and kneel to pray and the music stops. After the prayers, at a musical signal, the men rise and begin executing complex choreographic manoeuvres. *Baris tunggal* dancer makes his entrance and dances carrying a weapon.
Sanghyang (**sanghyang dedari** in particular)	There are many varieties. They are performed at irregular intervals when required to ward off or alleviate an epidemic or other disaster. The best known is the *sanghyang dedari*.	For the *sanghyang dedari*, four or five dancers each between 9 and 12 years old are required to be present at the ritual. However only two dancers get to dance in a single performance.	There are three main stages. First the *penudusan*, or purification by incense smoke during which goddesses are invited to descend as the girls inhale pungent incense. Next, the dancers fall back into a state of possession in the *kerawuhan*. They walk on red hot coals and are paraded throughout the village. Finally, the dancers are brought out of their trance by holy water, prayers and presentation of offerings.
Legong	A secular dance performed at the temple's anniversary, but increasingly performed for tourist entertainment.	Altogether, three dancers in the entire repertoire.	There are three parts. The *pengawit* is short and performed by one girl, the *condong*. The *pengawak* is the longest and is danced by two dancers in unison. Finally, the *pengecet* during which the gamelan doubles its tempo and the two dancers face each other and dance vigorously.

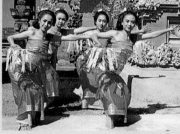
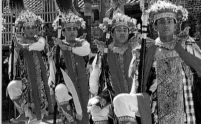
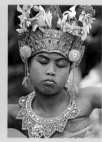
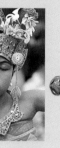
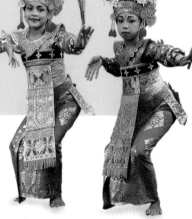

found in certain villages. In the mountainous region of North Bali, there are no less than 20 different versions which are usually identified by either the weapons used or the props carried by the dancers.

Sanghyang
Sanghyang is one of Bali's best known trance dances. It is believed that the dancer, a young girl or an elderly man, may be possessed by divine spirits, heavenly or wild animals, and other spirits. Since many villagers maintain a strong belief that the *sanghyang* has a spiritual power of protection, as ascribed in the old palm-leaf manuscript, *Lontar Kacacar*, this ritual dance can still be seen in many villages.

Traditionally, the *sanghyang* is performed in the event of an epidemic or other abnormality in the local village. Today, some villagers stage secular versions for tourists. There are at least ten different kinds of *sanghyang*. The name of each is based on the spirit which possesses the dancer or medium.

Legong and *cak* (*kecak*), two of Bali's most admired art forms, have been inspired by and are based on the *sanghyang*.

Legong
In the 19th century, I Dewa Agung Made Karna, ruling prince of Sukawati, while deep in meditation, saw two beautiful nymphs in elaborate costumes performing an elegant dance. When he woke up, the king called for the headman of Ketewel village to create some masks to replicate the faces of the nymphs and a new dance to resemble his vision. The newly created art form became known as *topeng dadari, sanghyang legong* or *legong topeng*. The new dance inspired artists from Blahbatuh village to create a similar type of dance called *nandir*, which subsequently inspired many artists of Gianyar, under patronage of the King of Gianyar, to develop a new *legong* dance similar to the one seen today.

The *legong* has been frequently regarded by outsiders as the symbol of the beauty of classical Balinese culture. Some adore the *legong* because of its performers — from two to three pre-adolescent girls with colourful and elaborate costumes and splendid headdresses full of flowers — or because of its artistic beauty, which lies in the harmonious interplay of movement and gamelan music.

(Above left to right): The gabor, baris tumbak, sanghyang dedari *and* legong.

The origin of the legong *is unclear, but the most widely accepted tradition expounded by the late I Ketut Rinda, an artist and expert on old Balinese manuscripts, is that it is based on a genealogical chronicle of the Princes of Sukawati, the* Babad Dalem Sukawati.

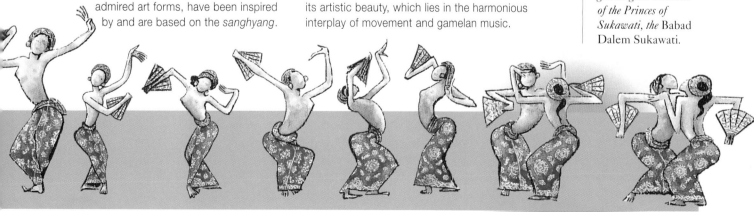

West Java: Ketuk Tilu and Tayuban

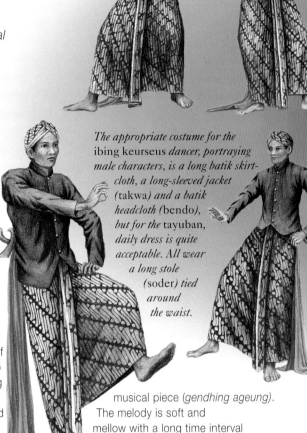

*T*here are two traditional genres of social dance in West Java. The focal point of these dances is a group of professional performers, called ronggeng, *whose duty is to encourage men from the audience to come out and dance with them to the accompaniment of a gamelan orchestra. The* ketuk tilu *belongs to the rural community and is, or was, generally danced outdoors with minimum musical accompaniment. The* tayuban, *on the other hand, was a more up-scale performance conducted indoors with fuller gamelan accompaniment.*

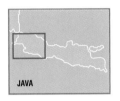

Tayuban

The *tayuban* featured the *ronggeng*, who danced for and with a generally male audience. In a closed environment, these indoor parties unfortunately fell into disrepute. The art of the dance, however, was not allowed to die. Early this century a nobleman from Sumedang, Raden Bantjakusuma, re-choreographed the movements into a more refined dance. Some years later one of his students, Raden Sambas Wirakusumah, made an attempt to systematise the classical elements of the dance, which resulted in a group of four solo compositions expressing four definitive types of male characters. They could be performed on social occasions, such as public performances with a full classical gamelan orchestra.

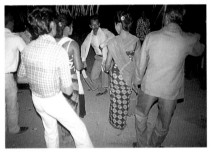

The earlier tayuban *dancer was the* ronggeng *who danced for mainly male spectators.*

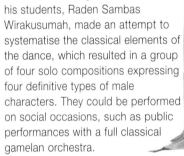

The appropriate costume for the ibing keurseus *dancer, portraying male characters, is a long batik skirt-cloth, a long-sleeved jacket (*takwa*) and a batik headcloth (*bendo*), but for the* tayuban, *daily dress is quite acceptable. All wear a long stole (*soder*) tied around the waist.*

Ibing Keurseus

R.S. Wirakusumah disseminated his concept through his dancing school, Wirahma Sari. The four dances evolved into the basis of Sundanese dance education and became known as *ibing keurseus* (literally 'course' dances or 'dances for teaching').

1. **Leyepan:** The *leyepan* is a refined dance executed in slow tempo in conformity with the staid and sedate character which it depicts. The movements are smooth, flowing and distinguished by a soft rolling of the head and a continual downward gaze. It is accompanied by a long

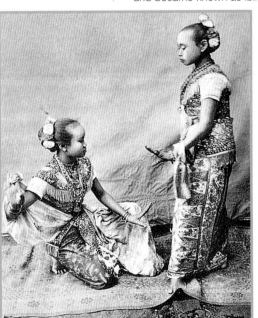

The ronggeng *wore a plain top, with a long batik wrapped around her body and a stole draped over her shoulders.*

musical piece (*gendhing ageung*). The melody is soft and mellow with a long time interval between gongs, which punctuate the end of each phrase.

2. **Nyatria:** The *nyatria* is another refined dance, but the tempo is faster and the movements are accentuated and rapid. Head movements are cleanly executed and quick. The dancer holds his head high, presenting an alert, accessible countenance. The *nyatria* is said to typify the character of the Sundanese people. Only two musical compositions are used, *Gawil* and *Kakacangan*, both bright and clear.

3. **Monggawa:** (Please see the opposite page).

4. **Ngalana:** The *ngalana* is also a strong dance but executed at a faster tempo than all the others. The movements are similar to the *monggawa*, but performed at a more rapid pace. The gaiety expressed in music and dance is accentuated by a movement known as *pakblang*: the dancer flips the long ends of his stole alternately above his head while taking short jumps and nodding his head in sharp, clear movements; or, instead of flipping the scarf ends, he may clap his hands over his head. The *sepak soder* is another possible movement in the *ngalana* dance.

Ketuk Tilu

The *ketuk tilu* derives its name from its accompanying music ensemble: three (*tilu*) kettlegongs (*ketuk*) that produce a steady, fixed

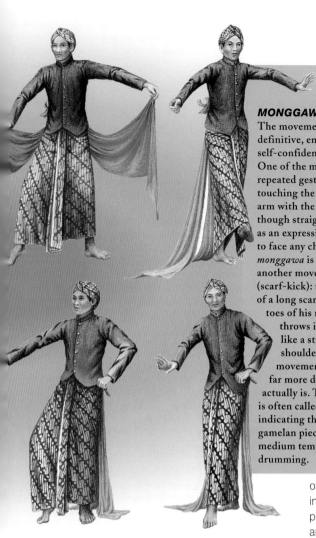

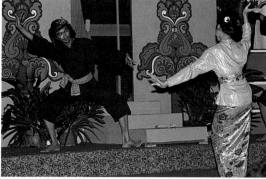

MONGGAWA DANCE

The movements are vigorous and definitive, emphasising directness, self-confidence and strength. One of the most frequently repeated gestures is the *capang*: touching the middle of the upper arm with the opposite hand as though straightening the sleeves, as an expression of being ready to face any challenge. The *monggawa* is distinguished by another movement, the *sepak soder* (scarf-kick): taking up one end of a long scarf (*soder*) between the toes of his right foot, the dancer throws it (or kicks it: *sepak*) like a streamer over his shoulder. It is an exciting movement, appearing to be far more difficult than it actually is. The *monggawa* dance is often called *kring dua*, indicating that the accompanying gamelan piece is short, with medium tempo and loud drumming.

Movements Vocabulary
The movements of the *ketuk tilu,* and the drumming, intensify as the performance progresses climaxing in the energetic display delivered by the male dancer in the fourth and final component of the show. His movements, derived from the *pencak silat,* are vigorous, masculine and proud; they are exaggerated to cause amusement. Each phrase of music is accentuated by a drumbeat. The tempo increases as the music nears the end, stimulating the performer to greater heights of display. The drummer and the audience add encouragement with skillful drumming, rhythmic vocal sounds and hand-clapping.The dancer climaxes with an ostentatious and dramatic drop (*depok*) with arms outstretched. The audience responds with applause and cheering. Satisfied with his success, which has been greatly enhanced by the *ronggeng*'s simple movements, the dancer is quite happy to give her a large tip.

A well-known and recent adaptation of the ketuk tilu *is the* jaipongan *which has spread widely into many parts of Indonesia.*

rhythm, one large *kendhang* drum and two smaller *kulantor* drums which produce a rich combination of drum patterns, a two-stringed lute (*rebab*), and sometimes a singer (*sinden*) and *kerek* (small metal plates struck with a wooden mallet) to accentuate the drum patterns.

The performance takes place in the evening in an open space. An oil lamp (*oncor*) set high on a pole marks the centre of the arena. Arranged at a four-metre radius around this arena are the orchestra and the audience, who have been attracted by the *tatalu,* a specific gamelan melody played to announce the show.

At a signal from the leader of the group, the gamelan stops playing. The leader prays for a successful party after which the dancers (*ronggeng*) open the show with the *jajangkungan* dance. They move in a circle around the lamp, raising themselves up on their toes in time with each gong beat. At the end, they move into the *wawayangan* dance, now facing the audience. The movements and music are derived from the *wayang* theatre. At the conclusion of this segment, the *ronggeng* invite the men in the audience to dance with them, for which the men will pay a small fee, dropped into a container beside the lampstand. Finally, the *ronggeng* stop for a rest, while a male dancer takes over to entertain the audience with the *panjak* dance. The beauty of the soloist's more sophisticated performance is usually so challenging, that some man is sure to jump into the ring at the end of it and ask one of the *ronggeng* to join him in a dance.

(Below) The ketuk tilu *is an exciting social dance form and since the 1960s has undergone many refinements and simplifications to make it an acceptable national dance form not only for young men and women, but also for formal stage performance. One of the best-known and recent adaptations is the* jaipongan, *which has spread beyond the borders of its homeland in West Java. The* ronggeng's *purpose is to entice men in the audience to dance with her, for which they will pay a small fee. She 'dances the night away' constantly changing partners so as to leave no one out. The men are challenged to demonstrate their skill, each trying to outdo the other.*

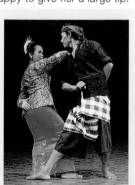

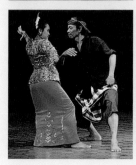

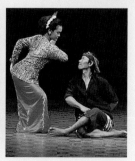

Dances of West and South Sumatra

The dances from West and South Sumatra range from combination of martial arts and dance such as the alau ambek *to graceful female dance like the* gending sriwijaya. *Unique forms of dances such as the* alau ambek, alang suntiang *and* gending Sriwijaya *are particular to the area but West and South Sumatra also possess dances which are shared with other parts of Sumatra and Indonesia such as the* pencak silat *and* tari piring.

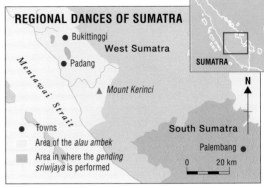

REGIONAL DANCES OF SUMATRA

- Bukittinggi
- **West Sumatra**
- Padang
- ▲ Mount Kerinci

SUMATRA

N

• Towns
▢ Area of the *alau ambek*
▢ Area in where the *gending sriwijaya* is performed

South Sumatra

Palembang ●

0   20 km

The tari piring *(plate dance) is one of the dances of the Minangkabau. West Sumatra.*

Alau Ambek

Alau ambek is a traditional dance from the Minangkabau culture of West Sumatra which is based on martial arts movements. It is said to have originated in the period when the kings of ancient kingdoms conducted battles to expand their hegemony: the kingdom sponsoring the losing fighter would be obliged to surrender its territory to the winner. Today, the dance is merely an exhibition of skill in the martial arts, but it retains a spiritual nuance and thus cannot be performed without the permission of the highest traditional authorities, the *ninik mamak* (male elders of the matrilineal clan), since improper performance could have disastrous consequences for the community. The *ninik mamak* are identified at the performance with the display of valuable paraphernalia owned by them such as ceremonial hangings and banners (*tirai, candai, tabie*), announcement gongs (*canang*), and three ceremonial betel quid containers (*carana bapaga*).

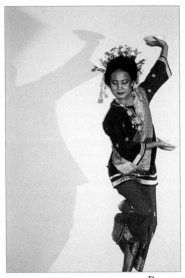

Presentation

An *alau ambek* performance resembles a martial arts duel supervised by two arbiters, *janang*. Movements

consist of such motions as shaking hands, attack and defence, four steps, and stealing a step, all delivered in slow motion. Arm movements include crossing the arms like 'scissor points', various symbolic gestures (*imbur*), and baiting (*batuah*). The musical accompaniment, *dampeang*, has male and female tones. The male *dampeang* is high-pitched, signalling an imminent attack, while the lower-pitched female *dampeang* directs the steps to attack or defend. Costumes consist of wide *galembong* pants, black shirt, belt and headcloth (*destar*).

Alang Suntiang

The *alang suntiang,* also called *alang suntiang panghulu*, which means 'eagle dance, the adornment of the *panghulu*', is a traditional dance form from Padang Lawas in the Agam regency of West Sumatra. Replicating the skilful and rapid movements of the eagle, the dance is said to have once been famous all over the three original Minangkabau regions of settlement (*luhak nan tigo*) as the pride of the *panghulu* (traditional leaders). Having fallen into disuse long ago, the *alang suntiang* was revived in 1964 as a part of traditional ceremonial life and is today performed at weddings, an infant's bathing ritual (*turun mandi*), and to welcome important visitors. It has also become the learning material for dance students. It continues to appear only with the permission of the *ninik mamak*, basically to accompany the bearers of the *sirih* (betel quid) container (*carano*) required at all traditional ceremonies. Formerly staged inside the *rumah gadang* (the traditional 'great house') within the area framed by the *tonggak nan ampek* (four posts), the *alang suntiang* may now be presented inside a building or outside, according to the wishes of the *ninik mamak*.

Costumes and Musical Accompaniments

Traditionally, the performers are an even number of men. Musical accompaniment is provided by

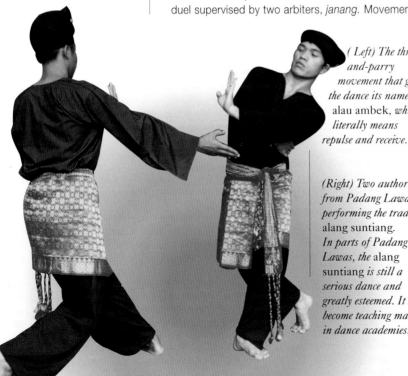

(Left) The thrust-and-parry movement that gives the dance its name, alau ambek, *which literally means repulse and receive.*

(Right) Two authorities from Padang Lawas performing the traditional alang suntiang.
In parts of Padang Lawas, the alang suntiang *is still a serious dance and greatly esteemed. It has become teaching material in dance academies.*

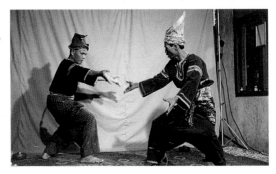

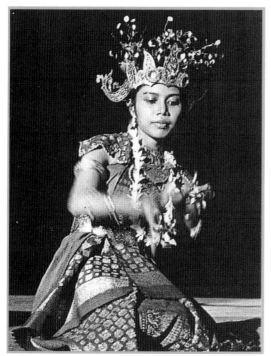

(Above) The gending Sriwijaya *is reminiscent of old court dances.*

In its present form, it is composed in the 1940s.

the *adok* (frame-drum), *talempong jao* (set of kettlegongs), *saluang* (bamboo flute), *pupuik beranak* (reed) and frequently also the vocalisation of songs like *pasalaman, tanduak buang, dok dinandong, si kumbang cari, awan bentan, si junda*. Costume consists of long pants in the wide and loose *sarawa lambuak* or *gunting enam* style, a shirt and a *destar palangi* (headcloth) interwoven with gold thread, a dagger slipped into the waistband and, once upon a time, a sword as well.

Gending Sriwijaya

Inspired by the glory of the ancient kingdom of Sriwijaya in South Sumatra, the *gending Sriwijaya* is today considered to be a traditional court dance of the Palembang region. The *gending Sriwijaya*'s music and lyrics, however, were only introduced in the early 1940s, during the Japanese occupation of Indonesia. They were subsequently united with the dance and reworked by Suhainah Rozak and Masnun Toha into dance suitable for performance to honour and welcome important guests.

Performance

The *gending Sriwijaya* is a stately dance performed by an even number of women dressed in lavish costumes of gold-threaded brocades and masses of gold jewellery. The movements are gracefully languid and simple, stressing the beauty of the fingers which are extended by long golden finger-covers. Little flicks of the fingers cause chains of little gold discs on the underside of the finger-covers to tremble exquisitely. The chorus of dancers is led by a group of three young women carrying the equipment for betel-chewing, an age-old welcoming tradition throughout Southeast Asia; but the dance is performed as pure entertainment.

ALANG SUNTIANG PERFORMANCE

Dance patterns consist of the ❶ *tapuak pasalaman*, which is a request for forgiveness directed at the audience, closing with the *rantak pasalaman* (greeting by footwork); ❷ *tanduak buang*, describing the buffalo's horns; ❸ *awan bentan*, 'waves of clouds blanketing the sky', which once involved sword-play in which the wielder of the sword cleanly sliced a banana leaf bound to the other's forehead without touching the person; ❹ *dok dinandong*, which describes the movements of an eagle eyeing its prey; ❺ *tari gandang*, or dance of happiness, with the audience participating with rhythmic handclapping; ❻ *adau adau*, depicting a rice-straw mat weaver as a symbol of community prosperity and the skill of the youth in working the ricefields; ❼ *barabah pulang mandi*, the 'ducks return home to bathe', flapping their wings in all directions; and finally the conclusion, in which the performers again beg the forgiveness of the audience.

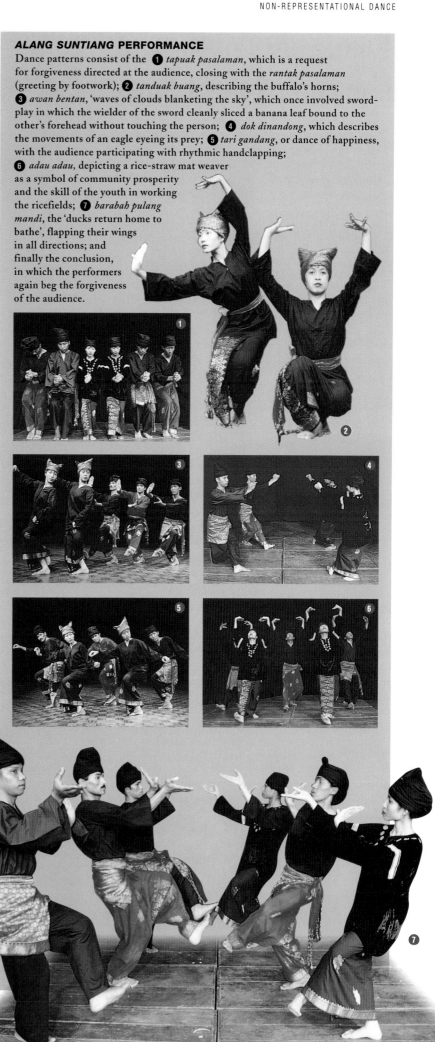

East Kalimantan and Coastal Malay Dances

*T*he dances of the Dayak of East Kalimantan and the coastal Malay areas constitute two of the more prominent groups of dances which exist outside the more conventional and popularly known dances of Java and Bali. The coastal Malays inhabit the east littoral of North Sumatra along the Straits of Melaka.

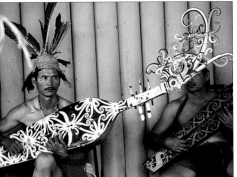

(Above) The sampe' or three-stringed lute is a wondrous object to behold, with its swirling and curling ornamentation.

⤹*The* kanjet temengan *is similar to the* kanjet teweg.

Crouching low, the kanjet pepatai *dancer, emulating a warrior, turns smoothly to the left then right, pivoting slowly on the balls of their feet, abruptly springing up with a loud war whoop and lunging in attack.*

Dances of East Kalimantan

Kanjet, giring-giring and *mandau* dances represent three kinds of dance native to the Dayak peoples of inland East Kalimantan. The first dance refers to performances held outdoors to welcome guests and as a ritual complement. The main musical instrument used in accompaniment is the *sampe'* (lute).

Kanjet

Dance steps in the *kanjet* are simple, and this has permitted continued adaptation and widespread practice. In the traditional context are the *kanjet teweg* (gong dance), *kanjet temengan* and *kanjet pepatai* (sword dance). New adaptations include *kanjet lasan*, a modification of the *kanjet teweg,* and *kanjet liling* or *leleng*.

Feet are kept close together with heels raised. Movement is one of constant turning, pivoting on the balls of the feet. Strong calf muscles and heel control are used to keep balance. The torso is lowered on deeply bent knees as it is turned as far as possible to one side without losing balance, and then to the other side, one movement flowing into the next with great fluidity. All the while, the hands rotate incessantly and delicately. Movement is slow, controlled and graceful.

Giring-giring

The *giring-giring* is a long ribbon of bells worn just below the knees. The dancer may also carry a long staff in the left hand which is knocked against the ground to coincide with the fourth footstep. In the right hand, a 30-centimetre-long bamboo stick filled with beans is shaken rhythmically to

The kanjet teweg *is performed by a bride as part of her wedding ceremony. She dances on the face of a small gong, holding strung hornbill feathers in each of her hands.*

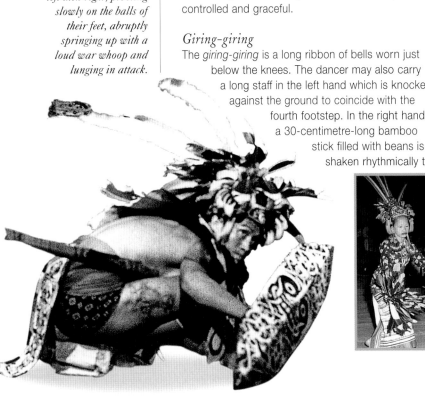

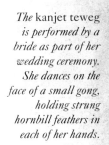

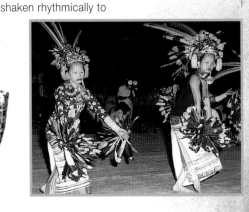

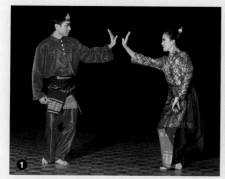
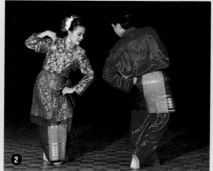
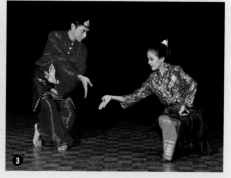

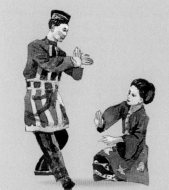
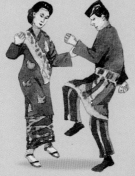
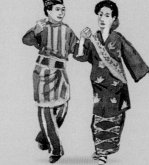
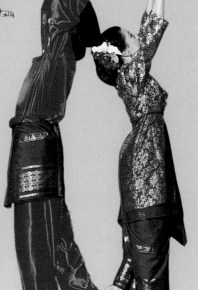

SERAMPANG DUA BELAS

In this dance the *tari lagu dua* tempo has been so accelerated that vocalised *pantun* accompaniment is impossible. This tempo is called *pulau sari* or *terancang*. The *serampang dua belas* emphasises eye-play, lithe foot movements and jumps, plus limbre body and hand gestures. The lack of regulated structure in the *pulau sari* inspired a school-teacher, Sauti, to construct a set of 12 patterns based on movements found in such Malay dances as the *mak yong* and *zapin*.

The arranged *serampang dua belas* consists of three parts: *mak inang*, *tanjung katung* and *lagu dua*. Each with different rhythmic patterns. The dance was widely spread through competitions mostly among students.

produce a shuffling sound. Musical accompaniment is provided by *kangkanong* (large drum) and *gandang* (double-headed drum). The zig-zagging pattern of the dance is said to replicate the motions of villagers planting rice in the fields.

Tari Mandau

The *mandau* is a very sharp bushknife. The *mandau* dance is normally performed by men and sometimes also by women. It describes the training in the use of the *mandau* for self-protection. Music accompaniment is provided by the *sampe'*.

Coastal Malay Dances

By the mid-20th century, the traditional Malayan music and dance of theatre genres such as the *mak yong, menora, mendu* and *bangsawan* had almost vanished. A few purely entertaining dances remained, among which were the *senandung, lagu dua, mak inang* and *serampang dua belas* dance.

Malay dance are transferred as part of oral tradition, in which young aspirants watch and imitate the teacher. This quartet of dances serves as the basis for teaching dance.

The Senandung (Drifting) Dance

The *pantun nasib* lyrics accompanying the dance bewail bad luck (*nasib buruk*) rendered in a repeated four-bar rhythm. Guitar- and cello-plucking have been successfully used by modern bands to imitate this beat generally produced on the *ronggeng* drum and gong.

Tari Lagu Dua

The musical accompaniment for this dance is gay, with a rather fast rhythm and some 12 variants of drum-beating. The tempo displays early Portuguese influence. Dance steps are executed with grace.

Tari Mak Inang

This dance has a slow 'walking'-like rhythm. The *pantun* lyrics are generally 'cheerfully comical' (*pantun jenaka*). Around the 1930s, the tempo was doubled, resulting in the *cek minah sayang* song-and-dance, which includes 12 movements and makes use of a handkerchief. The dance is reminiscent of the West Sumatran *kaparinyo*, probably due to Minangkabau migrants, and this in turn is derived from the Portuguese-African *capriol* dance.

❶ *The* senandung *beat is sometimes referred to as the* lagu berhanyut *(drifting melody), because it recalls the crackling of the sea-breeze and the fisherman leaving his proa to drift with the sea or river current.*
❷ *Male dancers* mengebeng *(lower one shoulder while circling the female dancer) and* menyentak *(lunge for partner, taking small running steps and stopping short of touching).*
❸ *The* Mak Inang *dance is a social dance performed by male and female couples.*

Dance Forms in South Sulawesi

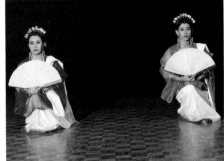
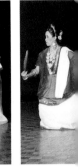

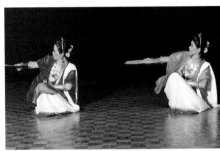
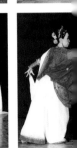

*T*he Province of South Sulawesi is inhabited by many ethnic groups. The largest of these are the Bugis, Makasarese, Mandarese and Torajans. Each has its own language and its own specific dance style. Nevertheless, when they go abroad, all travel under the general Bugis-Makasarese label.

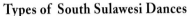

(Above) A pajaga dancer.

(Below) Mamasa's dances follow circular and linear floor patterns.

Types of South Sulawesi Dances

South Sulawesi boasts some 316 traditional dances, of which 98 belong to the Bugis, 66 to the Makasarese, 116 to the Mandarese and 36 to the Sa'dan Torajans. The Makasarese call their ritual dances *sere* and entertainment dances *pakarena*. To the Buginese these are *pajaga* or *jaga* and *pajogeq* or *katia*, respectively. Up-river Mandarese refer to dances as *malluya* or *sayo* and *bondesan*, while coastal Mandarese use *tudduq*. The Torajan word for dance is *gelluq, pagelluq* or *burake*.

The Dances of Makasar

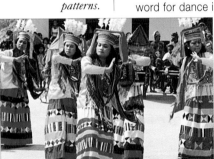

(Below left) Dancers at a ceremony, South Sulawesi.

(Below right) The pagelluq began as a dance of praise to God for His beneficence. Today, it serves as the basis of new choreographers for pure entertainment.

Makasarese dances are characterised by a contrast between movement and rhythm: female dancers move independently from the tempo of the *genrang* (double-headed) drum. Torso movement is rare: the dancer's body must remain firm throughout the dance. Feet must remain fixed to the ground, eyes focused on the ground in front. Arm movements, and the dancers' concentration, are directed at heaven and earth. Likewise, the design of musical instruments, costume and adornment follow a vertical line. Examples are the dancer's long-sleeved blouse, the very long necklace and the unique *simpoleng patinra* hairknot that stands upright.

Mandarese Dances

The special characteristic of Mandarese dances is a 'roundness', perceived in make-up, dress and floor

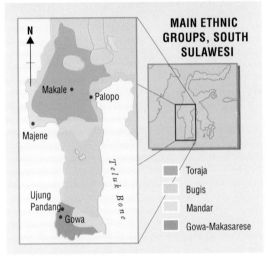

MAIN ETHNIC GROUPS, SOUTH SULAWESI

Makale
Palopo
Majene
Ujung Pandang
Gowa

Teluk Bone

☐ Toraja
☐ Bugis
☐ Mandar
☐ Gowa-Makasarese

pattern. The ideal dancer's face is round, too. This is echoed by the cut-off *baju pokko* blouse, large round 'pomegranate' earpins (*subang dalima*) and very round hairknot. Dance themes in upstream Mandar come from the world of fowl, buffaloes and insects, whilst dances on the coast derive from marine life: crabs, fish, prawn and fowl. The theme of the dance is reflected in the name, movements and lyrics of the dance, and costume and adornment.

Torajan Dances

The predominant feature of Torajan dances is the foot movement. The dancer takes steps so short that progression is almost imperceptible. Her feet seem anchored to the ground, while body, and especially arms, appear to stretch sideways and upwards. Each movement constructs an inverted triangular form.

Buginese Dances

In general, the movements of the Buginese dancer are more fluid and dynamic compared to those of the Makasarese, and the floor pattern expands, rises and falls in wave-like motion. Expansion, verticality and waviness are reiterated in the design of the dancer's costume and make-up. The dancer's *baju bodo*

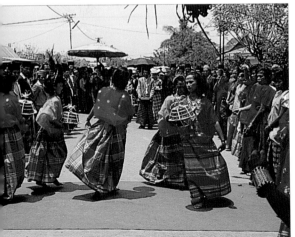

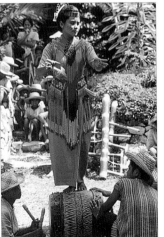

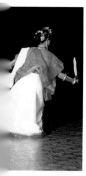
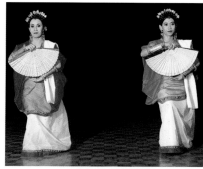
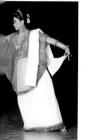
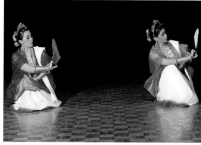

(short-sleeved blouse) is starched to inflexible rigidity (*tokko*), and her hairline extended with an application of a black paste (*daddasa*) so that it curves and waves above her eyebrows.

Pajogeq Dance

The *pajogeq* dance is known throughout the Bugis region, but especially in Watampone and vicinity on the east coast of the province. Its name derives from the root *joget* which means 'to dance'. The *pajogeq* has many variations, amongst which are the *pajogeq makkunrai* danced by women, and *pajogeq calabai* performed by transvestites. The *pajogeq makkunrai* has two sub-divisions, one danced exclusively in the palace by daughters of the aristocracy (*pajogeq andi*) and another performed outside the palace by slaves (*pajogeq ata*) or transvestites. The most developed versions are the ones danced by slaves and transvestites.

In the past, local celebrities, who were aristocrats and the wealthy, were invited to *majogeq* performances. When the dancers moved into the *ballung* segment, anybody in the audience interested in a dancer (*pajogeq*) could ask her to rise and perform in front of him. If he was sitting, she would bend her body, as she sang and danced, so that her hairknot would touch him. Then she would be handed a payment for services which could be money, a handkerchief, or expensive perfume. This scene could be repeated as often as the man continued to pay. Sometimes the dance would begin at 7:00 p.m. and end at 6:00 a.m. the next morning.

A *pajogeq* performance begins with a dance performed in unison by several pairs of dancers led by an elderly woman, *indok pajogeq*. One or more male members of the troupe, *pengibing*, then join(s) them. After this comes

the *ballung* accompanied by singing. The final act is the *mappasompeq* or *mengibing* in which the audience is permitted to join the dancing or request a dance and song by a favourite dancer who is rewarded with gifts.

The dancer may also initiate dancing with a member of the audience, *mengibing*, by handing him a scarf (*cinde*). The recipient of the invitation is referred to as *nalejjak tedong* (trod on by a buffalo). The competition for a dancer's favour, always rewarded with a gift, is sometimes quite heated and in the past not infrequently ended in fighting and blood-spilling.

Outside the palace, the *pajogeq* dance is generally performed as entertainment at wedding parties, fairs, and so forth. Performances are rare today because the Buginese aristocracy consider this social dance undignified.

THE *PAJAGA* OF LUWU

Twelve teenaged girls 12 to 15 years old are used to perform the lovely *pajaga* dance to entertain the court on ceremonial occasions. Their low-flowing skirts and floor-length scarves served to emphasise the grace of their movements. Music is provided by the dancers' own singing and drumming. It is not permissible to change or adapt the *pajaga*.

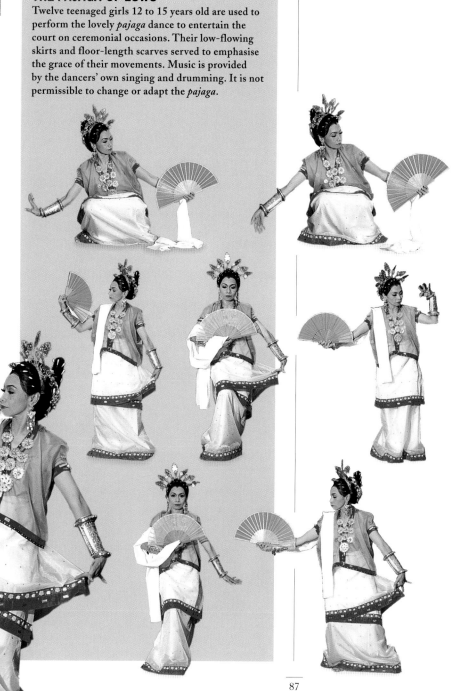

《《*The* pakarena *of Gowa-Makasar was introduced to the royal court by angels who came to earth to teach the feminine arts to the women. It became a dance of worship to thank the deities for having taught them the way of life. Three to five pre-pubescent girls would sing as they performed the elegant, slow-motion dance to the accompaniment of two throbbing drums.*

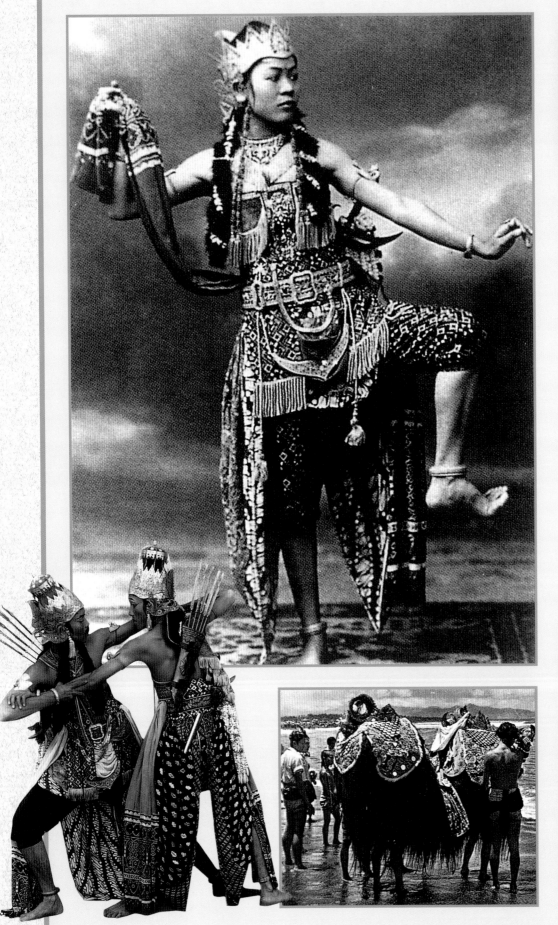

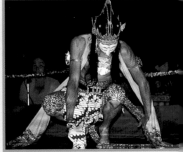

(Main picture) Nyai Bei Mardusari, a famous dancer-singer in traditional Javanese langrendiyan theatrical performance of the Mangkunagara court.

(Above) The Javanese wayang topeng performance is one of the better known forms of traditional theatre in the royal courts of Surakarta and Yogyakarta.

(Below extreme left) The Javanese wayang wong drama theatre is perhaps one of the oldest forms of performing arts in Indonesia.

(Below left) The sacred and mythical barong ket represents an important character in the traditional Balinese theatre of barong/calonarang and newly created forms such as the kecak ramayana. The barong ket is also used in religious rituals such as village cleansing rituals.

(Below) A dancer acting the role of a princely figure in the Balinese arja dance-drama.

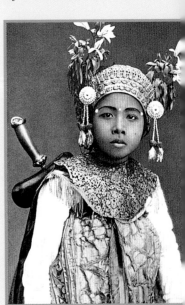

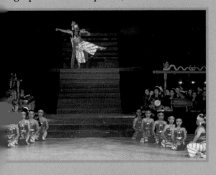

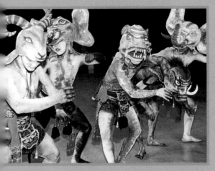

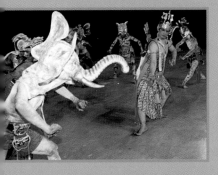

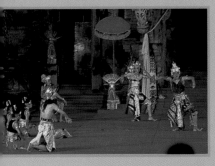

TRADITIONAL THEATRE

Many places in Indonesia are the cradles of specific cultures with their own languages and traditions. In some of them traditions include one or more theatrical art form. A theatrical art form can be defined as a performance in which there is a story to be enacted by *dramatis personae*, either played by living actors and actresses, or by puppets manipulated by a puppeteer. Some ethnic cultures, such as Bali and Java, have a complex system of theatrical performances, whereas some others hardly possess any theatrical art under the same definition. In these places the theatrical genre is replaced by the performance of oral literature or story-telling. The art of story-telling is indeed a rudimentary theatre, since the narration is always done in a specific style. The story-teller often accompanies himself by playing an instrument. In West Java he, the *tukang pantun*, accompanies himself with a *kecapi*, a stringed instrument.

Stories presented in either story-telling or theatrical performance comprise a variety of subjects: genealogies; myths and legends; stories of heroes from local chiefdoms combating ogres; stories of the royalties of ancient kingdoms; stories taken from the Mahabharata and the Ramayana, mostly in localised versions, and also other stories originating in foreign countries, such as the Amir Hamzah (Menak) cycle of stories from Persia, and the 'Sam Pek - Eng Tay' story from China. The local 'colouring' of these adapted 'foreign' stories is done in several ways. First, there is the transformation through the use of the local language with its own conceptual biases due to the specificity of words and terms. Another aspect is the reinterpretation of the story itself, in which the leading message, or the peripheral ones, may divert from the original. A greater measure of transformation is found whenever a story of foreign origin is superimposed on or amalgamated with local stories.

Examples of the last instance can be found in the Javanese *wayang purwa* cycle of stories which basically narrates the exploits of the characters from the Mahabharata and Ramayana epics. Nevertheless, in many stories it may be found that their characterisation, their speech and deed, and their attitude as well as philosophy of life, may deviate a lot from the Indian version.

Another prominent feature of traditional theatre forms is a conventional set of characters for each theatrical form. For instance, in the *mak yong* play of Riau, Sumatra, the set of basic characters comprises the young princess, the queen mother, the young prince, the older king and the attendant/jester.

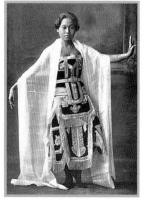

Folk Theatre of East and West Java

The ludruk *and* srimulat *are two forms of popular theatre which originate from East Java.* Ludruk *is a specifically East Javanese form of popular theatre and its stories are built around the vicissitudes of daily life.* Srimulat *was established in Surakarta in 1950 and moved to Surabaya in 1961.*

(Above) In Malang, East Java, the ludruk *performance in the 1930s opened with the* tari beskalan *danced by women. This evolved into the* tari ngremo Putri Malangan, *in which a long scarf hanging from the neck is essential. Malang is the only area where the opening dance is performed by women.*

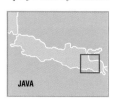

JAVA

(Below) The ngremo *dancer performs with feminine grace and sings a song asking the audience's forgiveness for mistakes that may be made during the show.*

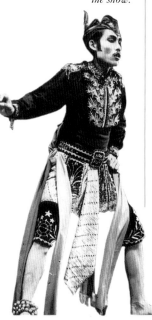

Lerok Ngamen (1907-1915)

The *lerok ngamen* began with a farmer, Pak Santik, from the Jombang region of East Java. To augment his income, he would go 'on the road' *(ngamen)* as a one-man show using comedy and ballad interspersed with the sounds of gamelan music imitated by mouth. To keep his identity private, he powdered and painted his face thickly, and dressed in clown-like attire. Thus evolved a *kesenian barangan* (travelling show) referred to locally as *lerok*.

With time, the one-man show grew into a three-man show. The monologue became a lively dialogue, and the ballads could be sung in dialogue form.

Lerok Besutan (1915–c.1920)

The three-man *lerok ngamen* with its comedy and songs grew so popular that troupes were often invited to entertain guests at parties. Quality was improved and a live gamelan introduced, composed of the *kendhang* (double-headed drum), *saron* (metal xylophone), *kempul* (small hanging gong), gong, *siter* (zither), and the musicians.

The core drama continued to be enacted by three actors, each with a designated role. There were Besut, a common man, the *wedokan* (man in woman's role) as Besut's wife Asmunah, and Man Jamino, an elderly man.

The metamorphosis of the *lerok ngamen* into the *lerok besutan* paralleled the development of the religious-ceremonial traditions of Java. The actors assumed symbolic characters, visualised in attire. Besut became conspicuous for his odd costume. Clad in a red Turkish fez and long black trousers under a white skirt-cloth *(bebed lawon)* and bare-chested, Besut symbolised the common man, unsophisticated, with an inherent spiritual purity. In contrast, Asmunah was very fashionable in *kebaya*-blouse and batik skirt-cloth, representing a woman of the times. The elderly Man Jamino astutely kept harmony between the two extreme poles of life.

The *lerok besutan* was usually performed in the front yard of the host's home. In the evening, Besut would appear carrying a torch, followed by Asmunah, eyes covered with a white veil, a wad of tobacco stuck in the corner of her mouth. Behind came Man Jamino. Hands pressed tightly together, the three would bow deeply to the four points of the compass *(kiblat papat)*. Asmunah would then remove her veil and discard the wad of tobacco; the lamps were lit,

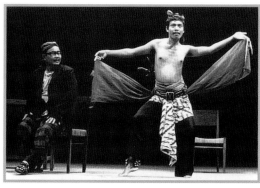

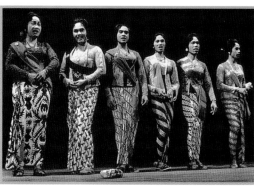

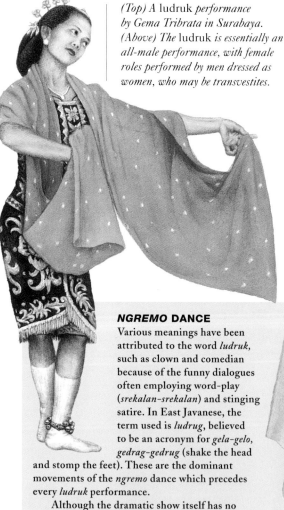

(Top) A ludruk *performance by Gema Tribrata in Surabaya. (Above) The* ludruk *is essentially an all-male performance, with female roles performed by men dressed as women, who may be transvestites.*

NGREMO DANCE

Various meanings have been attributed to the word *ludruk*, such as clown and comedian because of the funny dialogues often employing word-play *(srekalan-srekalan)* and stinging satire. In East Javanese, the term used is *ludrug*, believed to be an acronym for *gela-gelo, gedrag-gedrug* (shake the head and stomp the feet). These are the dominant movements of the *ngremo* dance which precedes every *ludruk* performance.

Although the dramatic show itself has no relationship whatsoever to the *gela-gelo gedrag-gedrug* movement, the performance is incomplete without the *ngremo* dance.

Gamelan instruments accompanying the ngremo dance are either in the *pelog* or *slendro* scale.

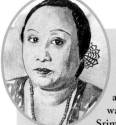

RADEN ADJENG SRIMULAT

Raden Ajeng Srimulat (1905-1968) was born in Solo to an aristocratic family. Her father was district chief of Bekonang. Srimulat's love of art led her to abandon her background for the world of theatre. She was disowned by her family, because performing in a travelling *ketoprak* group was considered a disgrace.

Together with the artist Teguh, whom she married, Srimulat established the Gema Malam Srimulat travelling theatre group, in 1950. Based at the Taman Sriwedari Park in Surakarta, Central Java, the group performed all over Java, and even in Medan (Sumatra) and Balikpapan, Banjarmasin and Palangkaraya (Kalimantan). When the Dagelan Mataram clowns Joni Gudel, Bandhempo and Atmonadi joined the group, clowning became a dominant feature.

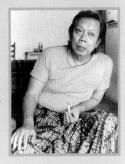

and the performance began. Besut represents man seeking enlightenment, *pepadhanging urip*. The actions prior to the play are symbolic of the blossoming of consciousness.

Ludruk (1920-present)

The *lerok besutan* evolved into the *ludruk*, which enacts scenes taken from life and presented with even more realism.

The *ludruk* opens with a welcome expressed in the *ngremo* dance.

Before the main presentation is a comedic intermission (*dagelan*) carried out by a pair of comics as well as the *tandhakan* or *bedhayan ludruk* dance performed by a number of transvestites. Indeed, one of the main characteristics of the *ludruk* is that it is an all-male cast.

Srimulat

Srimulat performances are humorous, with clowning strongly emphasised. Horror stories were directed with humour rather than fear. Plays such as *Mayat Hidup* (Living Corpse) and *Dracula* were presented by comically satirising man's behaviour instead of frightening the audience.

(Above) A srimulat performance in Jakarta in 1995.

(Bottom left) Longser *and an archival image of* ubrug *(right).*

HISTORY OF *SRIMULAT* THEATRE

1950 — Srimulat established Gema Malam Srimulat. They performed music and songs with a Javanese tone and *keroncong* (a hybrid music style) beat, mixed with clowning.

1950s — Clowning became dominant when the Dagelan Mataram clowns Joni Gudel, Bandhempo and Atmonadi joined the group. The group performed in Java, parts of Sumatra and Kalimantan.

1961 — The group moved to Surabaya under the name of Srimulat Review.

1968 — Srimulat passed away. Teguh took over and retained the name Srimulat.

1970s — The group enjoyed great popularity.

1977 — Teguh and second wife, Djudjuk Djuwariah, moved to Surakarta.

1978 — Aneka Ria Srimulat was formed at the Bale Kambang Amusement Park.

1981 — Srimulat Solo flourished and the Srimulat Jakarta was established at the Taman Ria Remaja Senayan park. Another branch was established in Semarang.

1987 — Srimulat Jakarta reached the apex of its success. Decline was accelerated by the deaths of three senior clown artists.

1989 — Srimulat Jakarta and Srimulat Semarang closed down. Srimulat Surabaya, led by Djudjuk's brother, Bambang Tedjo, suffered a drop in audience numbers.

mid-1994 — Teguh and Djudjuk established travelling theatre groups in Kediri and other regency capitals.

LONGSER AND *UBRUG*

Two of the better-known folk theatres of West Java are the *longser* and *ubrug*. The *longser* is often considered older and more indigenous in character than the *ubrug*. The theme of the *longser* expresses the dreams, hopes and fears of the villagers and the urban poor. The *longser* was originally an outdoor theatre. It was usually performed in an arena in the middle of which stood the *oncor* (a coconut-oil lamp fixed to the top of a bamboo pole).

The *ubrug* contains more foreign elements than the *longser*. There are four categories of stories: the *babad*, the sheik, the *wayang* and the folk story or romance. The *babad* is a mix of literature and history; the sheik stories are based on Middle Eastern sources; the *wayang* derives sources from the Mahabharata and Ramayana; and the folk stories deal with daily life. The *ubrug* is melodramatic and relies on caricature. Though the *ubrug* is more suited to a formal theatrical stage with backdrop, it can be performed in an open field or arena.

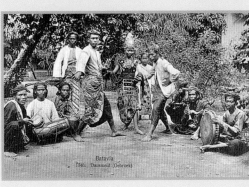

Drama Gong

Drama gong, the vernacular theatre of Bali, is essentially spoken drama accompanied by gamelan gong orchestra. Drawing its performance elements and techniques from traditional Balinese performing arts and modern (Western) drama, drama gong is one of the very few newly created performing art forms by modern Balinese artists which are warmly welcomed by the local community members. In this regard, drama gong has become one of the best models of art innovation in Bali utilising art elements of traditional and modern cultures.

(Above) A manuscript drawing of the character, Turas, in the Balinese arja *dance-drama.*

»»A portrait of a Balinese arja *dancer playing the role of Praba. Painting by Rudolf Bonnet.*

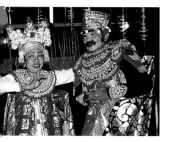

*(Above) The refined prince (*putra manis*) and one of his two servants (*penasar manis kelihan*).*

A Form of Popular Theatre

Drama gong is produced as communal effort by using all artistic materials and talents of the populace, and its activities rely very much on the public support. More importantly its plays speak to all members of the community instead of selected audience members. Drama gong shares these unique features with Javanese ketoprak.

Among major Balinese popular theatres, drama gong is the youngest. Although some productions of modern drama sandiwara accompanied by gamelan gong have taken place around the early 1960s, drama gong appeared for the first time in 1966. The creator of this new dramatic form was Anak Agung Gede Raka Payadnya, an actor-dancer of Abianbase village of Gianyar who is an artist from the Konservatori Karawitan Indonesia (KOKAR) (Conservatory of Indonesian Traditional Music). Mr Payadnya created this new theatrical form by combining performance elements and techniques of various forms of traditional Balinese performing arts including gong kebyar, modern Balinese sendratari, and arja drama, with that of modern drama (sandiwara).

The most important influences of Balinese traditional performing arts nurtured in drama gong include the domination of gamelan music, the prominent use of the vernacular Balinese language, and the presence of stock-characters who are usually stereotyped as refined (alus or manis) and coarse (keras or buduh). Some influences of Western drama can be seen from the use of proscenium stage with static decor, painted scenery, modern lighting, and realistic acting throughout the play.

(Left) The prince and princess in the arja. *In recent decades principal roles, especially the romantic ones, are taken over by female artists. Comical roles are still performed by men.*

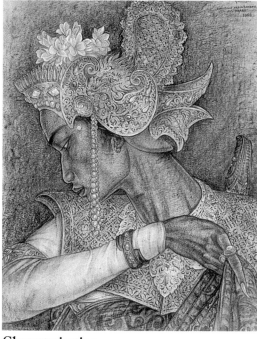

Characterisation

There are normally about 12 leading actors featured in drama gong play. These include a king (raja) and his queen (permaisuri), with two ministers (patih) of different character (wise and greedy). The favourite roles are the refined princess (putri manis) with her servant (dayang), the refined prince (putra manis) with a pair of male servants (penasar), the coarse prince (putra keras) with his two buffoons, and the ugly princess (putri buduh). Farmers (dukuh) are also important personalities in the play. The appearance of these roles in the play follow no fixed orders as the structure of drama gong performance is very much determined by the story line of the play. Sometimes the play begins with the appearance of the king and his wise ministers, many plays start with the appearance of the refined princess with her loyal servant, and in most drama gong performances, the male servants of the refined prince begin the play.

Stories

Drama gong plays are primarily derived from Panji stories or Malat. Well-known Balinese legends including 'Jayaprana', Chinese love story 'Sampik Ingtai', and some stories from the Mahabharata, are also commonly performed in the drama gong. Like most Balinese theatrical forms, the central theme of drama gong plays (lakon) is the struggle between good and evil, and at the end the good usually overcomes the evil. The plays, which are tragi-comedic in nature, contain moral teaching and other messages in addition to the romantic and endless comical scenes. It is important to note that all stories were originally told in the national language, Bahasa Indonesia, but now the entire drama gong play uses the Balinese language.

The structure of drama gong, as one presently sees it in Bali, follows that of the arja dance-drama; however it is informal, rather flexible or adaptive to change. There are normally four main scenes in the drama gong plays which feature the king and his queen, the refined prince or princess, the coarse prince, and the farmers. The appearances of characters depend on the improvisation of the actors themselves since there is no play script. *Drama gong* actors can freely improvise on their acting and dialogue.

Apart from dialogue, singing is also used to create the mood and atmosphere of a particular scene. The *tembang semarandhana* is, for instance, sung by ladies in sad situations while the men sing the *tembang sinom wug payangan*.

Rise and Fall

Shortly after its creation, *drama gong* became one of the most popular performing art forms on the island. In fact, around the mid-1970s, during the peak of its popularity, nearly every village in Bali had a *drama gong* group. There was almost no big *odalan* ceremony on the island without at least one *drama gong* performance, and every Saturday night there were about five *drama gong* performances in different locations around Denpasar city. It was during these years *arja* dance-drama lost its importance as their public turned away and embraced *drama gong*.

Now the popularity of *drama gong* is declining. There are no more than three active groups on the island at present, and *drama gong* performance is not easy to find. Despite these facts, *drama gong* performances continue to draw the largest crowd. During the Annual Bali Art Festival, for instance, between 6,000 to 7,000 people attended the *drama gong* performances at the Ardha Chandra open stage at the Bali Art Centre in Denpasar. In the villages, there are about 500 to 1,000 people attending its performance. While this clearly shows that many people still love this form, it brings hope

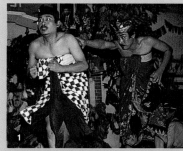
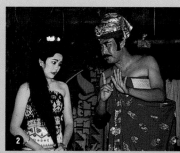
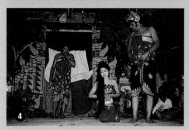
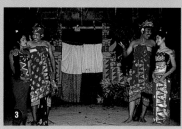

that *drama gong* will continue to survive for many more years to come.

Ritual Aspects

Although the Balinese frequently perform the *drama gong* for various religious ceremonies, it belongs to the secular *balih-balihan* arts. It is staged primarily to entertain the ritual participants, and to add to the festivity of the event. However, like most Balinese performing arts, *drama gong* performances also require offerings (*sesajen*). Simple backstage ritual is usually conducted by a temple priest (*pemangku*) before any one of the performers enter the performance space. This is to consecrate the performance arena and to bless the sets, the actors and the musicians. This ritual practice is also intended to transform all 'raw' materials of the drama into a 'live' art production. The primary aim of this ritual is to attain *taksu*, the spiritual power needed for stage appearances. It is believed that the presence of *taksu* will transform the actor into the character he or she plays, and this condition will enhance the artistic quality of the entire performance.

❶ *The king, performed by A.G.A. Payadnya, pushing one of his servants in a comical scene.*
❷ *The king conversing with the beautiful and amusing princess.*
❸ *The young prince with his lover (the princess's servant) and the king with his lover, a princess.*
❹ *The king is angry with the princess.*

«« *The punakawan characters in the* drama gong *play,* Aji Saka. *This feature was broadcast on Indonesian television on 9 April 1997.*

MUSICAL ACCOMPANIMENT AND PERFORMANCE

The entire *drama gong* performance is accompanied by *gamelan gong kebyar* orchestra. This gamelan ensemble is often used to accompany the *kebyar duduk* dance which was popularised by I Mario after the 1920s (see right). This is a large gamelan orchestra composed of percussion instruments including *gangsa* metal xylophones and gongs of different sizes, drums, cymbals and bamboo flutes. There are between 20 to 25 male musicians in the orchestra playing different instruments to provide non-stop accompaniment for the play. The music is played to indicate changes of scenes and dramatic moods, as well as to illustrate all stage actions. Among the most commonly used musical forms in the performance are the fast two-beat *batel* to accompany fighting scenes, the four-beat *bapang* or the eight-beat *bapang gede*, both in medium tempo, to accompany the entrance of the male servants, the 16-beat *palayon* to signify the entrance of the refined prince and princess, or the slow *legodbawa* to accompany audiences and sad scenes.

In the old days, a *drama gong* performance took all night to complete. Normally it started around 10:00 p.m. and went on until 6:00 a.m. the next morning. Nowadays, a *drama gong* performance

may take between four to five hours, and it usually begins around 9:00 p.m. and ends around 2:00 a.m. The change of this performance duration, as experienced by all major art forms in Bali, is due to modernisation and industrialisation which make the Balinese more time-conscious. As a result, they tend to avoid going to a long performance if they have to work the next morning.

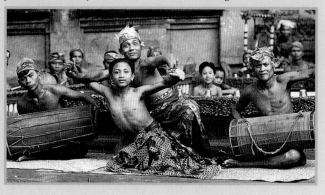

Bangsawan, Mendu and Wayang Gong

Bangsawan, mendu *and* wayang gong *are three genres of traditional theatre which share the same Malay cultural background.* Bangsawan *originated in the Malay culture, and is derived from oral Malay literature which is written in* pantun *(quatrain poetry) style. The* wayang gong *has been influenced by the* bangsawan, *especially in presentation techniques, as well as some visual aspects of performance.*

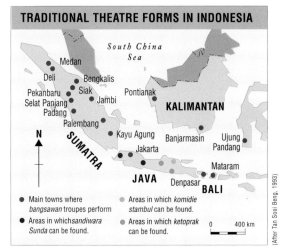

TRADITIONAL THEATRE FORMS IN INDONESIA

South China Sea

Medan
Deli
Pekanbaru • Bengkalis
Selat Panjang • Siak   Pontianak
Padang • Jambi   **KALIMANTAN**
Palembang
N • Kayu Agung   Banjarmasin   Ujung
Jakarta   Pandang
SUMATRA
Mataram
JAVA   Denpasar
BALI

● Main towns where   ● Areas in which *komidie*
  bangsawan troupes perform   *stambul* can be found.
● Areas in which*sandiwara*   ● Areas in which *ketoprak*
  Sunda can be found.   can be found.

0   400 km

(After Tan Sooi Beng, 1993)

Bangsawan and Other Forms of Theatre

Bangsawan is generally found in northern Sumatra, but its strong influence has spread throughout the whole island. In other areas, similar theatre forms developed under various names such as *dulmuluk* (Abdul Muluk), and *indera bangsawan* of South Sumatra, and *dardanella*,

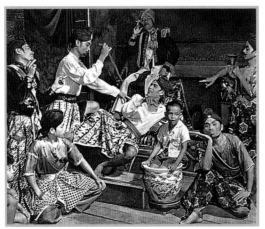

opera/komidi stambul and *komidi bangsawan* on Java. The Sundanese drama form, *sandiwara sunda*, also reflects *bangsawan* influence. The *ketoprak* of Central Java, especially that on the north coast, has evolved in the *bangsawan* style. *Bangsawan* elements are also visible in the *mamanda* or *tanta-yungan* of Kalimantan.

Mendu is found in the Riau area, the source of the old Malay language. For this reason, the cultural background of this theatrical form is old Malay.

Wayang gong originated in Java and has become a part of South Kalimantan cultural tradition and it manifests strong ethnic overtones from this region. It is the local version of the *wayang* theatre.

The sandiwara sunda *was very popular with the West Javanese earlier this century. As in all the folk theatres of Indonesia, only the plot outline was determined before the show; everything else was left up to the actors.*

Bangsawan

Bangsawan is a traditional theatre form generally found on the island of Sumatra, with the Malay culture as its dominant cultural background. It has been known by various names: *komidi bangsawan*, *dardanella*, *opera/komidi stambul*, all of which adopted many Western theatre techniques. This is reflected by its performance style which always uses a stage, even when presented outdoors.

It has been noted that *bangsawan* was first introduced in Malaya around the year 1870, by an all-male theatre group from India. It was called *wayang parsi*, because the stories performed were derived mostly from the Middle East and India. It spread southwards and across the Straits of Melaka into Indonesia. It was given the name *bangsawan*, which means aristocrat, because the stories were originally about a royal family.

The main distinguishing characteristic of the *bangsawan* theatre is the manner of presentation. Dialogue is in four-lined *pantun* verse, because this is the style of oral Malay literature which is the source of the stories. Words are sung by the actors, both dialogue and narrative. Themes are also extracted from Middle Eastern tales, legends and folk stories. They may be presented according to the original, but are often adapted to the local ethnic culture or fused with local folk stories.

The Malayan influence is evident in both the style of dances and the music. Instruments used include the violins, *kendhang* (double-headed drums), *tambur* (single-headed drum), *seruling* (flute), guitars, the clarinet-like *serunai*, and accordion.

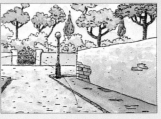
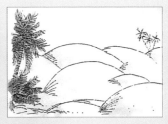
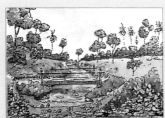
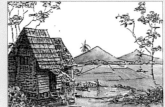
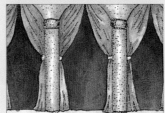

BACKDROPS AND STAGE PROPS

Stage props and backdrops play essential roles in creating a realistic setting for the story portrayed. The modern street scene (*strit*) is used for a story based in the present. An *istana* (*istana tebuk*) is a place for court audience, kampong (*kampung*) represents village scene, landscape (*padang pasir*) is used for depicting desert settings, the forest (*hutan*) is used for hunting scenes, and the garden (*taman*) is used for love scenes.

Other main backdrops include the sea (*laut*), heaven, a cave (*gua batu*), clouds (*awan*), black cloth (*kain hitam*). All these props and backdrops are used in Malaysian *bangsawan*. (After Tan Sooi Beng, 1993)

Music is an inseparable component of the *bangsawan*. Introductory music at the commencement sets the atmosphere for the show as it attracts spectators. Music played during the performance creates the mood of the story, accompanies singing and opens and closes scenes.

A performance always begins with a prelude in the form of song(s) or dance(s). The feature story follows, consisting of many scenes and several acts. An intermezzo of jokes and comedy divides the feature into two parts. For a finale, all the actors return to the stage to sing and perform the audience's favourite songs. *Bangsawan* is sometimes referred to as a Stambul comedy (*komidi stambul* (Istanbul)), because of the emphasis on humour. Most traditional Asian theatres do not separate 'comedy' from 'tragedy'. Regardless of whether the story is serious or funny, the humour comes out strongest; the actors cry and laugh at the same time. Joking clowns are an important part and they are given roles as servants or retainers.

Costumes are always shiny and sparkling, like those of the *1001 Nights*. The idea is to give the impression of a Middle Eastern kingdom, no matter how simple the equipment and props may be. *Bangsawan* is an example of traditional theatre that has been influenced by Western techniques in its performance. It uses a stage, complete with backdrop painted to suggest the setting.

Bangsawan elements are also very evident in the mamanda *theatre of South Kalimantan. Stories are entertaining and simple. Each performance begins with a dance and song. Costumes are based on local traditional fashion adorned with accessories such as epaulettes that vibrate as the male main characters move.*

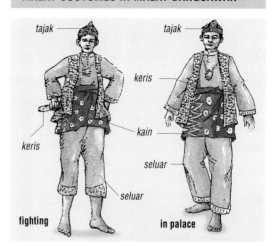

MALAY COSTUMES IN MALAY *BANGSAWAN*

tajak

keris

keris

seluar

fighting

tajak

keris

kain

seluar

in palace

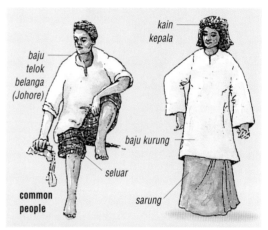

baju telok belanga (Johore)

seluar

common people

kain kepala

baju kurung

sarung

JAVANESE COSTUMES IN MALAY *BANGSAWAN*

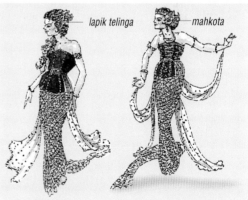
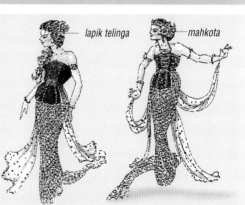

lapik telinga

mahkota

Bangsawan is influenced by the Western theatre and film as it seeks to enact fictional reality. This is achieved through measures which include lavishly made costumes representing the rich and wealthy in the ancient Malay world which are contrasted with the simple costumes worn by ordinary folk such as people living in kampongs.

Sources for stories are also found in other historical periods and areas such as old Javanese stories from the *wayang* repertoire including *Panji Semirang* (right).

***orang muda* (hero)**

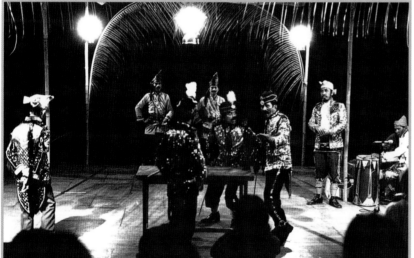

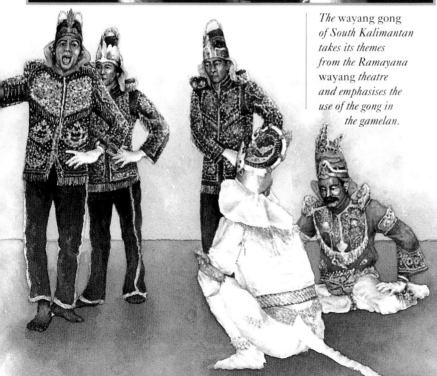

The wayang gong *of South Kalimantan takes its themes from the Ramayana* wayang *theatre and emphasises the use of the gong in the gamelan.*

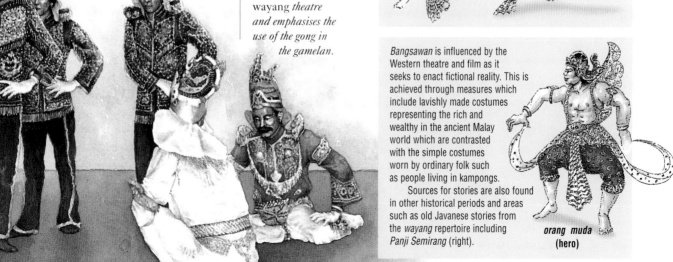

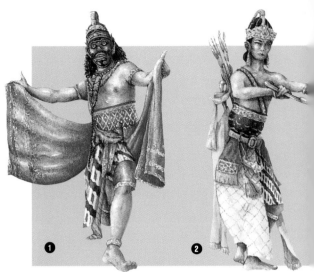

① ②

Forms of Traditional Theatre in Central Java

*T*he Javanese theatre is characterised by dance-drama which has experienced a history of court patronage. In many ways court dance-drama seems to be a theatre based on an amalgamation of stories adapted from the shadow play and dance movements from court dances such as the serimpi and bedhaya.

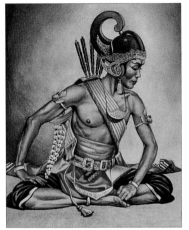

(Top) A member of a Javanese court military unit, bugisan, *performing a dance from the* langendriyan. *(Above) A* wayang wong *character,* Laksmana, *with the characteristic headdress taken from the* wayang wong *theatrical genre.*

(Below) Some basic dance movements in the wayang wong *performance.*

Wayang Wong

Wayang wong literally means human *wayang. Wong* is the Javanese word for person or human being. *Wayang* means puppet or a dramatic performance which uses either puppets or human beings as actors. Although some scholars believe that *wayang wong* was in existence as early as the 12th century in East Java, the invention of today's *wayang wong* is traditionally ascribed to either Sultan Hamengkubuwana I (1755-1792) of Yogyakarta or Mangkunagara I (1757-1795) of Surakarta, in Central Java. Both the Yogyakarta and Mangkunagara courts considered *wayang wong* not just a form of royal entertainment but also an adjunct to state rituals such as weddings, circumcisions and the welcoming of state guests.

Many performance conventions in *wayang wong* are borrowed from the *wayang kulit* (shadow puppet theatre). The *wayang wong* is based on the Javanese versions of two Indian epics, the Ramayana and the Mahabharata. A *wayang wong* performance is divided into three sections defined by the modal designations of the gamelan music: *pathet nem, pathet sanga* and *pathet manyura* if a five-tone *slendro* scale gamelan is used; or *pathet lima, pathet nem* and *pathet barang* if a seven-tone *pelog* scale is used. *Wayang wong* make-up, costumes and characterisation are also drawn from shadow-play conventions.

History

Wayang wong has become highly developed and standardised in the courts of both Surakarta and Yogyakarta. Court *wayang wong* reached its peak in the first half of the 20th century. In Yogyakarta, Hamengkubuwana VIII (1921-1939) produced 11 full-scale *wayang wong* performances. Some employed 300 to 400 male dancers and took three to four days (6:00 a.m. to 11:00 p.m.) to complete. In Surakarta, the popular *wayang wong panggung* was created by order of Susuhunan Pakubuwana X (1893-1939) for nightly performance at the Sri Wedari recreational park. This kind of *wayang wong*, performed on an elevated stage complete with curtains and props, is still found in some Javanese cities.

Golek Menak

Hamengkubuwana IX (1940-1988) inspired a major development of *wayang wong*: the *golek menak* dance-drama. The *golek menak* takes its themes from the Menak stories which are an adaptation of Persian tales found in many parts of Southeast Asia.

Wayang wong *performances are increasingly held in public theatres for the pleasure of tourists and Indonesians alike today. The backdrop usually represents the interior of a palace or the royal garden.*

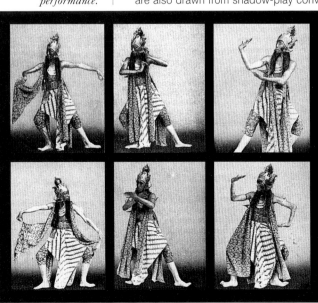

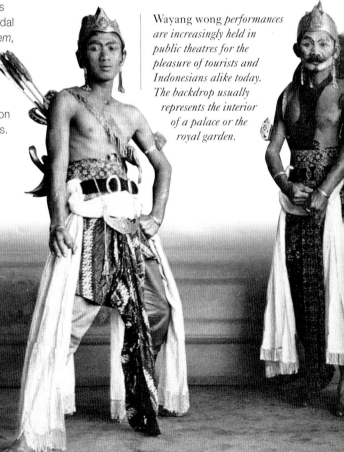

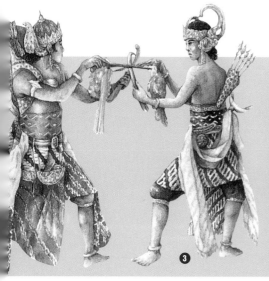

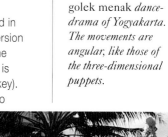

DANCE STANCES IN THE *WAYANG WONG*

❶ *Pondhongan* ('the carrying of a woman by a man'): the pose is representative of a desire to embrace a woman and carry her away. The arms are extended forward to the sides and the body is inclined forward with the arms and the gaze projected forward. The character depicted here is Klana.

❷ *Nylekenthung* ('to turn the hands inward'): the arms are held in front of the stomach, at a distance of about two handspans from the body. The elbow is flexed and palms of the hand turned outward, so the back of the hands are facing each other.

❸ *Nyuduk nangkis* ('to thrust and parry'): represents a battle in which each character attempts to stab the other. The character on the right is Arjuna; and Karna is on the left.

Rengganis from the golek menak *dance-drama of Yogyakarta. The movements are angular, like those of the three-dimensional puppets.*

Many performance conventions in *golek menak* were developed from the *wayang golek,* a puppet theatre popular in the rural areas of Yogyakarta that uses three-dimensional rod-puppets and enacts Menak stories. *Golek menak* dancers imitate the movements of the rod-puppets in great detail, such as the stylised 'breathing' of the puppets.

In 1990, as part of the 1990-1991 Festival of Indonesia in the USA, *wayang wong* and *golek menak* of the royal courts of Yogyakarta were major performances.

Langendriyan

Another important Javanese dramatic form is the *langendriyan*. This operatic dance-drama was created during the second half of the 18th century in both Surakarta and Yogyakarta. Raden Mas Haria Tandakusuma, son-in-law of Prince Mangkunagara IV (1853-1881), created the Surakarta version, while Raden Tumenggung Purwadiningrat and Prince Mangkubumi created the Yogyakarta version in 1876.

Langendriyan uses the story of *Damarwulan*, an historical romance about the struggle of Queen Ratu Ayu Kencanawungu of Majapahit in East Java to suppress the rebellion led by Menakjingga,

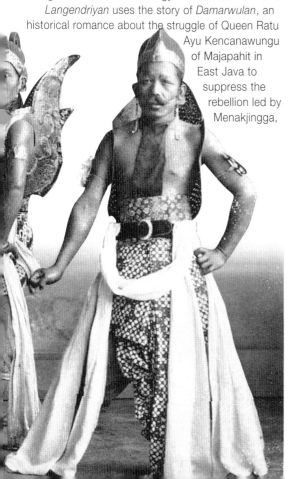

regent of Blambangan. As with other Javanese dramas, the *langendriyan* is accompanied by a gamelan orchestra, but the dialogue is rendered in Javanese singing, *tembang*. The Yogyakarta version takes the Ramayana stories, and because of the many characters within them, the performance is called *langren-mandra-wanara* (*wanara* = monkey). It used to be performed by an all-male cast who danced in the squatting position. In the 1970s and 1980s, Javanese choreographers Sardono W. Kusumo, Retno Maruti and Sal Murgiyanto combined the *langendriyan, wayang wong* and *bedhaya* dance to create another dramatic form called *langenbeksa*. Some episodes of *golek menak* were also reinterpreted.

Sendratari

In 1961, Gusti Pangeran Haria Djatikusuma, son of Susuhunan Pakubuwana X who was in charge of tourism within the Indonesian government, together with Dr Soeharso led a team in the planning of a huge open theatre to be built in front of the Lara Jonggrang temple in Central Java. A special government committee assigned a group of performing artists from Yogyakarta and Surakarta to create the dance genre which was later named *sendratari* (*seni* [art], drama and *tari* [dance]). Initially, he called the newly created dance-drama a ballet.

Well-known traditional performing artists involved in the creation of the *sendratari* were choreographer Raden Tumenggung Kusumakesawa, and gamelan player and composer Raden Lurah Martopangrawit from Surakarta; Kanjeng Raden Tumenggung Wasitodipura from Yogyakarta; and the painter-designer Kusnadi.

Initially, the *sendratari* was created as a tourist attraction. More than 150 dancers were recruited from Yogyakarta, Surakarta and Prambanan to perform on the huge amphitheatre stage. Surakarta and Yogyakarta styles of dancing were blended and new movements created to fit the new setting and audience. In Bali, a smaller-scale Balinese version of *sendratari ramayana* was created.

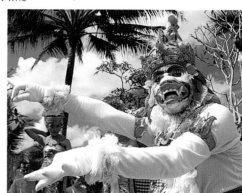

Hanoman, the white monkey, in the sendratari ramayana *in Bali.*

A scene in the wayang wong *theatre in which Petruk appears to be advising a saddened* ksatriya *prince who is also being consoled by a princess.*

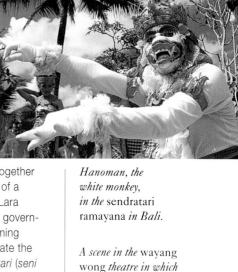

Cak, Barong, Gambuh and Prembon

The Balinese theatrical art is characterised by various genres of dance-drama which have taken their structures from traditional or ritual sources. Whereas the gambuh *presumably derives its roots from the Majapahit era, the others are either modern mixture and assimilation of dance and drama such as the* cak *and* barong *and* calonarang *or a medley composed of different forms such as the* prembon.

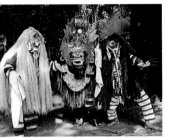

(Above) The barong ket *is a mythological animal, who in the* barong *and* calonarang *play represents good against evil represented by Rangda, the witch.*

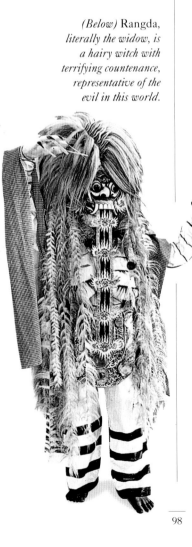

(Below) Rangda, literally the widow, is a hairy witch with terrifying countenance, representative of the evil in this world.

Cak

The *cak* was once an all-male chorus that accompanied the exorcistic *sanghyang* dance, dating back to pre-Hindu times. Its song was a rhythmic repetition of the words *ecak-ecak-ecak*.

The song of the *cak* also included songs of praise and prayers, inviting the spirits to join in the festivities. Their arrival was manifested in the entrancement of the *sanghyang* dancers.

The *cak* today is a distinct performance built around the Ramayana story cycle. It is believed to have evolved in the village of Bedulu in Gianyar in 1935. Arising from the interest of two European artists living in Bedulu, the new *cak* was carried by the rushing current of tourism and transformed into a favourite form of entertainment. A dramatic episode from the Ramayana was included in the new *cak* and in 1969, the single episode was lengthened into a whole epic story.

The *cak* performance is very simple in all respects. The dancers, who can number more than a hundred, sit in a series of concentric circles focused on a torchlamp planted in the centre. They are dressed in calf-length skirt-cloths (*kamben*) with bared chests and three white dots (*wina*) painted on each temple and between the eyebrows. The Ramayana figures, who

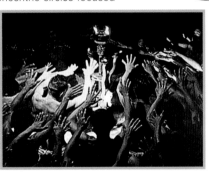

enact the story in the central space nowadays, wear splendid traditional Balinese dress but formerly they wore simple costumes not unlike the chorus. Conversations are spoken in the Kawi language by the Ramayana figures and in Balinese by comic counsellors or *penasar*.

Nature provides the inspiration for movement in the *cak* dance: the flickering flames of fire, the blowing wind, waving palm trees, the rush of waves, animal movements, jumping, and clapping hands. Each motion is emphasised with hissing or shouting *ecak-ecak-ecak* in an endless variety of rhythms bound together in melodic compositions taken from gamelan music. The Ramayana figures, on the other

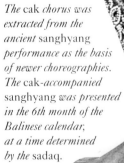

The cak *chorus was extracted from the ancient* sanghyang *performance as the basis of newer choreographies. The* cak-*accompanied* sanghyang *was presented in the 6th month of the Balinese calendar, at a time determined by the* sadaq.

hand, perform stylised movements derived from other dramatic forms.

Barong and Calonarang

The *barong* seems to be the Balinese version of the Chinese lion. It is a 'lion-faced' animal, *barong ket*, depicted through a large mask with a cloth 'body' which conceals the two men who wear the 'mask' to 'bring it to life'. Their legs thus become the legs of the mythical creature.

Calonarang is a classic Balinese dance-drama presenting a semi-historical story, although the name itself is not known in history. A minimal performance presents the characters of Rangda (whose name literally means widow), who represents the black magic of Calonarang; Matah Gede, manifestation of Calonarang before she took up black magic; several *sisya*, students of black magic under the tutelage of Calonarang; Pandung, representing Airlangga's prime minister ordered to dispose of Calonarang; and the *leyak-leyakan*, who represent the black magic worked by the students of Rangda.

The *calonarang* dance-drama came into being some time in the 19th century. It is a composite of existing performing-art forms and has a ritual aspect — a small shrine is placed in one corner of the stage and the stage is consecrated before the performance. A few performers must also possess special protection against the *leyak*, and Pandung must be consecrated beforehand. At the peak of the battle, Pandung really does try to kill Rangda, but is deflected by the magical power of both Rangda's mask and its wearer.

In the 1930s, the *calonarang* drew the attention of Walter Spies who was doing research on Balinese dances and he often arranged performances for tourists. In Ubud where he lived, there was also a *barong* performance that included a demonstration of magical protection in which performers stabbed themselves, but were not hurt. In time, the *barong* performance was assimilated into the *calonarang* dance-drama and the new arrangement became a much-loved form of tourist entertainment.

GAMBUH

Gambuh — archaic, highly stylised, by turns raucous and exquisitely stately — is said to be Bali's oldest surviving ritual theatre, comparable to Noh theatre in Japan, and Kathakali in India. Its music, literature and very specific dance vocabulary are thought to originate from Java of the Majapahit era.

While *gambuh* is said to be the archetype of all Balinese dramatic genres which ensued, it has declined in importance since the beginning of this century, although it is still staged in the temple in celebration of important holy days, or in palaces on other ceremonial occasions. Nowadays a performance generally takes up to three hours and illustrates sequences from the long cycle of tales called the *Malat*, revolving around the heroic mythical prince Panji.

For the Westerner who is used to clearly marked boundaries between dance, drama and certain forms of music, *gambuh* is a novel theatre language and form. The heart of this spectacle is neither a plot unfolding, nor the narration of any drama, but a continuous presentation of dramatis personae, accompanied by attendants who translate the dialogues in the archaic Javanese literary language known as Kawi into Balinese vernacular language.

The characters who make an appearance while dancing are led by the extraordinary music underlined by a chorus of long, bamboo flutes. The *gambuh* gamelan orchestra is an ensemble of a spiked lute called *rebab*, together with drums, gongs, bells and flutes, accompanied by one or more *juru tandak* singers intoning verses in Kawi. (Kunang Helmi)

Prembon

Prembon (composition) refers to a form of dance drama consisting of various elements taken from various Balinese theatrical arts. It was composed in the 1940s by order of the king of Gianyar, I Dewa Mangis VIII, who wanted all the favourite characters of the various theatrical genres brought together in a single presentation. In the *prembon* one will find the clowns from the *topeng*, the dancer-soldier of the *baris*, the princess and her maidservant from the *arja* drama, the strong prime minister from the *gambuh* dance-drama, and the semi-histories of the kings of Bali and excerpts from the Hindu epics.

Performances are presented in the Kawi language (main personalities) and Balinese (clown attendants). Balinese is also used to transmit the content of the Kawi speech to the audience. Music is provided by the *gamelan gong kebyar*.

Prembon is also used now to refer to a revue-style presentation of a mixture of traditional Balinese dances performed within the settings of hotels.

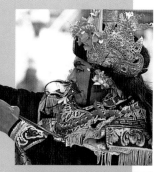
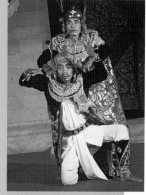
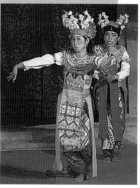

(Above, top to bottom) The gambuh *is staged in the temple to celebrate important holy days and in the palaces at times of marriages, and on other ceremonial occasions. A performance takes one to six hours and continues over several days, during the day. More recently the* gambuh *is performed for tourists.*

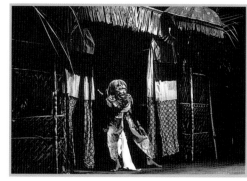

(Left) The combined drama of topeng prembon *includes the old man from the* topeng panca *repertoire. Known as the* Tua *(old man), he is also found in the ritualistic* topeng pajegan.
(Right) The topeng prembon *is usually held on stage and is aimed at foreign tourists.*

Mak Yong and Randai

M ak Yong *and* randai *are two prominent forms of traditional theatre in mainland Sumatra and the Riau Islands.* Mak Yong *is a traditional Malayan theatre style which began in the Malay Peninsula around the 17th century. It arrived in the Riau islands about the 19th century.* Randai *is a traditional West Sumatran narrative dance-drama from the Minangkabau region.*

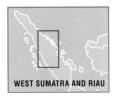

WEST SUMATRA AND RIAU

»»*The garuda-bird holding a papier mâchè chicken in its beak.*

(From top left, clockwise) The late Mak Timah (Fatimah) as Makyong executes the buka tanah *ritual that precedes the* makyong *performance. She is assisted by an apprentice. Makyong performances are still being held although they are not as popular as before.*

Mak Yong

The *mak yong* theatre is believed by some to have been influenced by the Hindu-Buddhist Thai and the Hindu-Javanese culture. The name, *mak yong*, is perhaps a derivation of *Mak Hyang*, another name for *Dewi Sri*, the rice goddess.

Theme

There are a dozen or so original *mak yong* stories. Others are developed from the *menora* theatre of Thailand, the Malayan *wayang kulit* (shadow-play) and *bangsawan* theatre, and the Javanese Panji tales.

The *mak yong* stories relate how a young crown prince struggles to achieve his goals, enduring hard-ship, disaster and suffering with the help of the gods. The essence of the story is the struggle between good and evil, with good emerging triumphant.

The many *mak yong* characters include Pak Yong (king), Pak Yong Muda (young prince), Mak Yong (queen), Puteri Mak Yong (young princess), Ci Awang (elderly male attendant/counsellor), young attendants (servants), Mak Inang (counterpart of Ci Awang), Inang Bongsu (youngest *inang*), Tok Wak, the gods, giants and genies, people from 'the west' or villagers, elements of nature (stars, birds, elephants, snakes), ladies-in-waiting, and *pembatak* (villains). The elderly

male character is a wise person, the king's guard, advisor and attendant. He is portrayed by a man wearing a red mask and in many stories, is also Mak Inang's husband. Tok Wak is the astrologist, or the king's orderly. Generally all roles are played by women, except those requiring masks, which are played by men. In Malaysia, there are no masks and hence, no male performers.

Presentation

The *mak yong* theatre uses songs and dances to convey specific meanings. There are songs for walking, war, love, dialogue preludes, etc. Instruments include a two-stringed lute (*rebab*) in Malaysia and a clarinet-like *sarunai* in Riau, a pair of long double-headed drums, a pair of *tetawak* gongs, a pair of *gedombak* drums, two *talempong* (sets of kettlegongs), one *breng-breng* (flat gong) or a *canang* (hanging gong), and several pairs of bamboo clappers (*ceracap*).

A ritual expert, the leader of the actors opens the performance with the *buka panggung* (open the stage) or *buka tanah* (open the earth) ritual. This ritual is for driving away ghosts or earth goblins who might disturb the show. This is followed by *betabik* (opening songs and dances), the *menghadap rebab* (face the lute) ceremony, and a round dance called *sedayung mak yong*. After a song in walking tempo, the feature begins. The show was previously used to pass on social and religious values and concepts of government administration; today the *mak yong* is played purely for entertainment.

Randai

The *randai* was influenced by early popular forms of theatre such as the local *basijobang*, Dutch *tonil* plays, and especially the *komidi bangsawan*. It is said that in 1932 in the Payakumbuh area of West Sumatra a *komidi bangsawan* group decided to

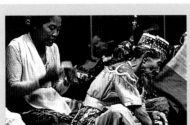
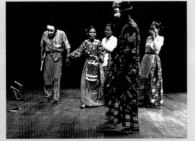
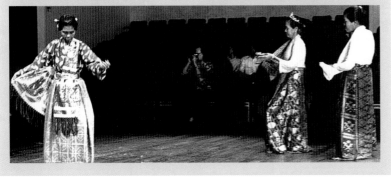

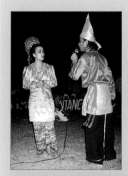
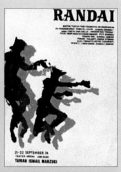

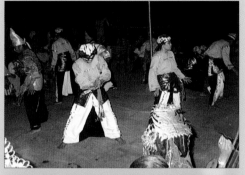

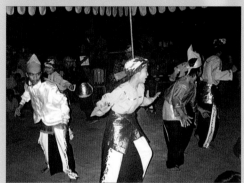

Randai *performances held at Padang Panjang, Sumatra. (Top right) Poster announcing the holding of a* randai *performance at TIM Centre.*

conclusion, as well as during fighting scenes.

The performers stand in a large circle five to eight metres across. Before each scene, they dance in a ring, singing and keeping the rhythm with hand-clapping and leg-slapping. The song serves as a narration, a scene opener, an opening salute and/or a closing item. Dialogues are presented by actors who sit or stand in the middle of the circle; the rest of the players squat on their haunches in a circle around the outer perimeter to define the boundaries of the performance area. When the players dance in a circle, the sound 'hep ta' is heard, which is the signal to begin the next movement of song. The 'hep' sound is uttered simultaneously with hand-clapping and the 'ta' sound with leg-slapping. As these movements are taking place, the words 'hep' and 'ta' are vocalised by the performers.

Randai is a form of folk entertainment performed after harvest, during wedding and other parties. Show-time is in the evening; it can take several days or a week to complete a story.

Costumes consist of black or white low-crotched trousers, black long-sleeved mandarin-collared shirt, fringed and beaded head-cloth, and a large handkerchief wrapped around the waist. The leading man and the *dubalangs* (district chiefs) carry a knife or a *keris* (dagger).

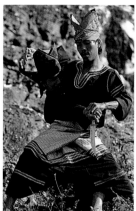
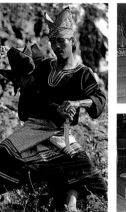

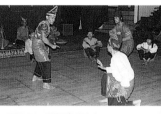

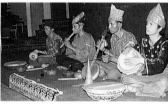

(Above left) Local Minangkabau pencak silat *forms the basic movements in the* randai.
(Above top) Martial arts movements.
(Above) The randai *musical ensemble consists of a lute, flute, small gongs and various drums.*

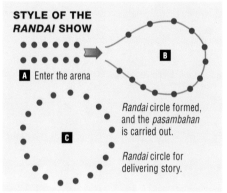

STYLE OF THE RANDAI SHOW

A Enter the arena

B

C

Randai circle formed, and the *pasambahan* is carried out.

Randai circle for delivering story.

Special Characteristics of the *Randai*

Randai has evolved into a conventional stage performance, but it retains certain special folk-play characteristics. These are the circle formation, the martial arts, and the use of the *kaba* stories. Even with the development of new stories outside the *kaba* repertoire, they stay within the framework of dramatised *basijobang* (*sijobang* recital) or *bakaba* (*kaba* recital).

(Below) As the story is being played out, the randai *dancers sit cross-legged in a ring around the performance arena.*

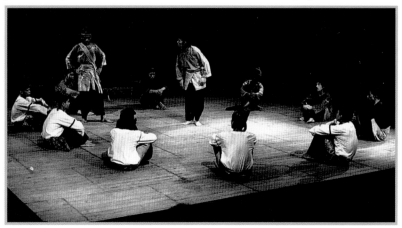

improve the *basijobang* with elements from the Dutch *tonil* play and local *pencak silat* martial arts. The stories were expanded with other *kaba* stories and several new scripts were written. The *randai*, as it was named, quickly became a favourite with the Minangkabau people. Various troupes appeared, taking their names from the stories or the *kaba* characters. *Randai* is freely explained to mean 'having fun while forming a circle'.

Theme
Randai presents historical events, Minangkabau tradition, and lessons passed down from parents to children to prepare them for life. The most interesting part is the eternal wisdom of the traditional advice transmitted to the audience in the dialogue.

Presentation
A *randai* group may have between 14 and 25 players, depending on the story. Once performed outdoors, it is now often presented in a theatre. Basic movements are taken from the *pencak silat*, and executed at the beginning of the play, when making the transition between scenes, and at the

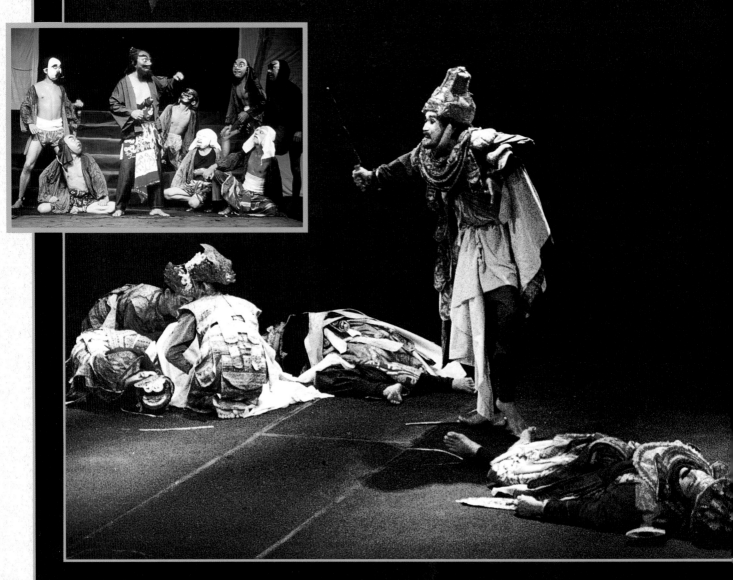
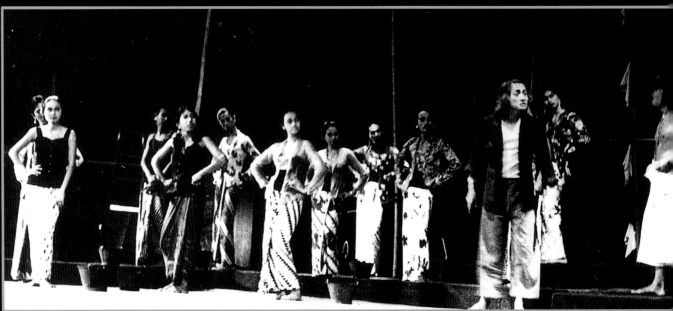

MODERN INDONESIAN THEATRE

Indonesian theatre today is the response of a society challenged by deep and rapid change, and the expression of its experience in coping with that change. Indonesia entered the 20th century and came face to face with three historical facts. First, it was divided into hundreds of ethnic groups, living on thousands of islands; secondly, it was a Dutch colony; and thirdly, there was a growing idea of freedom and the nation-state. These challenges moved the pens of the first Indonesian playwrights and sent actors to the stage.

When Indonesia came under Japanese occupation (1942–1945), the spirit of nationalism that had been expressed in the 'Youth Pledge' of 1928 became more intense and widespread. The turbulence and suffering caused by World War II seemed to enhance the aspiration to freedom and the determination to be free. These three-and-a-half years of occupation were productive in terms of playwriting and performances. In the 1950s, the first decade of national independence, playwrights expressed their reflections on the physical struggle for independence (1945–1949). They depicted the disappointments and frustrations of a nation that had to watch its high hopes clash with the realities of independence. These aspirations, disappointments, frustrations and the fighting spirit were well expressed by both playwrights and theatrical artists.

The flourishing Indonesian theatre has been sustained by traditional and Western sources. Since Indonesian culture itself can be defined as a mixture of traditional ethnic elements and Western ones, Indonesian theatre fuses these elements for its idioms.

Since its birth around 1925, modern Indonesian theatre has produced a kaleidoscope of works by many outstanding artists. Rustam Effendy, Sanusi Pane and Armijn Pane are representative of playwrights evoking the experience of a nation aspiring to independence. Utuy T. Sontany, Usmar Ismail, Emil Sanosa, Kirdjomuljo and Nasjah Djamin are artists who have expressed so well the hopes, the frustrations and that never-dying spirit of a young nation's struggles.

When the nation entered a new epoch, the epoch of industrialisation, the painful but promising process of development was portrayed by such artists as Jim Lim, Teguh Karya, Suyatna Anirun, W.S. Rendra, Arifin C. Noer, Putu Wijaya and N. Riantiarno.

Studiklub Teater Bandung (STB)

The amateur theatre group, Studiklub Teater Bandung (STB — Bandung Theatre Study Club), was founded in Bandung on 13 October 1958 under the leadership of Jim Lim and Suyatna Anirun. Its first manager was actress Srie Kartini, with a staff of three. Members of the group were mostly highschool students and students of the Faculty of Art of the Bandung Institute of Technology.

(Below) The influence of the Sundanese theatre is very strong in most STB performances, especially the longser *theatre, and the* wayang, *and in the use of masks. Masks are employed in many STB performances.*

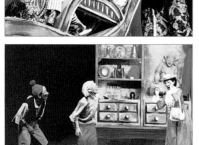

(Above) Karto Loewak (Volpone), *an adaptation of the work by Ben Johnson by director Suyatna Anirun. The play was presented in 1973, 1982 and 1988.*

»Scenes from Shakespeare's King Lear *with the director, Suyatna Anirun, playing the role of Lear. The play was presented by STB in Bandung, Yogyakarta and Jakarta in 1986, 1987 and 1988 respectively.*

The History of STB

Until the fall of the Old Order government in 1965, the Bandung Theatre Study Club annually presented three or four plays, which were mostly American, British or Russian, as well as some by Indonesian authors. Performances were always directed by Jim Lim, who emphasised the theatrical angle, and Suyatna Anirun, who concentrated on the artistic aspects. Suyatna was a student of ITB's Art Faculty. The theatrical passion of these young people was very prominent in Bandung, because it was the only group of its kind. Their theatrical guides were foreign-language theatre books (English, Dutch and French) that members happened to own. Jim Lim's role as a philosopher in the theatre was remarkable, because he mastered all three languages.

The Pioneer Theatre

The STB established a basic acting course in 1962, which developed into an educational academy in the following year. The Film and Theatre Academy, as it was named, was managed by Jim Lim, Enoch Atmadibrata, Srie Kartini and Saini K.M.

In 1966, under the New Order government, Jim Lim established a new theatre group, Teater Perintis (Pioneer Theatre). The emphasis was placed on artistic reformation within the group. Jim Lim's choice of plays was contemporary European drama, such as the works of Eugene Ionesco, F. Durenmatt, Tennessee Williams and Jean Giraudoux. Jim's ideas were broad because he maintained an interest in overseas theatre through subscription to a French theatrical magazine. Teater Perintis closed when he moved to France in 1967. STB was then led by Suyatna Anirun.

Repertoire

In the post-1970 era, plays already presented in the past have been re-staged with a new approach. In all, STB has staged more than

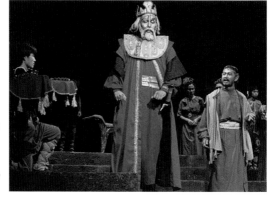

60 dramatic works, including those translated from plays by W. B. Yeats, Anton Chekov, Nikolai Gogol, Robert Anderson, Tennessee Williams, Shakespeare, Eugene Ionesco, F. Durenmatt, Goethe, David Storey, Bertoldt Brecht and Albert Camus.

The STB often collaborates with the Goethe Institute, Alliance Française and the British Council in Bandung, church and other religious organisations, and military personnel. This co-operation is primarily in the form of funding performances and choice of plays. Although STB often presents foreign plays adapted to the Indonesian cultural environment, it also performs original Indonesian plays, especially the works of Saini K.M., Utuy Tatang Sontani, Ajip Rosidi, Kirdjomuljo, Kadarusman Achlil and Motinggo Busje. Altogether, 19 original Indonesian plays have been performed.

Organisation

The original STB, established in 1958 and legalised on 22 May 1959 as an official organisation, has seven board members: Adrin Kahar, Jim Lim, Suyatna Anirun, Sutardjo Wiramihardja, Srie Kartini, Soeharmono Tjitrosoewarno and Thio

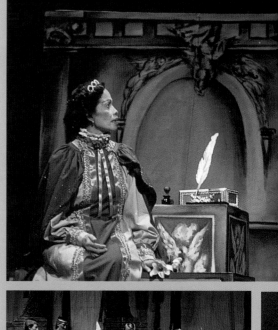

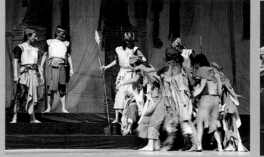

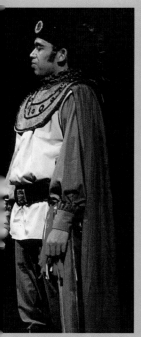

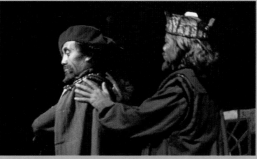

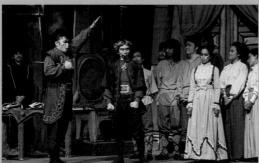

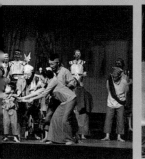

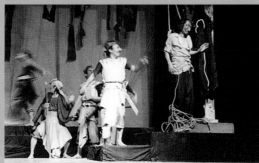

STB is Suyatna Anirun

The name of Suyatna Anirun is inseparable from the history of the Bandung Theatrical Study Club. Up into the 1960s, Suyatna was artistic director and actor. Since the 1970s, his job has been more as director, with artistic matters handled by the younger generation. His ability as an experienced actor was still evident when he played King Lear in 1986.

Besides working as actor and director, Suyatna translates foreign scripts and has written a few plays. It is clear that his participation in STB is multi-faceted. His style, too, has been imprinted on performances since 1967 when he took over from Jim Lim. Suyatna also works as a newspaper editor and teaches acting and directing techniques at the Indonesian Academy for Dance and Theatre in Bandung.

Two or three plays are performed annually, mostly from Western repertoire. STB is the oldest theatre group still actively performing. This is enabled by the determination of Suyatna Anirun and friends to maintain the group's existence.

(Extreme left and near left) Scenes from Friedrich Schiller's Don Carlos *presented by STB under the direction of Suyatna Anirun, in Bandung and Jakarta in 1993.*

(Left, second row) Scene from Yevgeny Schwarz's work, Sang Naga, *directed by Suyatna Anirun, presented in 1988 in Bandung.*

(Left, bottom row, three pictures) A Suyatna Anirun adaptation of Bertoldt Brecht's work, Lingkaran Kapur Putih, *was directed by Suyatna Anirun and presented as a masked drama in 1978 and 1989.*

Tjong Gie (Gigo). The same board members still manage the organisation, except for Jim Lim, and Gigo who has passed away. Suyatna Anirun manages theatrical matters, while the others handle funding and marketing. Performances are sponsored, while rehearsals are mostly covered by the organisation when there is money in the treasury, and the rest is taken care of by the STB members. Profit, if any, is divided amongst performers and the rest deposited in the treasury. STB tries to maintain regular customers by distributing information on performances by post. The audience is mostly artists, lecturers, students and other intellectuals.

With this type of organisation, STB tries to sustain itself, but this demands tremendous sacrifice from members. Only those who really love the theatrical art would be able to endure such pressure. Some help does come from certain committees which continue to provide funding assistance because of the club's good reputation.

STB Performance

The Bandung Theatre Study Club (STB) is known all over the country for its high theatrical quality. Every performance is creative, even when plays are presented several times. As 70 per cent of the scripts are translations of foreign plays, there is always a creative challenge in the process of adaptation: they are always performed with an Indonesian cultural basis. *Romeo dan Julia* (Romeo and Juliet), *Romulus Agung* (Romulus the Great), *Kuda Perang* (War Horse by Heinrich von Kleist) are all presented with backgrounds of ancient Indonesian kingdoms.

The distinctive quality of STB performances is their visual beauty and accuracy, and sometimes a classical imagery in their lighting, blocking of stage space, costumes and settings. The actors' placement in scene arrangements (*mise-en-scène*) can be considered almost perfect in the conventional classical sense. The theatrical approach tends to be realistic and romantic, employing a Stanislavskian acting technique, where actors strive to convey the subtleties of roles using emotion in a natural manner, a style that Suyatna Anirun brings from his 1950s days.

Every STB performance is a 'cultural event', at least to Bandung society, and becomes a topic of discussion in local as well as Jakarta newspapers. Although they have established a unique theatrical style, and are quite well-known, they still receive heavy criticism for being conventional, academic, established and under-developed.

The Studiklub Teater Bandung (STB) performing Shakespeare's Romeo dan Julia *at Taman Ismail Marzuki in 1982.*

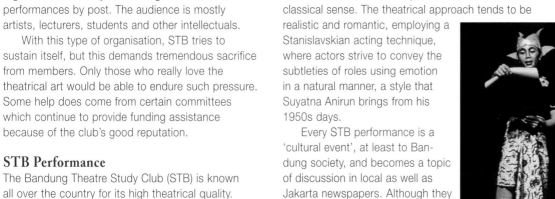

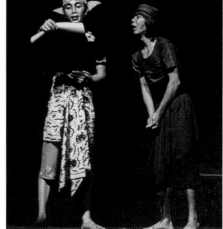

Modern Indonesian Theatre Groups

*I*ndonesia has produced a number of theatre groups which have developed in an environment of rapid social, economic and political change. This change has provided a fertile source of inspiration for the work of the artists from these troupes.

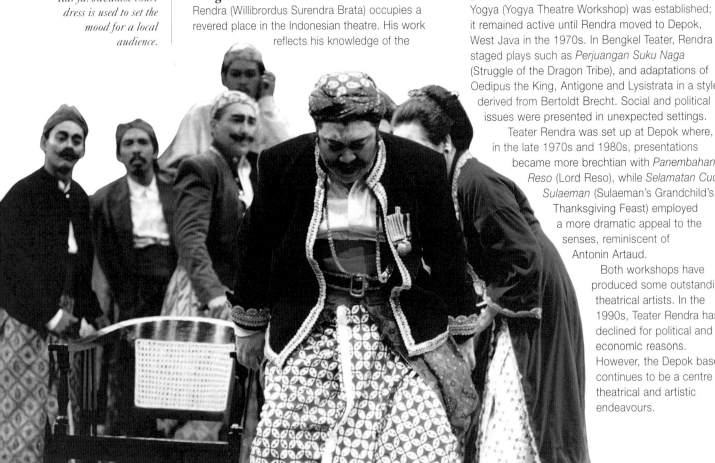

»» Oidipus, a better-known production by Bengkel Teater in which Rendra directed and played the role of the main character in the story. (Top left) Rendra playing the lead role in the production as Oidipus. (Top right) Posters. (Bottom) Oidipus and Iocasta, the two main characters in the play.

Inspektur Jenderal, written by Nikolaj Gogol, a 1993 Teater Populer production directed by Teguh Karya. Javanese court dress is used to set the mood for a local audience.

Teater Populer

Teater Populer (Popular Theatre) was founded by Teguh Karya on the philosophy that 'theatre is a serious art; theatre is a science; theatre is a skill. It needs idealism, the right environment and facilities.' Teguh's study at the National Academy of Theatre (ATNI) in Jakarta contributed to his belief that theatre is a serious science.

After studying abroad, Teguh spent several years (1961-1972) as head of the Art and Culture section of Hotel Indonesia where he established the Teater Populer which performed monthly. The quality of performances attracted a regular audience of 3,000 who paid monthly subscriptions. The group soon began to work apart from the hotel, and its idealism and seriousness established it as a kind of educational force in the field of theatre.

Teguh Karya is the soul of the troupe. He studied under the followers of European idealism and rationalism, and realism becomes the dominant style of Teater Populer. Teguh himself directed 22 performances, including works by Ibsen, Molière, Lorca, Pinter, Tennessee Williams and Bertoldt Brecht.

Bengkel Teater

Rendra (Willibrordus Surendra Brata) occupies a revered place in the Indonesian theatre. His work reflects his knowledge of the oppressiveness of a court culture that he detected in the policies of the New Order regime. To combat this, Rendra formed a counter-culture, *urukan* (disrespect for polite or conventional things). This attracted negative attention from the government and Rendra's performances have been restricted since 1975.

Like other artists of the 1950s and 1960s, his first works were realistic. This conventional realism continued until his return from three years in the USA, when he experimented with Teater Mini Kata (Minimal-Word Theatre). In 1967, Bengkel Teater Yogya (Yogya Theatre Workshop) was established; it remained active until Rendra moved to Depok, West Java in the 1970s. In Bengkel Teater, Rendra staged plays such as *Perjuangan Suku Naga* (Struggle of the Dragon Tribe), and adaptations of Oedipus the King, Antigone and Lysistrata in a style derived from Bertoldt Brecht. Social and political issues were presented in unexpected settings.

Teater Rendra was set up at Depok where, in the late 1970s and 1980s, presentations became more brechtian with *Panembahan Reso* (Lord Reso), while *Selamatan Cucu Sulaeman* (Sulaeman's Grandchild's Thanksgiving Feast) employed a more dramatic appeal to the senses, reminiscent of Antonin Artaud.

Both workshops have produced some outstanding theatrical artists. In the 1990s, Teater Rendra has declined for political and economic reasons. However, the Depok base continues to be a centre of theatrical and artistic endeavours.

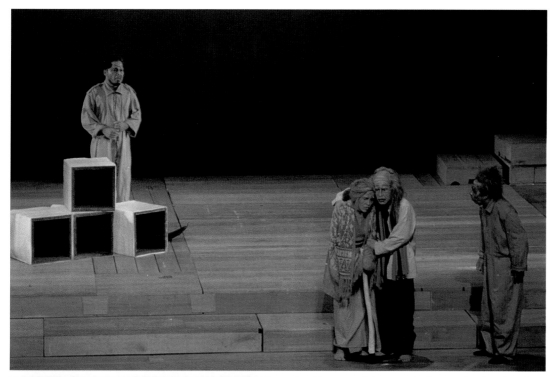

(Top) Performances by Putu Wijaya's Teater Mandiri are meant to be mental torture — to shock, disturb and upset the audience to think about problems and consider solutions.

(Middle) The performance of Konglomerat Buriswara by Teater Koma in 1990.

(Bottom) Ozone by Arifin C. Noer. Arifin turned to his home traditions of the Cirebonese masres folk theatre for his idiom, contorting characters and events to present a viewpoint more effectively. A strong feature of Teater Kecil is its sympathy for the poor and powerless, the victims of development and modernisation.

(Below) The late Arifin C. Noer directing the film Rembulan dalam Baskom (Rembulan in the Washbasin).

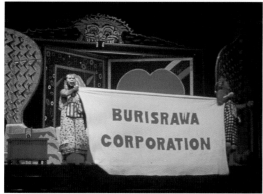

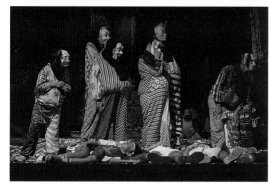

shocking anecdotes, acrobatics, and a drumband, etc. These scenes are presented as spectacles (*tontonan*), full of colour, movement and music which is both dynamic and monotonous.

Teater Kecil

One of the most outstanding troupes in Indonesia is Teater Kecil (Little Theatre). Established as an experimental theatre in 1968, its founder, Arifin C. Noer (1941-1995), attempted to meet the challenges of the post-1965 era by using theatre to expose the truth. He knew that the theatre had been used as a medium for political propaganda, and that language had been distorted to suit the ideological need. That is why the troupe's first plays and performances tended not to rely on words, but on action, music or musicality and visual effects.

FROM THEATRE TO FILM — DOMESTIC FILM PRODUCTION

The domestic movie industry enjoyed a boost of activity during the late 1970s when foreign movies from the USA and other Western countries were restricted. Many theatrical producers such as Arifin C. Noer and Teguh Karya soon ventured into film production to meet the demands of the local film industry. Competition has grown increasingly in the domestic film industry, Asian film market and international film industry. The quality of Indonesian films has also improved as a result. Today Indonesian films are not only shown in numerous countries in the Southeast Asian region but are also entered into prestigious film festivals such as the Asian Film Festivals. In 1997 a big-budget Indonesian film, *Fatahillah*, was released all over Java.

DOMESTIC FILM PRODUCTION

NUMBER OF FILMS (Non-government)

150 / 120 / 90 / 60 / 30 / 0

1945 1950 1955 1960 1965 1970 1975 1980 1985 1990 1994

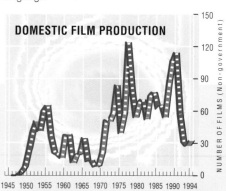

Teater Mandiri

A product of Bengkel Teater Yogya, Putu Wijaya was fascinated by the word *mandiri* which in Indonesian means to be socially independent and responsible. Based on this philosophy, Putu formed the Teater Mandiri (Independent Theatre) in Jakarta in 1977. He also applied the Balinese concept of *desa-kala-patra* (place-time-situation) to his theatre group's creativity and operation.

Putu Wijaya, as a Balinese, has a style reminiscent of traditional Balinese paintings which are characterised by lack of perspective and a plethora of anachronisms. It is no wonder that his theatre is full of bizarre events, broad humour,

Modern Theatre Groups in Yogyakarta

*Y*ogyakarta is a centre of Javanese culture and its theatre has a strong cultural base in the wayang kulit, wayang wong, ketoprak, langendriyan, srandul *and* ketek ogleng. *Modern, Western-style theatre was introduced by intellectuals of Yogyakarta, a university town. Development of modern theatre in Yogya can be traced back to 1936.*

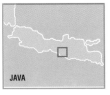

JAVA

»»Poster promoting a performance of the play, Dor, *by Teater Mandiri in 1979.*

(Below and inset) The ketoprak ongklek *is a folk theatre of the Yogyakarta area. It is obviously influenced by the Arabian Nights-type* bangsawan *and* stambul *theatres, and also by the all-male* ludruk *theatre.*

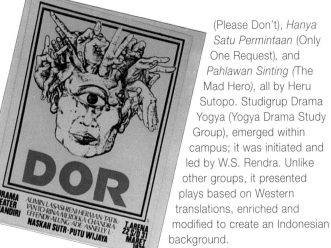

Traditional Influence on Modern Theatre

Despite the appreciation of Western theatre, strong traditional and popular theatre forms have continued to influence the development of modern theatre and they became more pronounced after the national capital was moved to Yogyakarta in 1946. In 1950 the capital was reinstated at Jakarta and most theatre 'notables' moved with the capital. An interested few kept modern theatre alive in Yogyakarta and at the beginning of the 1950s a school of dramatic art was established. It was up-graded in 1954 to the Indonesian Academy for Dramatic Art and Film (ASDRAFI). Graduates include Maroeli Sitompoel, Chaerul Umam, B.M. Hutomo, Ali Shahab, Teguh Karya and Tatiek Malyati.

Early Theatre Groups

Many early theatre groups were established by students and artists. The earliest was Teater Indonesia (Indonesian Theatre) set up in 1955. Its main aim was to foster the appreciation of modern theatre by Yogyakarta audiences. In the same year, Teater Pusara (Graveyard Theatre) was established. It presented a theatre programme on Radio Republik Indonesia (RRI).

Himpunan Komidi Kalang Kabut (Association of Chaotic Comedy) was set up in 1955. Its repertoire included *Janganlah Jangan*

(Please Don't), *Hanya Satu Permintaan* (Only One Request)*, and Pahlawan Sinting (*The Mad Hero)*, all by Heru Sutopo. Studigrup Drama Yogya (Yogya Drama Study Group), emerged within campus; it was initiated and led by W.S. Rendra. Unlike other groups, it presented plays based on Western translations, enriched and modified to create an Indonesian background.

In 1961, Teater Muslim was formed and it staged its own religious scripts. One of its more famous plays was *Iblis* (Devil) by Mohammad Diponegoro. Members included Amak Baldjun and Arifin C. Noer, the latter contributing scripts including *Aminah* and *Telah Pergi Ia, Telah Kembali Ia* (She Has Gone, She Has Returned).

The most outstanding figure of modern theatre in Yogyakarta is W.S. Rendra, with his innovative ideas based on his autodidactic study of the theatre. Two of Rendra's most memorable plays of this time were *Oidipus Sang Raja* (Oedipus the King) and *Paraguai Tercinta* (Beloved Paraguay).

Bengkel Teater and After

Teater Sanggar Bambu (Bamboo Studio Theatre), Teater Antasari (Antasari Theatre) and Teater Sriwijaya (Sriwijaya Theatre) were set up by Rendra's protegés while he was studying in the US. After

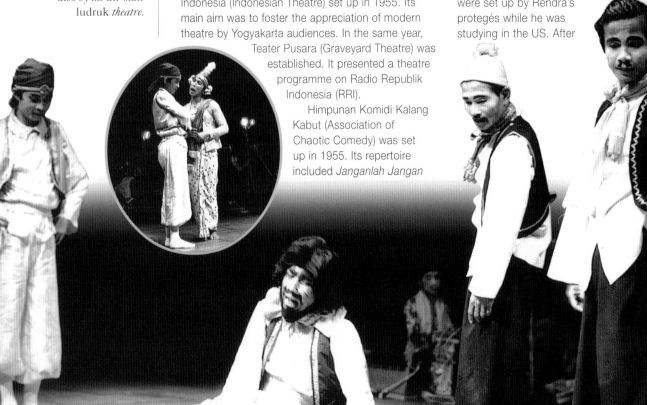

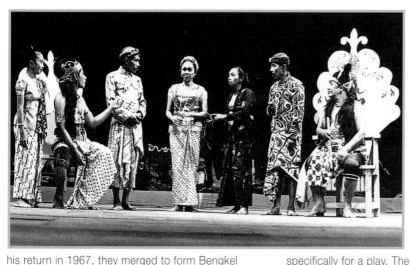

Teater Dinasti and Teater Jeprik

Former Teater Alam members Fajar Suharno, Azwar A.N., Moortri Purnomo and Gadjah Abiyoso formed Teater Dinasti (Dynasty Theatre) in 1978. Teater Jeprik emerged at the same time under the leadership of Noor W.A. These expanded the *sampakan* theatre concept to include some humour and musical accompaniment arranged specifically for a play. The *sampakan* ethic was evident in the presentation of *Jenderal Mas Galak* (Ferocious General) in 1978.

Conventional theatre were also developed in the 1970s. Groups included Teater Stemka, Teater Puskat and Teater Arena which staged plays based on Western dramas.

Teater Gandrik

Another outstanding group, Teater Gandrik (Good Grief! Theatre), was formed in 1983 by Kasiharto to participate in the Festival of Popular Performing Arts (Yogyakarta). They performed *Gambar* (Picture) written by Fajar Suharno and won first prize.

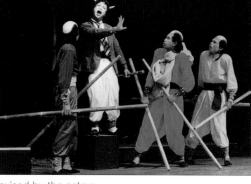

The *sampakan* style reached its ultimate form in Teater Gandrik. The plays are developed and improvised by the actors. Dialogue, music and dance are used to portray current social issues, balancing criticism and humour in an attempt to create an intimacy with the audience. Teater Gandrik uses *plesedan* (double-meaning) and not satire or sarcasm to present issues which are often not resolved at the end of the performance. Teater Gandrik performances included *Pensiunan* (Retirement) and *Dhemit* (Ghost).

Dhemit is a production by Teater Gandrik in Jakarta in 1990. It is written by Heru Kesawa Murti and directed by Jujuk Prabowo.

his return in 1967, they merged to form Bengkel Teater (Theatre Workshop) under Rendra's leadership, assisted by Moortri Purnomo, Azwar A.N. and Bakdi Sumanto. The name 'bengkel' was chosen because the aim was to 'overhaul' Yogyakarta's theatre groups and restore their popularity. Rendra believed that Indonesian theatre was too Western-oriented and wanted to establish his own creative environment with Bengkel Teater. Western scripts were adapted for an Indonesian audience and Rendra's own work, full of current socio-political issues, was also presented. His play, *Bip Bop,* led to the reform of Indonesian theatre aesthetics during the 1970s.

Bengkel Teater performed mostly in Jakarta and theatre activities in Yogyakarta declined. Concerned with this situation, some members began to form their own groups. Teater Alam (Natural Theatre) was set up in 1971 and Teater Mandiri (Independent Theatre) was established by Putu Wijaya.

Teater Alam

Conscious of the lack of funding and small audiences, Teater Alam looked for a 'new' style to suit the atmosphere prevailing in Yogyakarta. Azwar found this in the traditional *srandul* theatre. A small group of five could handle an entire performance, each person fulfilling several functions. An actor, when not on stage, would take over the musical accompaniment, freeing the former player to go on stage or perform some other necessary function.

This system was adopted by Teater Alam in the presentation of *Dunia Terus Berputar* (The World Keeps Turning) in 1972 and was gradually developed as a means of overcoming high costs and maintaining a flexible 'people' approach. In 1974, Teater Alam initiated Teater Arisan (Rotation Theatre) comprising 46 young people's theatre groups. Teater Arisan performed plays in villages on a rotational basis, following the presentation style of Teater Alam, the *sampakan* style. In 1982, Teater Alam Foundation was established to extend theatre activities to film, television and cultural education.

Other theatre groups continued to follow the 'Western realism' model. One was Teater Arena led by Fred Wibowo.

Isyu, a play which was written by Heru Kesawa Murti and directed by Jujuk Prabowo for Teater Gandrik.

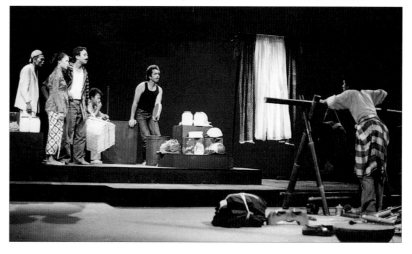

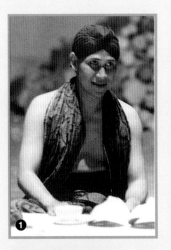

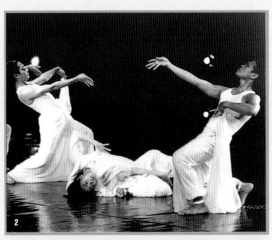

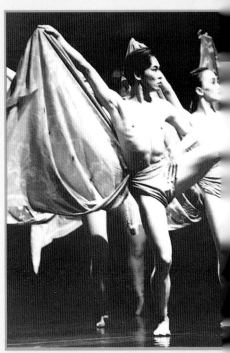

1 *Sulistyo S. Tirtokusumo, a promising young choreographer who is also very much involved in the traditional theatre scene.*

2 Bulan Berkaca, *a dance by Wiwiek Sipala who incorporates a variety of contemporary and ethnic elements in her work.*

3 *Sardono Kusumo draws inspiration from various cultural and ethnic groups in Indonesia*

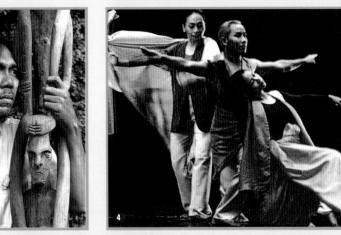

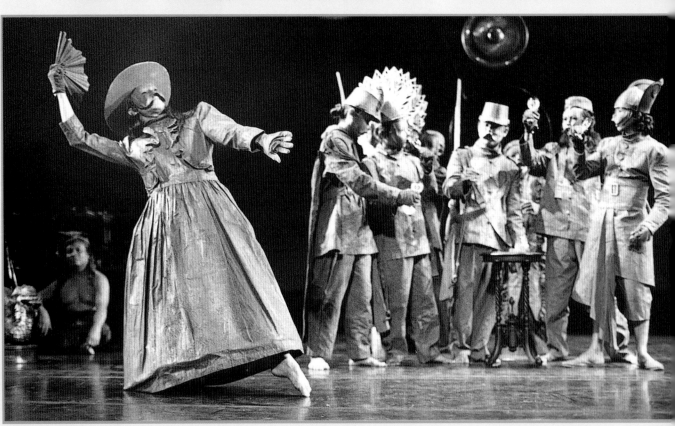

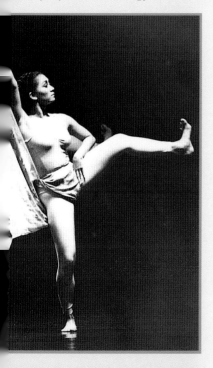

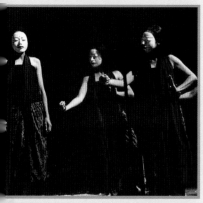

CONTEMPORARY INDONESIAN DANCE

The term 'contemporary dance' has been used to signify dances more recent than 'modern dance'. Modern dance came about as a reaction against the established classical ballet. The exponents of modern dance regarded classical ballet as having reached a stagnant stage of technical development, aside from its themes that always seemed to involve beautiful tales and did not allow a free interpretation of real-life problems.

The modern dance movement itself has been conceived as having three subsequent generations, the first one is concerned with the personal impression as well as style of each choreographer, the second constitutes a generation of choreographers trying to find new foundations in dance techniques, and the third generation consists of choreographers who will always run after new ideas for each of their works.

Many are influenced by the innovations of dance elsewhere in the world, although the majority started out working in a certain traditional dance style. One of these pioneers was Jodjana. Together with other modern choreographers of the same generation, Jodjana created works that were entirely choreographed to realise his personal impression of certain themes.

The echo of the second generation of modern dance, as represented by the Martha Graham studio, was particularly captured by the Indonesian choreographers Wisnoe Wardhana, Bagong Kussudiardja and Seti-Arti Kailola. Seti-Arti presented the concentrated style of Martha Graham, while Bagong and Wisnoe employed some Graham elements but further developed their own ways in rehearsing and composing their works.

Sardono W. Kusumo is a choreographer belonging to a younger generation. He has never looked for a special expressive style or dance technique, but tries to explore new possibilities in each of his works. In the development of new choreographies, we ought to take into account dance works that utilise the treasury of tradition as source. Among these are works by Retno Maruti, Tom Ibnur, Deddy Luthan, Gusmiati Suid, Wiwiek Sipala and Julianti Parani.

This panorama is completed by new dance works based on ballet techniques. These works used ballet as a starting point and often bring out the Indonesian image through the use of certain movements which borrow techniques and inspiration from the dances of the ethnic groups in Indonesia or through their costumes and music.

The Pioneers of Modern Indonesian Dance

*T*he three pioneers of modern Indonesian dance are Seti-Arti Kailola, Bagong Kussudiardja and Wisnoe Wardhana. All spent some time training with the Krida Baksa Wirama (KBW classical Javanese) dance association established by the Sultan of Yogyakarta outside his court wall in 1918.

Semar, a recent production by Bagong. It was Bagong's aim to provide a practical (praktis) dance program combined with the family spirit (kekeluargaan).

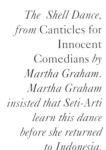

The Shell Dance, from Canticles for Innocent Comedians by Martha Graham. Martha Graham insisted that Seti-Arti learn this dance before she returned to Indonesia.

Seti-Arti Kailola

Born in Selat Panjang, Sumatra, on 7 November 1919, the daughter of a widely travelled physician, Seti-Arti attended school outside Java, including three years in the Netherlands. She returned to Indonesia in 1934. Seti-Arti next studied classical Javanese dance under the guidance of G.P.H. Tedjakusuma at the KBW (Krida Baksa Wirama) studio in Prince Tedjakusuma's Yogyakarta home for two years (1937–1938), then realised that Javanese dance was not what she wanted to do. 'There is no expression of emotion, no way to express yourself in the classical dance of Java,' she said.

Seti-Arti moved back to Jakarta in 1942 and studied what was called in those days 'interpretive dancing' from Ms. Adele Blok de Neve, a dance teacher of Dutch origin. In 1950, she read an article in the *Christian Science Monitor* about Martha Graham, the well-known modern choreographer, and in the following year found herself studying with Ms. Graham in New York for 11 months. Back in Jakarta in 1952, Seti-Arti

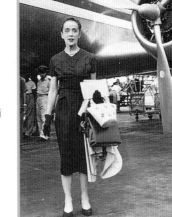

opened a dance school named Sutalagati, meaning 'The Art-of-Movement School'. Boys and (mostly) girls of the Indonesian middle class, wealthy Chinese and children of Euro-American diplomats enrolled in her school. In December 1955, the Martha Graham Dance Company performed in Jakarta, and there was a reunion between Seti-Arti, Ms. Graham and members of her company.

Two years later, with a grant from the Rockefeller Foundation, Seti-Arti went back to study at the Graham School in New York. In fact, two other young Javanese choreographers from Yogyakarta, Bagong Kussudiardja and Wisnoe Wardhana, also received Rockefeller grants to study with Graham for a brief time. It was at the Graham School in New York and the Summer School of Dance in Connecticut College that Seti-Arti met Bagong and Wisnoe.

Returning to Indonesia in 1958, Ms. Kailola continued teaching at Sutalagati Dance School, which had attracted more than 300 students. She taught the Graham technique, but created her own repertoire for her students: *Aku, Rhythm of Life* and *There is No Real Freedom Without Discipline* are some of her creations. *Aku* was a group dance inspired by the poem by

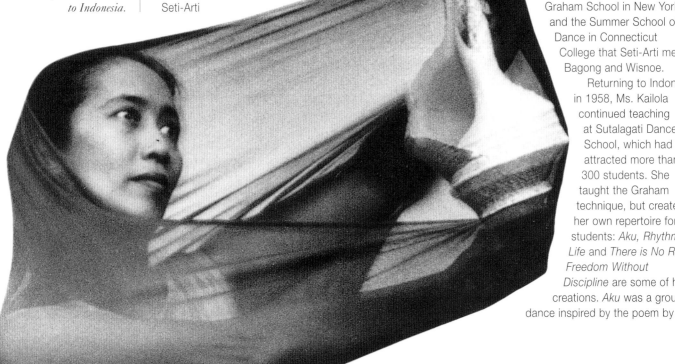

famous Indonesian poet Chairil Anwar. At the end of the piece, Seti-Arti danced a solo with a poetry-reading of *Aku* as background.

Seti-Arti Kailola wanted to instil into her students a respect for strict discipline, but they were not ready for it. Most came to study dance as amateurs, not to become professional dancers. In 1964, following the death of her husband, Seti-Arti closed her school and went to live in New York. Twenty-five years later, she returned to Jakarta. Among hundreds of her former students are Ibu Wuriastuti Soenario, now Executive-Director of the Indonesian Tourist Promotion Board, the late Rahadian Yamin, the late Wim Tomasoa and Pia Alisjahbana. For a short while, Farida Oetoyo and Julianti Parani also studied with Seti-Arti Kailola.

Bagong Kussudiardja and Wisnoe Wardhana

Bagong Kussudiardja and Wisnoe Wardhana trained for years as classical Javanese dancers at the Krida Baksa Wirama studio in Yogyakarta before their short training with Martha Graham. Bagong had even created new dance pieces, such as *Kuda-kuda* (Horse Rider) and *Layang-layang* (Kite Flyer). Bagong's strong creative drive comes partly from his study at ASRI, the Western-oriented Indonesian Academy of Visual Arts in Yogyakarta.

Like Seti-Arti, Bagong also had mixed feelings about his study of classical Javanese dance.

"From the time I started painting in 1946 and during the years of my study at the Indonesian Academy of Visual Arts (ASRI), I found complete freedom in exploring the various processes in the art of painting and in expressing my own mood and spirit without being fed technical norms. Then why, I thought, can't this freedom of expression be applied to the art of dancing?

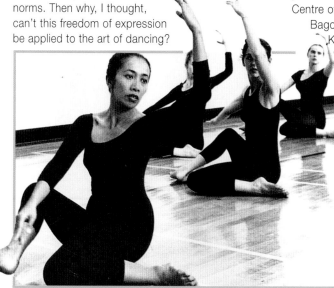

What would be wrong with resisting complacency and further developing cultural themes already in existence?"

Bagong and Wisnoe established their own modern dance schools in Indonesia in 1958: the Bagong Kussudiardja Training Centre for Dance (Pusat Latihan Tari, commonly called PLT Bagong Kussudiardja) and the Wisnoe Wardhana Contemporary Dance School.

Both are known as excellent teachers and

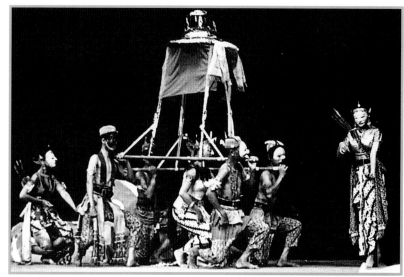

choreographers and have created hundreds of dances and dance-dramas. Later in his career, Wisnoe affiliated himself more closely with teaching and education. He earned a doctoral degree from the Indonesian Institute for Teaching and Education (IKIP) in Yogyakarta, where he continues to teach. He also directs the Wisnoe Wardhana Institute of the Arts, and a non-formal educational forum in art and culture for the general public called Puser Widya Nusantara (Nusantara Centre of Learning).

Bagong founded the Padepokan Seni Bagong Kussudiardja (PSBK) in 1978 in the village of Kembaran, Bantul, on the outskirts of Yogyakarta. The school attracts students from Southeast Asia, Australia, America and Europe, and from all over Indonesia.

After his return from study in the USA, Bagong created works with a Graham influence. *A Bird in the Cage* and *The Sufferer* are examples. The latter piece, resembling Graham's *Lamentation*, was a solo in which the dancer wore a cylindrical piece of cloth that exposed only hands and feet. In his later works, Bagong combined dance and musical elements from three distinctly different areas: Central Java, Bali and Pasundan (West Java). Many pieces have a narrative theme and are accompanied by an expanded gamelan orchestra (*Arjunawiwaha* and *Ratu Kidul*).

The founding of the PSBK brought in many students from throughout Indonesia and other Asian countries with diverse cultural backgrounds. Bagong was inspired to create 'national' works, like *Echo of Nusantara* and *Village Festival*, in which he combined various dance steps and musical elements from different parts of Indonesia, to mirror the cultural wealth of the country.

(Top) Kris Mpu Gandring, *masked-drama choreographed by Wisnoe Wardhana, 1971.*

(Above) The three pioneers in front of the Summer School of Dance, New London.

«*Seti-Arti in class at the Graham School. Seti-Arti's persistent effort to create a new dance form attracted the attention of the late President Soekarno, who once asked her, "Do you want to change traditional Indonesian dances?" "No," she replied, "I want to teach the young people a new movement vocabulary so they will be able to express themselves."*

Sardono W. Kusumo

Sardono W. Kusumo plays an important role in the development of modern Indonesian dance. Well-trained in the classical dance of Java, Sardono spent his early career as one of the main dancers in the Ramayana Prambanan dance-drama at the Prambanan Temple outside Yogyakarta. This group was a new concept set up to present Javanese culture to tourists in a purpose-built theatre. Later, Sardono studied with Jean Erdman, an exponent of American modern dance in New York, in 1965.

Sardono's work 'represents the essence of all things ... stirs our deepest feeling and touches the essential'.

(Right and below) Sardono W. Kusumo gains inspiration from Indonesia's historical remains.

Sardono and His Works

Sardono's work is a modern vehicle of expression which makes creative use of traditional dance elements. Many of his experimental pieces candidly (and sometimes contradictorily) incorporate Indonesia's rich cultural traditions. A New York critic, Deborah Jowitt, remarked that "Sardono's enigmatic, strangely fascinating if structurally unbalanced blend of Indonesian dance-theatre with personal vision and contemporary theatrical devices aligns him more with radical directors like Peter Brook".

Early Works

Sardono began creative work in Jakarta in 1968. At the Taman Ismail Marzuki Arts Centre, he initiated a dance workshop to try out what he had learned in New York: creative movement exploration and improvisation. Interestingly, he did not teach any particular Western/modern dance technique. Instead, he let workshop participants make use of what they already possessed: ballet, Javanese, Balinese, West Sumatran dance techniques.

In his early career, Sardono experimented with various traditional Javanese dance forms. He maintained a narrative theme and what he calls the spirit of Javanese tradition, but trespassed the standardised movement forms of the classical Javanese dance. *Ngrenaswara* (1972) and *Menak Cina* (1976), Javanese dance-dramas he directed for the Jaya

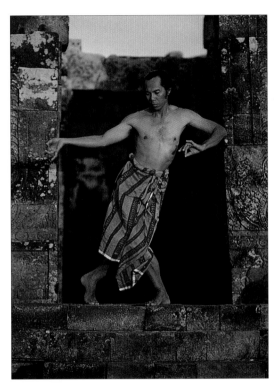

Budaya dance group, are two examples. In these works, Sardono blended refined movements of the *bedhaya* dance (Javanese court dance performed by women), narrative singing of the *langendriyan* drama (in which characters dance and sing), and the Javanese *wayang wong* (theatre with human dancer-actors) dramatic plot. One of his experiments, *Samgita* (1971), went 'too far' for traditional Javanese audiences, however. When it was performed in Sardono's home town of Surakarta, some of the audience threw rotten eggs onto the stage.

Intercultural Workshops

In 1972, Sardono conducted an intercultural workshop in Bali. Bringing along Javanese dancers, he worked with the villagers of Teges, in Ubud, to explore the Balinese *kecak* dance. Teges villagers were delighted with his experiment, but local authorities were upset and banned performances of the piece on religious grounds. As a result, *Cak Tarian Rina* (1973), which was commissioned by the Jakarta Arts Council, failed to appear in the annual Arts Festival at Taman Ismail Marzuki Arts Centre. In 1974, however, following his successful performance at the Nancy Festival in France, Sardono revisited

THREE DECADES OF SARDONO'S WORKS

Traditional Dance Drama:

Sumantri Gugur	(1971)	Kethek Ogleng	(1972)
Rama Bargawa	(1971)	Damarwulan	(1972)
Ngrenaswara	(1972)	Menak Cina	(1976)

Contemporary:

Komposisi Tiga	(1969)	Ten Minutes of Borobudur	(1987)
Melintas Ruang	(1969)	Elisa in Bali	(1988)
Samgita Pancasona I–XII	(1969-1970)	Mahabhuta	(1988)
Cak Tarian Rina	(1972)	Sanctum	(1988)
The Sorceress of Dirah	(1974)	Ramayana-ku	(1990)
Yellow Submarine	(1977)	Passage through the Gong	(1993)
Meta Ecology	(1979)	Detik..., Detik..., Tempo	(1994)
The Plastic Jungle	(1983)	Opera Diponegoro	(1995)
Lamenting Forest	(1987)	Ramayana Prambanan	(1996)

Bali. That year, he brought 33 Balinese and Javanese to perform *The Sorceress of Dirah* (1974), which incorporates Javanese and Balinese theatrical elements of music, dance and shadow play.

Sardono Dance Theatre

Sardono formed the Sardono Dance Theatre in 1973 to present traditional Javanese court dances intermixed with modern theatrical imagery. The dancers' movements are derived from the style of the traditional dance schools.

Environmental Explorations

In the second half of the 1970s, Sardono worked with the Kenyah and Modang, two Dayak sub-groups living in the interior of East Kalimantan. Frequent trips into the tropical rainforest awakened his interest in environmental issues. *Meta Ecology* (1979), *Plastic Jungle* (1983) and *Lamenting Forest* (1987) are products of Sardono's environmental exploration.

Meta Ecology was performed outdoors at the Jakarta Arts Festival in association with a performance by the Alwin Nikolais Dance Company from New York. In this piece, Sardono's dancers performed in mudpools to increase their sensitivity and to enhance the audience's awareness of the basic elements of nature: earth and water. In *Plastic Jungle,* Sardono used transparent plastic tubes as pillars and covered the stage with plastic trash, amongst which Dayak performers danced. His message was that even deep in the Kalimantan rainforest, trees were being replaced by plastic. In *Lamenting Forest*, Sardono let Dayak dancers not only perform in his piece, but also speak directly to the press about their burning forest.

Return to Java

During the late 1980s, Sardono's searching brought him back to his native Javanese spirit. *Mahabhuta* (1988), *Ramayana-ku* (1990) and *Passage through*

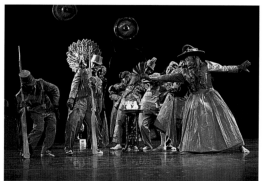

the Gong (1993) are the results. On seeing Sardono's performance at the Brooklyn Academy of Music's Next Wave Festival in 1993, New York critic Marcia B. Siegel wrote, "In Sardono W. Kusumo's meditative theatre-piece, *Passage through the Gong*, Indonesian cultural practice seemed to heal the wounds of modernism". The performance of *Mahabhuta* at Grutli Theatre in Geneva was described by *La Tribune de Genève* as "an endeavour to rediscover, through art, a balanced relationship between Man and Nature, between macro- and micro-cosmos, to revive their unity".

Ramayana-ku (My Ramayana) was composed in 1990 and first performed at the International Dance Festival in New Delhi, India, country of origin of the epic drama, Ramayana. Writing for *The Times of India*, Arshiya Sethi exulted:

"*Ramayana-ku* came as a breath of fresh air. Abandoning overt interpretation and a linear narrative structure, Sardono chose to distil the message and meaning of the epic, leaving vast vistas for individual impressions even in a minimal statement of dance ... In his stream-of-consciousness kind of choreography, he dismembers the familiar, to lay his finger on the essence. And then in the precious drop he shows the mysteries of the cosmos. His is the material great art is made of".

Siegel comments on Sardono's Passage through the Gong: "*...this piece was enthralling, from beginning to end. ...[it] had more than an engrossing theatricality. It showed us how traditional culture can be regenerated, and how it keeps spirituality. It even suggests what we've long forgotten, that art can make a difference in our lives*".

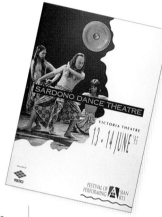

(Above) A brochure on the performance of Sardono Dance Theatre's Passage through the Gong *in Singapore in 1995.*

(Below) Scenes from the same work.

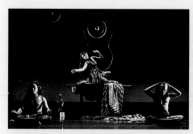

Eko Kadarsih exhibits fluid hand movement in her dance.

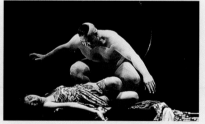

Sony Suharsono alternates between refined and frenetic movements.

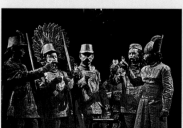

Dancers representing Dutch soldiers reenact a part of Indonesian history.

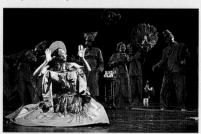

One of Sardono's roles in this performance is a masked woman.

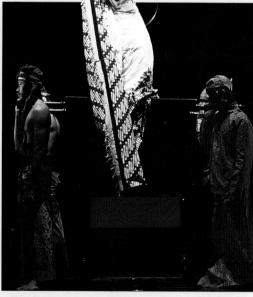

Eko Kadarsih is the embodiment of grace and elegance in her portrayal of Ratu Kidul.

TIM's Intercultural Workshop

*T*he establishment of the Jakarta Arts Centre Taman Ismail Marzuki (TIM) in 1968 provided a fertile ground for intercultural interaction, which stimulated the growth of modern Indonesian dance. Dance artists from different cultural backgrounds, Western ballet and local traditional Indonesian dance forms not only met and exchanged ideas, but also practised different dance techniques and jointly created and performed new works.

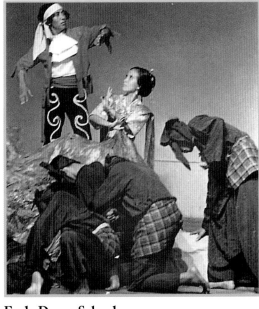

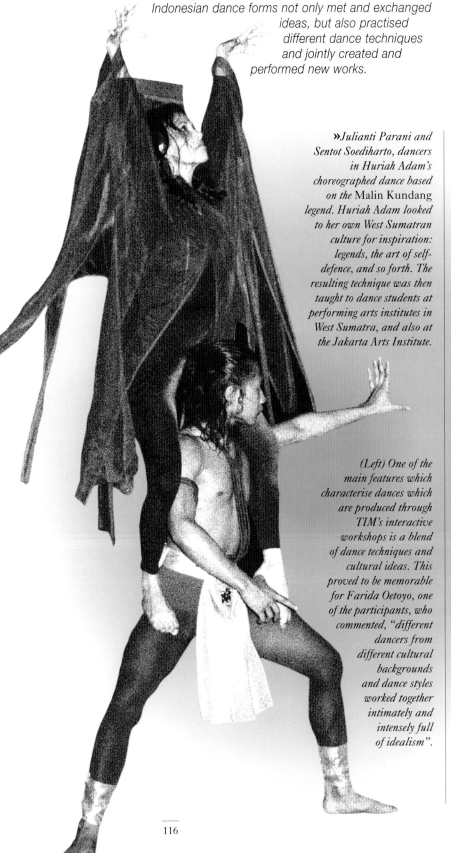

»Julianti Parani and Sentot Soediharto, dancers in Huriah Adam's choreographed dance based on the Malin Kundang *legend. Huriah Adam looked to her own West Sumatran culture for inspiration: legends, the art of self-defence, and so forth. The resulting technique was then taught to dance students at performing arts institutes in West Sumatra, and also at the Jakarta Arts Institute.*

(Left) One of the main features which characterise dances which are produced through TIM's interactive workshops is a blend of dance techniques and cultural ideas. This proved to be memorable for Farida Oetoyo, one of the participants, who commented, "different dancers from different cultural backgrounds and dance styles worked together intimately and intensely full of idealism".

Early Dance Schools

Prior to World War I, there were already ballet activities in Jakarta, but they were limited to Dutch families and wealthy Chinese. In 1945, when Indonesia proclaimed its independence, some ballet schools directed by Dutch dancer-teachers, such as Puck Meyer, Adele Blok de Neve and Fei Webenga, opened their doors to young Indonesians. From Puck Meyer's ballet school, Nani Lubis established Namarina (initially a gymnastics then a ballet school) in 1956 and Elsie Tjiok San Fang founded the Jakarta School of Ballet in 1957. When Ms. Tjiok left Jakarta in 1959, Julianti Parani and Farida Oetoyo took over the school, renaming it Nritya Sundara. Among other pieces, Nani Lubis choreographed *Joko Tarub, Nyi Endit* and *Asmara Dahana*. Early works of Julianti Parani included *Sang Kuriang, Rabanara, Petruk, Kesan Langgar* and *Pertemuan*, while Farida Oetoyo choreographed *Impression*.

Sardono's Intercultural Workshop

In 1968, Sardono W. Kusumo, a Javanese dancer who had just returned from study with Jean Erdman in New York, initiated a dance workshop at TIM Arts Centre. He was joined by Julianti Parani and Farida Oetoyo. They met up with Sentot Sudiharto, a renowned Javanese dancer; Huriah Adam, a Minangkabau dancer-musician-painter; and I Wayan Diya, a Balinese dancer who had just returned from seven years of study in Kalakshetra (Madras) and Ajanta Kalamandalam (Assam) in India.

Sardono led workshop participants in the exploration and improvisation of movement. His process-oriented workshop stimulated intercultural contact amongst dancers from different Indonesian regions. Each represented not only his or her own individual artistic approach, but also a cultural area and values.

Legacy of the Workshop

As a result of this workshop, Huriah Adam established an important foundation for the further development of Minangkabau dance. Based on various local martial arts movements, Huriah created

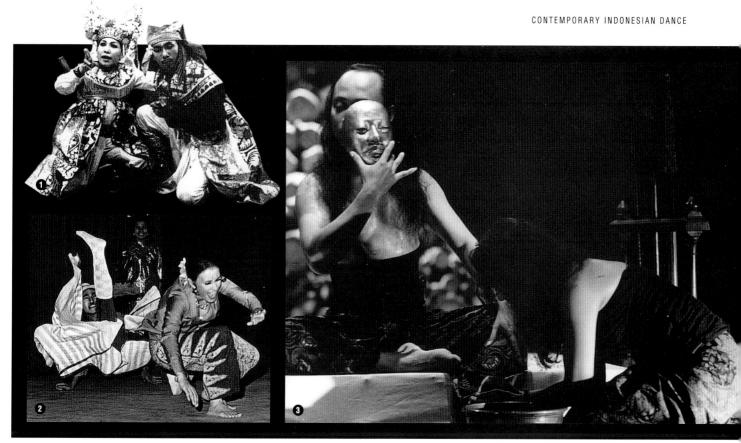

a 'new' Minangkabau dance technique which was then taught to dance students at the Indonesian Academy of Traditional Indonesian Music (ASKI) in Padang Panjang, the Indonesian High School of Traditional Indonesian Music (SMKI) in Padang, and the Jakarta Arts Institute. She choreographed several works such as *Barabah, A Couple of Fires* and *Malinkundang* dance-dramas. Unfortunately, Huriah Adam died in an aeroplane accident in 1971.

The Jakarta Arts Institute was opened in 1970 by the Jakarta Arts Council. Many of TIM's workshop participants became dance teachers at the Institute. Julianti Parani incorporated many local elements from the Betawi Jakarta culture into her later works, *Garong-garong, Bajidoran Angklung,* and many others. Betawi influence can also be seen in Farida Oetoyo's work of the 1970s: *Minang Variations, Rama and Sinta* and *The Explosion of Mount Agung*. In 1976, Farida Oetoyo founded her own ballet school, Sumber Cipta, and continued teaching and creating new dance choreographies.

During the 1970s, the Jakarta public saw many new works created by other choreographers from the Jakarta Arts Institute. In 1973, I Wayan Diya established his *Rasa Dhvani* dance group. Since then, he has choreographed many dance-dramas, including *Jelantik Bogol, I Jaya Prana Diterima* and *Tam-tam.*

Jaya Budaya

The Jaya Budaya dance group was established by the Jakarta Arts Council in 1971. Its purpose was to accommodate members of the disbanded Pancamurti (a Javanese *wayang wong* dance-drama group). Sardono, who was director in the early

1970s, invited the participation of old dance masters and young aspirants from Surakarta and Yogyakarta, the two centres of Javanese culture, and turned Jaya Budaya into a creative workshop. Some promising Javanese choreographers who emerged from the workshop are Sal Murgiyanto, S. Kardjono and Sulistyo Tirtokusumo.

Padneswara and Retno Maruti

In 1976, Retno Maruti established the Padneswara dance group within which she uses the conventions she considers appropriate for today's Javanese women as the basis for her creative process. Maruti believes in gradual change which is consonant with the past and greatly appreciated by many Javanese.

Retno Maruti's work incorporates various performance elements, dance movements, songs and music, which are based on the established Surakarta court convention.

❶ A scene from a production choreographed by I Wayan Diya.
❷ Plesiran-Cokek, choreographed by Julianti Parani inspired by the Betawi culture of Jakarta, and produced by Nritya Sundara.
❸ Panji Sepuh, choreographed by dancer Sulistyo Tirtokusumo.

Sulistyo as Panji in Panji Sepuh *(Panji the Elder).*

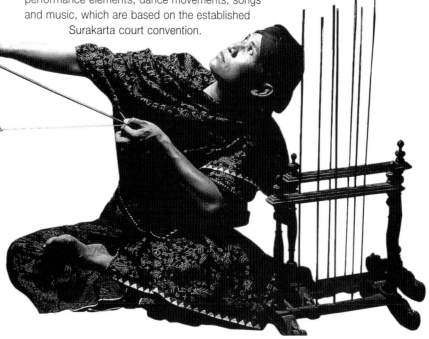

Young Choreographers' Festival

In 1978, the Jakarta Arts Council initiated a dance forum called the Young Choreographers' Festival. Held at the Taman Ismail Marzuki *(TIM)* Arts Centre in Jakarta, the festival was aimed at stimulating creativity amongst young dancers from all over Indonesia and at encouraging the creative flow in modern Indonesian dance. Members of the dance community of the Jakarta Arts Council had noticed that many tertiary dance schools, established by the Indonesian government in the 1960s and 1970s, had already introduced (Western-oriented) choreography courses in their curriculum, but there was no public forum for graduates to show new work.

The First Festival

The first festival was held on 9-11 November 1978 at TIM Arts Centre. Choreographers from five dance academies were commissioned to create new works. However, in a country where tradition has such a strong base, creativity cannot be entirely separated from traditional dance techniques and forms: many of the pieces presented used narrative themes and incorporated local dance and music vocabularies. Eight choreographers from five dance academies presented their works, individually and collaboratively.

In addition to presenting new work, the choreographers were asked to write down their creative process which would be shared and discussed with other choreographers, dancers and observers after the performance of each piece. Nine observers were specifically invited for this purpose: Edi Sedyawati, Sal Murgiyanto, S.D. Humardhani, Sardono W. Kusumo, Soedarsono, Julianti Parani, Farida Oetoyo, Cornelis J. Benny and Singgih Wibisono. Discussion was focused on, but not limited to, the aesthetic aspect of the performances. Exchange of ideas covered a wide range of topics, such as dance creativity, sources of choreography, the training of choreographers, and practical problems faced by the choreographers during their creative process. An earlier endeavour in criteria-setting in choreographic composition, however, was already made in 1972 by the Jakarta Arts Council.

At the end of the first festival, three important statements were issued by the observers. First, young Indonesian artists looked to traditional Indonesian arts as a rich source for creative exploration and development. Secondly, creative exploration was conducted not only in dance movement but also in music and visual arts. Thirdly, there was a strong base for the growth of modern Indonesian dance in the future.

> »*Young choreographers in Indonesia continue to refer to traditional stories and elements for ideas when composing new dances.*

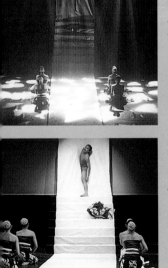

Legacy of the Festival

The Young Choreographers' Festival has made a significant contribution to shaping modern Indonesian dance. Since the second festival in 1979, choreographers with training outside formal dance academies were also invited to participate. From 1978 to 1986, seven festivals were held. The last, in 1986, was titled *Festival Karya Tari* or Festival of [New] Dance Work; 38 new works were presented by more than 40 choreographers from Java, Bali, Sumatra and Sulawesi. The forum culminated in the *Pekan Koreografi Indonesia* (Indonesian Choreographers' Week) which took place on 10-14 June 1987. In addition to the 14 works presented by 17 mature dance choreographers, a choreography competition was organised by the Council which attracted 30 participants.

Many of the country's modern choreographers participated in the Young Choreographers'

THE FUTURE OF YOUNG CHOREOGRAPHERS IN INDONESIA

Today, the 'young' choreographers are mature artists. The creative spirit of the younger choreographers is now making itself felt. In 1991, Sukarji Sriman's composition, *The Circle of Bliss*, based on Javanese dance, was applauded at the American Dance Festival's International Choreographers' Commissioning Program in Durham, North Carolina. Sukarji attended the Greenmill's Dance Project Choreography Workshop in 1992, performed in Tokyo in 1993, and restaged *The Circle of Bliss* for the Tanz '94 International Dance Festival in Vienna.

The ideas which gave birth to the Young Choreographers' Festival are now partly preserved by the Jakarta Arts Institute. In 1992, the Institute opened a creative dance forum called the Indonesian Dance Festival. The new forum differs from the previous one in two ways. First, it presents work by mature artists as well as young choreographers. Secondly, the work of Indonesian choreographers is complemented by the invited presentation of new work by Asian, Australian and American counterparts.

Festival early in their careers. They came from all over Indonesia, from Bali to West Java, Central Java, West Sumatra and many other places, and all had associations with the festival.

The length of a piece presented was set at 40 to 45 minutes; however choreographers were free to select movement styles and musical sources (traditional/non-traditional), as well as individual choreographic approaches. Despite this, many preferred to use traditional dance vocabularies.

International Experience

Some of these choreographers have represented Indonesia in various world forums. Their works have been well received by foreign audiences. In 1990, as part of the Festival of Indonesia in the USA 1990-1991, Endo Suanda directed a Sundanese dance troupe at the Symphony Space in New York. The following year in the same forum, Gusmiati Suid, Nurdin Daud and Marzuki Hasan's performance at Joyce Theater in New York won the prestigious 'Bessies' Performing Arts Award. In 1992, I Wayan Dibia performed at the Taipei International Dance Event with dancers from the Indonesian Academy of Arts, Denpasar. Deddy Luthan participated in the 1994 Triangle Art Program's choreography workshop organised by the Asian Cultural Council in New York. In this workshop, three choreographers from Indonesia, USA and Japan,

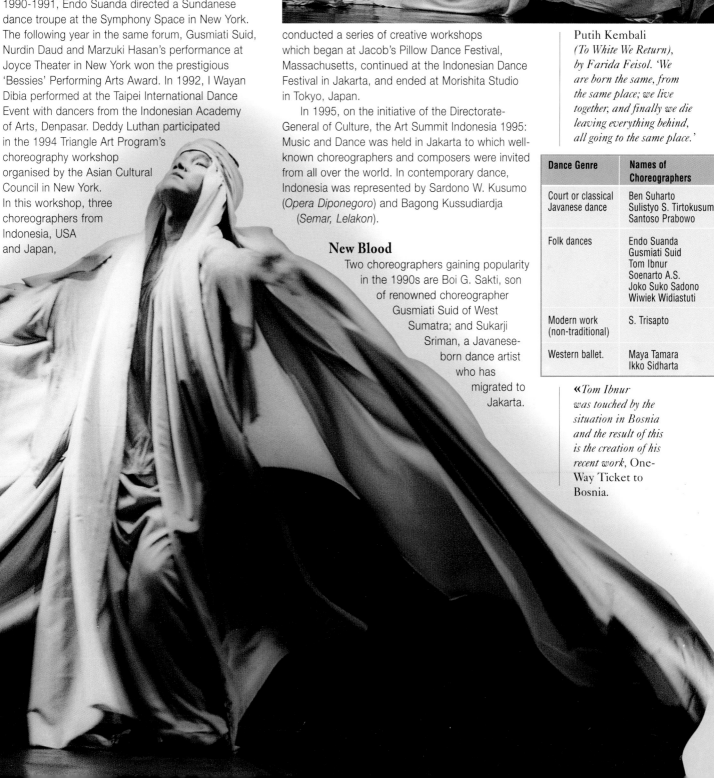

conducted a series of creative workshops which began at Jacob's Pillow Dance Festival, Massachusetts, continued at the Indonesian Dance Festival in Jakarta, and ended at Morishita Studio in Tokyo, Japan.

In 1995, on the initiative of the Directorate-General of Culture, the Art Summit Indonesia 1995: Music and Dance was held in Jakarta to which well-known choreographers and composers were invited from all over the world. In contemporary dance, Indonesia was represented by Sardono W. Kusumo (*Opera Diponegoro*) and Bagong Kussudiardja (*Semar, Lelakon*).

New Blood

Two choreographers gaining popularity in the 1990s are Boi G. Sakti, son of renowned choreographer Gusmiati Suid of West Sumatra; and Sukarji Sriman, a Javanese-born dance artist who has migrated to Jakarta.

Putih Kembali
*(To White We Return),
by Farida Feisol. 'We
are born the same, from
the same place; we live
together, and finally we die
leaving everything behind,
all going to the same place.'*

Dance Genre	Names of Choreographers
Court or classical Javanese dance	Ben Suharto Sulistyo S. Tirtokusumo Santoso Prabowo
Folk dances	Endo Suanda Gusmiati Suid Tom Ibnur Soenarto A.S. Joko Suko Sadono Wiwiek Widiastuti
Modern work (non-traditional)	S. Trisapto
Western ballet.	Maya Tamara Ikko Sidharta

≪*Tom Ibnur
was touched by the
situation in Bosnia
and the result of this
is the creation of his
recent work*, One-Way Ticket to Bosnia.

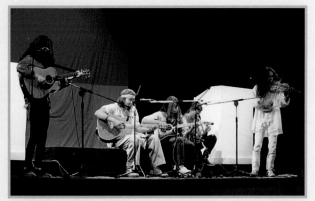

A concert performance by a group known as *Sawung Jabo* at the Taman Ismail Marzuki centre in Jakarta.

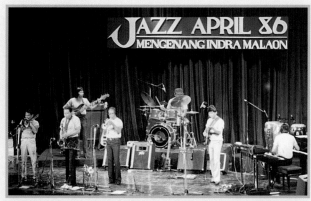

Ireng Maulana, one of Indonesia's top jazz groups, performing at the Jazz April 86 concert in Jakarta.

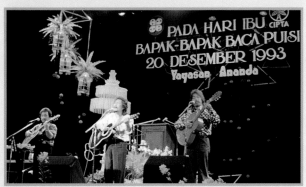

The group, Trio Bimbo, performing at a concert organised by the Yayasan Ananda on 20 December 1993.

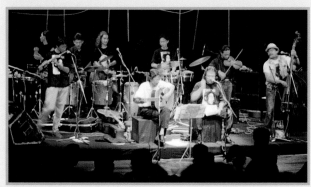

Harry Rusli, a popular Indonesian rock singer, sitting in front of the microphone in a concert held in Jakarta.

PHASES AND FACES OF MODERN MUSIC

The early 1900s were marked by a new enthusiasm. Younger educated Indonesians generated the nationalist movement, which would eventually lead to independence in Indonesia. They began to question the feudalistic system encouraged by colonialism and looked for alternatives in the Western models.

By the end of World War II, Western music moved from the home into public places. Instrumentalists, singers and composers mushroomed amongst the Indonesian community, some gained formidable reputations. Dance music based on jazz, the blues and other popular music became the trend. Nationalists were inspired to express their aspirations and patriotism in music; songs were created for children with lyrics they could relate to.

In the 1960s, Indonesia's first formally educated musician composed Indonesia's first orchestra music using Western instruments. Western classical music is taught throughout the country, and interesting experiments are being made not only with Indonesian themes and the insertion of local instruments but also through the exploration of the fundamental principles of Indonesian music expressed in ways to fulfil the new demands of expression.

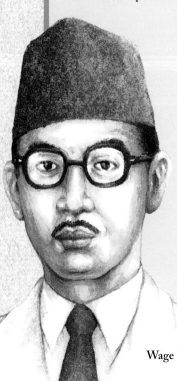

Wage R. Soepratman

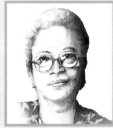

Ibu Soed

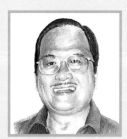

Pranajaya

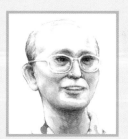

Pak Kasur

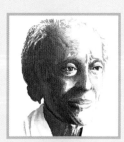

Kusbini

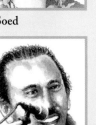

Iwan Fals

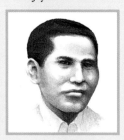

Cornel Simantjuntak

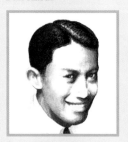

Ismail Marzuki

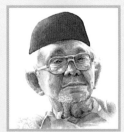

K.R.T. Wasitodiningrat

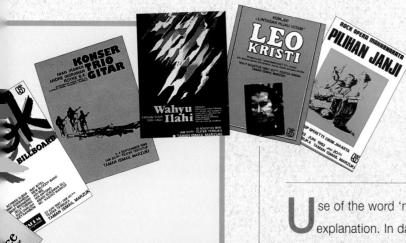

MODERN INDONESIAN MUSIC

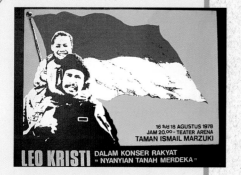

(Top, left to right) A musical show entitled, The Pirates of Penzance, *given by the Jakarta Players.*

A performance by Leo Kristi at Taman Ismail Marzuki's Arena Theatre, 1982.

Concert by three guitarists; Iwan Irawan, Andre Irawan and Royke B.K.

A poster promoting a billboard rock-action music concert at Taman Ismail Marzuki centre on 27 June 1982.

Wahyu Ilahi *(Inspired by God), a performance of poetry-reading to music at the Taman Ismail Marzuki Centre, 1978.*

A Mahabharata rock opera, Choice of Promises, *produced by Grup Operette Cikini Jakarta. The performance was held at the Taman Ismail Marzuki centre on 11-12 June 1982.*

(Above) A concert by Leo Kristi in conjunction with Indonesia's Independence Day celebrations.

Use of the word 'modern' in the context of Indonesian music, requires explanation. In daily Indonesian life, it refers to something entirely new, often antagonistic or opposed to the old or the past. It is often understood as having Western traits or originating from the West.

Then there is 'modern' in relation to the new Indonesia resulting from the rise of Indonesian nationalism early in the 20th century. Indonesians on all levels of this society disclaimed colonialism and fought for independence under the motto of 'one homeland, one nation and one language' as expressed in the Youth Pledge of 1928. This is perceived as the beginning of the awakening of 'modern' Indonesian culture; the proclamation of independence in 1945 is the historical line of demarcation separating the past from the present within the framework of a modern, unified state.

Finally, in the development of Indonesian music, the word 'modern' has no specific connotation. It has nothing to do with any particular movement or -ism. In Indonesia's music world, 'modern' signifies a marked difference from something of the past. Music in Indonesia is deemed to become modern most often because of the introduction of a new factor, a new approach which makes it different from other (past) traditional (original) art forms of Indonesia.

That there is often a misunderstanding of what we mean by 'modern Indonesian music' is not surprising. For instance, gamelan music is categorised as ancient, but is suddenly considered modern when the Western-classical music notation system is used (albeit very simply). At the same time, Western classical music is being perceived as modern music, as are *keroncong*, *dangdut*, *seriosa* and other forms of entertainment music, like jazz pop and rock.

These 'new', 'modern' Indonesian music are almost all the result of a long process of adaptation of foreign musical principles which entered Indonesia centuries ago. The development of 'new' forms took on a new momentum at the beginning of this century. It clearly constituted a new body of Indonesian art which was to become intimate in the second half of the 20th century, after the proclamation of Indonesian independence in 1945. In reality, in the dynamics of Indonesian culture, which is known to be open and adaptive, the development of new (modern) music has always walked hand-in-hand with old (traditional) music in Indonesia.

Music for the Nation: The Composers

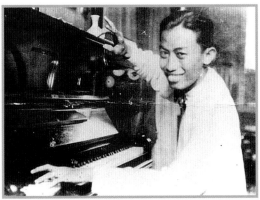

W hen the young journalist Soepratman wrote his song in 1928, his only desire was to dedicate it to the campaign to establish a sense of national unity amongst the youth of the Archipelago. He named it Indonesia Raya (Great(er) Indonesia). It was conceived as a national song, something for which Indonesian nationalist leaders had been waiting for some time.

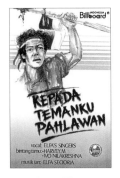

(Above) The cassette cover of a tape containing a number of national songs written by composers such as Ismail Marzuki and Kusbini.

♪ *Ismail Marzuki began to compose music when he was just 17 years old.*

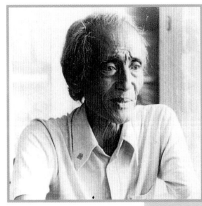

(Above) Kusbini, the buaya keroncong, *and a famous composer of national songs. Most of his compositions are* lagu keroncong

A National Anthem

In 1928, as a part of the same campaign, Indonesia's youth convened in a congress in Jakarta on 28 October where they pledged there was only 'one homeland, one nation, one language: Indonesia(n)'. *Indonesia Raya* was introduced at that same congress. It rapidly gained popularity amongst the younger generation involved in the national movement. Its lyrics, however, were so nationalistic that they were considered to be dangerous by the Dutch colonial authorities and it was soon banned, remaining silent until the years of the Japanese military occupation (1942-1945). In the context of promoting Indonesia as a part of the 'Greater East Asia Co-Prosperity Sphere', the Japanese en-couraged all nationalistic anti-Dutch sentiments. The nationalist leaders, national language, nationalistically inclined artists of all kinds and their nationalistically flavoured works were all put to use, and the strains of *Indonesia Raya* filled the air once again.

Shortly after the proclamation of independence on 17 August 1945, *Indonesia Raya* was unanimously chosen as the national anthem, but by then its composer had passed away (1938) and was unable to witness this proud event.

Wage Rudolf Soepratman

Wage Rudolf Soepratman was born in Purworejo in Central Java in 1903. He was named after the day on which he was born according to the Javanese calendar: Wage. At the age of 11, he went to live in Ujungpandang (South Sulawesi) with his sister, who had married a Dutch officer. To get into the local Dutch high school, he had to adopt a Western name; he took Rudolf, which was his brother-in-law's surname. Rudolf gained some success in school and with the diplomas he earned, was able to begin a career as a freelance journalist in Jakarta.

Other National Songs and their Composers

Music is very popular in Indonesia, in all its forms. The near-empty slate presented by the modern musical world in independent Indonesia inspired hundreds of people to write music, music for the nationalist 'cause', music for children, listening music, marching music, singing music. Some of the better known composers of national songs were Cornel Simandjuntak, Ismail Marzuki and Kusbini.

Cornel Simandjuntak

Cornel Simandjuntak was born into the Christian community of Pematang Siantar, North Sumatra, in 1921. He studied Western music at the Dutch seminary in Muntilan, Central Java, in 1937. With considerable musical skill, he composed an impressive list of songs, some of which were regarded as Indonesia's first art songs, in the 19th-century German *lied* style.

KUSBINI AND *BAGIMU NEGERI*

Kusbini wrote his masterpiece, *Bagimu Negeri*, in 1942. The song expresses the hopes and commitments pledged by young patriots of a nation that was just beginning to form. Though short compared to many other compositions, the simple but honest lyrics express and depict the vibrant spirit of a young nation struggling to attain its freedom from colonialism. Another composition by Kusbini is *Bersatu Padu*.

To you, [our] country, we pledge
To you, [our] country, we devote
To you, [our] country, we dedicate
To you, [our] country, our bodies and souls

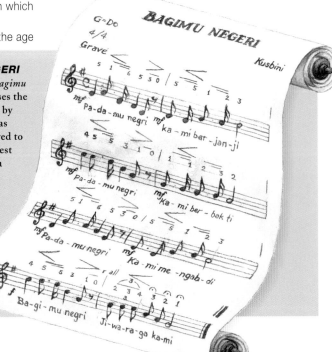

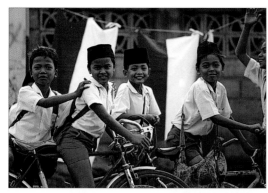

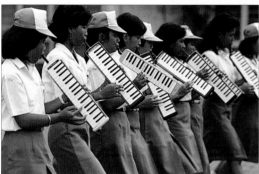

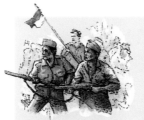

The war for independence, a source of inspiration for composers.

Raden Adjeng Kartini, the proponent for women's rights.

The general, crucial in the fight for independence.

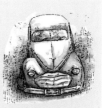

One of the main goals, building the economy.

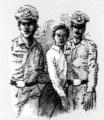

The youth of Indonesia and their education, an important issue.

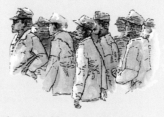

The celebration of National Day with parades and marches.

Pancasila, *the five basic principles of Indonesia.*

(Top) Indonesian school children making their way to school on their bicycles. In the background are several flags hung as part of the Independence Day celebrations. (Above) Schoolgirls marching as they play national songs on their pianicas.

Simandjuntak is best known for the lively *Maju Tak Gentar* (Onward, No Fear), which he wrote during the revolution for independence, which began in 1945. This strongly patriotic composition brought him wide respect. Both melody and lyrics are robust with an heroic power and the flavour of battle. His other works include *Citra, Kupinta Lagi, Mekar Melati, Mari Berdendang* and *O, Angin*. Simandjuntak died in 1946 in Yogyakarta. He was posthumously awarded a cultural medal by the Indonesian government in 1961.

Ismail Marzuki

Perhaps the most productive composer of national songs was Ismail Marzuki, who wrote more than 240 pieces. Born in Jakarta in 1914, Marzuki began to compose at 17 years of age. As a member of the Lief Java (Beloved Java) orchestra, he travelled around Java and to Malaya on concert tours. In 1937, he joined the colonial radio orchestra. He remained with the (Jakarta) radio orchestra in the post-independence period, until his death in 1958.

Ismail Marzuki left a vast repertoire of songs, one of which is the much-loved *Halo Halo Bandung*, a patriotic marching work composed when Bandung was engulfed in flames during a fierce battle in 1945. His other compositions include *Rayuan Pulau Kelapa, Kalau Anggrek Berbunga, Siasat Asmara, Jauh Dimata Dihati Jangan* and *Irian Samba. Rayuan Pulau Kelapa*, composed in 1944, received commendation and admiration from overseas composers.

In recognition of his dedication to his country and the arts, Ismail Marzuki was given the distinct honour of having his name put on the new Jakarta Arts Centre in 1968, which became known as Taman Ismail Marzuki. A bust was also made in his honour which now stands in the yard of the art centre.

Kusbini

Kusbini might just be the longest living composer on Indonesian record. Kusbini, whose name means *child from a special essence*, was born in Mojokerto, East Java, in 1906. His career began with (Jakarta) radio where he worked as conductor of the orchestra during the Japanese occupation. His special interest was *keroncong* music, a form of popular music that combines many ethnic and some foreign idioms. Kusbini was in fact known as the *buaya keroncong*, the *keroncong* crocodile. 'Buaya' is used here to refer to a person with a consuming passion, as Kusbini had for *keroncong* music.

Until his death in 1991, Kusbini was principal of his own music school in Yogyakarta. He was highly regarded for his work in developing music education amongst the younger generation, but his greatest contribution was the beautiful *Bagimu Negeri* (For You, My Country) written in 1942. *Bagimu Negeri* has become close to a second anthem, due to its simple and meaningful words.

(Above) Some of the more common symbols of Indonesia which have inspired national composers to write songs.

The bust of Ismail Marzuki.

The parade which is part of the 17th August celebrations.

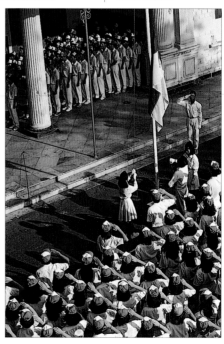

Music for the Children

*T*he growing 'national consciousness' of the early 20th century spread in many directions. The displacement of Dutch by the new national language, Bahasa Indonesia, left a vacuum that had to be filled. One of these was music. The children needed songs that were related to their environment which would also facilitate their learning the new language. Radio provided the perfect vehicle.

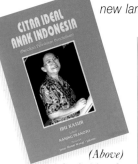

(Above)
A book citing the invaluable contribution of Ibu Kasur to children's music.

Choirs are popular with children, as well as adults. All organisations take pride in winning these contests.

(Below) Ibu Soed's children's songs are written based on common events and activities such as listening to falling rain, planting corn and going to school.

Development of Children's Music

In the late 1920s, children's songs in Bahasa Indonesia were already being aired on radio. These songs written by Ibu Soed were greatly appreciated by the Japanese who occupied Indonesia from 1942 to 1945. They assigned her to teach children's songs in Bahasa Indonesia on the radio, hoping to orient the Indonesians away from the West.

Many years after Indonesia had gained its independence, the radio network gradually opened up and spread across the Archipelago. A regular weekly program was set up which taught young children how to sing the songs written by Ibu Soed, Pak Kasur and A.T. Mahmoed.

The advent of television in 1962 gave a strong boost to children's music. Programmes were designed to teach children the art of music and singing. Children's singing competitions were introduced for individuals and school groups.

Music and the School Curriculum

Instruction of music leans towards vocalisation, particularly choral singing. The children are first taught to sing the song in the *do-re-mi* system and when they have mastered this, they learn the words. Songs are divided into two classes; obligatory and non-obligatory. Obligatory songs, or *lagu-lagu wajib*, consist of songs created as a form of nationalistic expression and are full of patriotic feeling.

IBU SOED (1908-1995)

Saridjah Niung Bintang, who married Soedibio and became known thereafter as Ibu Soed, was a precocious child. By the age of 20, her simple musical composition for children, written in Bahasa Indonesia, were being played on radio (*When I am Grown, When School is Over*). She had begun this work because she could not see why Indonesian school children should have to learn Dutch songs that sentimentalised about the tulips of Holland. Ibu Soed found inspiration everywhere, in rain dripping from a leaking roof, an act of heroism, a butterfly. Her songs are filled with gaiety and nationalism, and themes meant to encourage creativity and a sense of responsibility amongst the children of Indonesia.

A particularly outstanding moment in Ibu Soed's life occurred in 1928, when she played in the orchestra that introduced her country's future national anthem, *Indonesia Raya*. This was at the Youth Congress in Jakarta in 1928 that pledged 'one country, one people, one language : Indonesia(n)'. Wage Soepratman played the violin on that day.

During the Japanese occupation, Ibu Soed was assigned to work with Kusbini, the conductor, to teach Indonesia's children Indonesian songs via Japanese military radio. Compositions during this period include *Planting Corn*, and *I am a Hero*.

Ibu Soed wrote songs, music, plays and operettas for children, and also more serious music for adults, like *Sighing Jasmine* and *Some Years after Independence*. Near the end of her life, Ibu Soed received the ultimate recognition for her work, the coveted *Satya Lencana Kebudayaan*.

PAK KASUR (1912-1992)

K. Soerjono, fondly known as Pak Kasur by all and sundry, was educated as a teacher. His subsequent career included teaching, information officer, secretary of the national film board, guerrilla in the revolution and composer of children music. These involvement took him from Serayu village in Central Java where he was born, to Yogyakarta, Bandung and finally Jakarta.

Pak Kasur loved children dearly and in his free time would gather them together in a play group and teach them to sing songs which were composed by him. In Jakarta the little group evolved into a sizable playschool for children under official kindergarten age. Activities included playing, singing, dancing and poetry-reciting. From time to time the children would perform on Radio Republik Indonesia and after 1962, on TVRI, the new television station. After retirement from government service in 1968, Pak Kasur devoted his time to his playgroups, for whom he created a large volume of music (for example, *Riding the Horse-drawn Carriage* and *Getting Up in the Morning*) and stories, some of which were subsequently turned into short films for children (for example, *Amrin Plays Hookey* and *My Harmonica*). In all, Pak Kasur wrote some 140 song for children. His favourite teaching instrument was the native bamboo idiophone known as *angklung*.

In 1987, Pak Kasur suffered a massive stroke which left him paralysed. His work was carried on by his wife, Sandiah (Ibu Kasur), who continues to appear regularly on television with children.

LAGU-LAGU WAJIB	COMPOSITIONS BY PAK KASUR	COMPOSITIONS BY IBU SOED
Indonesia Raya (Greater Indonesia) by W.R. Soepratman	Naik Delman (Riding the Horse-drawn Carriage)	Hai Becak (Hey, Becak)
Maju Tak Gentar (Onward, No Fear) by C. Simandjuntak	Bangun Pagi (Getting Up in the Morning)	Kupu-kupu (Butterfly)
Halo-Halo Bandung (Hello, Hello Bandung) by Ismail Marzuki.	Harmonikaku (My Harmonica)	Tik-Tik-Tik, Bunyi Hujan (Sound of the Rain)
Ibu Kita Kartini (Our Mother, Kartini) by W.R. Soepratman	Amrin Membolos (Amrin Plays Hookey)	Menaman Jagung (Planting Corn)
Bagimu Negeri (For You, My Country) by Kusbini	Balonku Ada Lima (I Have Five Balloons)	Naik Kereta Api (Riding the Train)
Satu Nusa Satu Bangsa (One Country, One Nation) by L. Manik	Cicak Di Dinding (Cicak on the Wall)	Bila Sekolah Usai (When School is Over)
Hari Merdeka (Independence Day) by Hs. Mutahar	S'lamat Sore, 'Bu (Good Afternoon, Ma'am)	Bung Polisi (Mr Policeman)

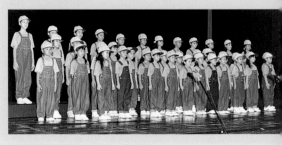

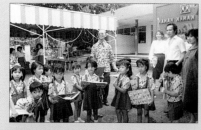
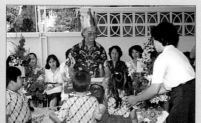
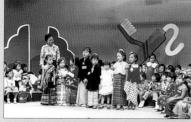
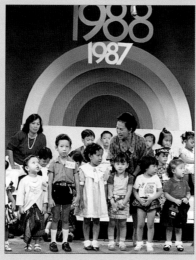
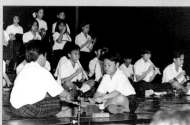

❷ BANGUN TIDUR

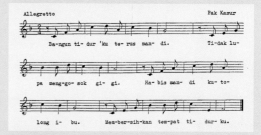

❸ MENANAM JAGUNG

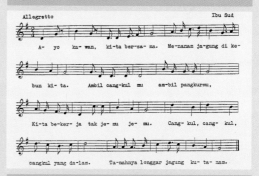

VARIOUS CHILDREN'S SONGS

❶ *Adik Menari* (Baby is Dancing): Look at baby dancing, swinging hands and feet, head swaying, dancing and laughing, head swaying, dancing and laughing.
❷ *Bangun Tidur* (Waking Up): Waking up, take a bath. Don't forget to brush [your] teeth. After bathing, help mother make bed. ❸ *Menaman Jagung* (Planting Corn): Come on friends, let's plant corn in the garden. Take your hoe, take the mattock, let's get to work. Dig, dig, dig deeply. The soil is loose, I 'll plant my corn. ❹ *Cinta Pada Tanah Air* (I Love [my] Country): I love [my] father and mother, I love [my] family, I love [my] friends and [my] abode. I love [my] country, my homeland, Indonesia. ❺ *Kasih Ibu* (Mother's Love): Mother's love for us [is] limitless, as long as time; just given, no return expected, like the Sun illuminating the world.

❹ CINTA PADA TANAH AIR

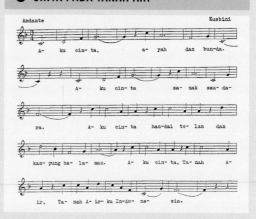

❶ ADIK MENARI

IBU KASUR AND CHILDREN MUSIC

After Pak Kasur's death, Ibu Kasur continued his work with children. She is an active speaker in forums and seminars on children education. She has also written many articles for newspapers and magazines. Pak and Ibu Kasur's work with children on television has led increasingly to the popularity of children's programmes and children's music in general.

❺ KASIH IBU

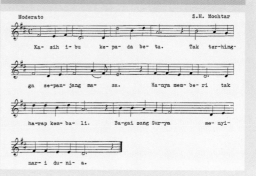

A concert by elementary school children in Jakarata. Various traditional and non-traditional instruments are used.

Modern and Experimental Indonesian Music

The emergence of Indonesian experimental music genre coincided with the development of Indonesian modern music early this century. The first generation of Indonesian composers, Soerjopoetro, R. Atmadarsana and R. Soehardjo, develop a concept of using gamelan elements and performance techniques in Western-style compositions.

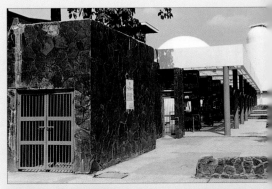

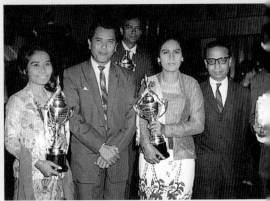

Early Developments

In 1951, two years after the country had gained independence, Indonesian popular music was given a significant boost through an annual singing competition by the government radio station, Radio Republik Indonesia (RRI) to determine *bintang radio* (radio stars) in the various categories of popular music; *keroncong*, *seriosa* ('serious') and *langgam*.

Growth of Indonesian Pop

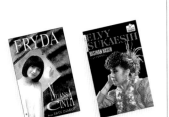

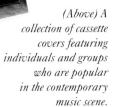

The 1950s marked the beginning of Indonesian popular music. In the next decade the local music scene received even greater stimulus with the installation of a government television network (TVRI) and programmes which allocated significant time to Indonesian pop music. An additional impetus was provided by a booming cassette industry.

(Above) A collection of cassette covers featuring individuals and groups who are popular in the contemporary music scene.

(Bottom right of box) Claude Debussy was the first European musician to adapt gamelan music into his compostions.

American and Latin Influences

The 1950s and 1960s saw the emergence of compositions which were based on American and Latin-American pop music rhythms such as the cha-cha and rock-and-roll, which were very popular in Indonesia during this period. American and Latin-American pop music was banned by President Soekarno in 1959 in an official government policy known as *Manipol-Usdek* which reinstated the 1945 Constitution and decried imported cultural idioms as being part of foreign cultural imperialism. (Manipol-USDEK is an acronym for <u>Ma</u>nifesto <u>Po</u>litik Undang-undang Dasar 1945; <u>So</u>sialisme Indonesia; <u>De</u>mokrasi Terpimpin; <u>Ke</u>pribadian Indonesia (1945 Constitution; Indonesian Socialism; Guided Democracy; Guided Economy; Indonesian Identity).

In spite of this, a number of pop music groups gained popularity during this period by creatively Indonesianising the Western music forms. Gumarang performed Indonesia's version of the cha-cha music, while Koes Bersaudara played Indonesian-style rock-and-roll. The era was also marked by the emergence in 1963 of the song *Patah Hati* (Broken Heart) which was the prototype of the Indonesian top-hit lamentation genre known as *lagu cengeng* (whining songs).

Creative Pop

In the 1970s, a group of young pop musicians endeavoured to provide an alternative to *dangdut* and *lagu cengeng*. Their compositions were oriented towards more original music treatments and lyrics of higher poetical value. Among these new young artists were Harry Rusli, Guruh Soekarnoputra, Chrisye and Eros Djarot. Their musical style became known as creative pop.

Music with a Message

In the 1980s, the Indonesian pop music scene became even more interesting with the emergence of songwriters

---

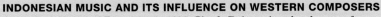

INDONESIAN MUSIC AND ITS INFLUENCE ON WESTERN COMPOSERS

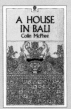

At the Paris Universal Exposition in 1889, Claude Debussy heard and saw performances of gamelan music and dance by a Javanese troupe. This exotic music had a profound effect upon him as documented in his letters. Gamelan influences in Debussy's piano compositions include his use of the whole tone scale (inspired from the five-toned *slendro* gamelan tuning), his passionate exploration of sonorities, harmonic colours, and above all, his piano style which is fundamentally percussive in style. Some of his compositions are *Pagodes* (from *Estampes*) and the preludes *Canopes* and *La fille aux cheveux de lin*.

The Canadian-American composer-pianist Colin McPhee (1900-64) was so attracted by the earliest published recordings of Balinese gamelan music that he journeyed to Bali, where he lived and studied for most of the 1930s. McPhee was however more well known for his musicological writings and biography than his own compositions. During the past decade there has been a great revival of interest in McPhee's music. His best known compositions are *Tabuhan-tabuhan* (1936), *Symphony No. 2* (1957), and *Nocturne for Chamber Orchestra* (1958).

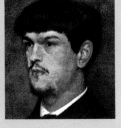

Neither Debussy nor McPhee ever learned to play the gamelan. Actual performance study in gamelan music by non-Indonesians only began after World War II at the Royal Tropical Institute in Amsterdam and the University of California in Los Angeles, featuring the traditions of Central Java, Sunda and Bali with instruction by Indonesian musicians. Since then, from 1960 to the present, the number of university and off-campus gamelan groups has increased almost geometrically. (Andy Toth)

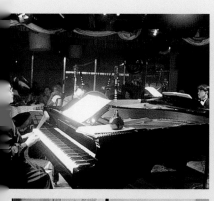
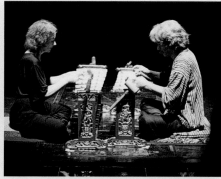
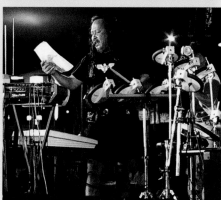
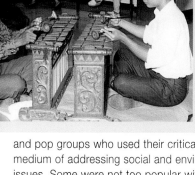

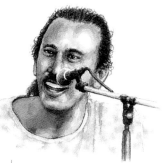

(From top left, clockwise) The Taman Ismail Marzuki Centre in Jakarta.

Trisutji Kamal performed her new composition at the Stage Cafe in Jakarta.

Paul Gautama and his wife playing an experimental duet on the Balinese gender.

Harry Rusli performing at a rock concert in Jakarta.

A student practising with his teacher on the gender *at the TIM Arts Centre.*

Masnun and Fetty Fatimah, golden-voiced keroncong *singers of the 1970s.*

Iwan Fals, a guitarist-singer from the popular rock group, Kantata Samsara.

(Below) Leo Kristi drumming on his guitar in his concert performance at the Jakarta Arts Council in Jakarta. The concert performance was held in conjunction with the National Day celebrations for three days beginning on 17th August, 1988.

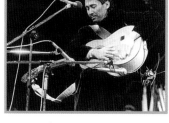

and pop groups who used their critical lyrics as a medium of addressing social and environmental issues. Some were not too popular with the authorities. Remy Sylado, a progressive pop-music figure with a background in literature, theatre, fine arts and theology, is considered a pioneer of this movement. Other composers and musicians include Leo Kristi, Dede Harris, Ully Sigar, Iwan Fals, Franky and Jane, and many others.

Experimental Indonesian Music

R. Soehardjo's work, *Birvadda Warawidya,* written in 1924 was based on three gamelan pieces named *Tarupala, Pangkur* and *Celuntang.* The notation used by the composer was derived from the Western classical system though the notes in the score are actually sung in a pentatonic (*slendro*) gamelan scale. In addition, the melodic phrases follow the traditional gamelan technique of improvisation called *cengkok-wilet.* As in the gamelan tradition, each female vocalist (*pesinden*) is identified by her individual improvisation technique, hence the piece sounds different each time it is performed.

Experimentation of the 50s

A new generation of composers emerged in the 1950s who sought to transform gamelan into a modern and national musical idiom. This has produced several new concepts in gamelan performance:
- Western instruments included in a new diatonic gamelan ensemble called *gentono*;
- the ensemble was directed by a conductor instead of the drummer;
- different classical gamelan ensembles were combined in the new works;

- various regional gamelan techniques were employed in the new compositions.
The latter three techniques can be identified in K.R.T. Wasitodiningrat's works. Wasitodiningrat was the most prominent experimental gamelan composer of the 1950s.

When East Meets West

The 1970s was noted for works composed by musicians with Western training in collaboration with traditional gamelan musicians. *Kemangan Masa Lampau* (Memories of the Past), composed in 1974 by Frans Haryadi (1930-1989), was an example of this interaction.

The music composed for the 1977 screenplay *November 1828* about the 19th-century national hero, Diponegoro, used the same concept of collaboration. In this work, Franki Raden collaborated with musicians from the Indonesian Conservatory of Traditional Music in Surakarta.

Composers who have worked with traditional musicians from other regions such as Bali and Sumatra include Slamet A. Sjukur, Rahayu Supanggah, W. Sadra, Sapto R., B. Pasaribu, Tony Prabowo and Otto Sidharta.

(Below, left) Pop singer-musician Harry Rusli in concert.

(Below) Ully Sigar, a vivacious pop singer and composer of songs totally focusses on environmental awareness in her songs.

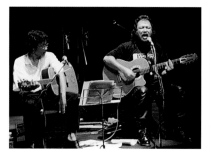
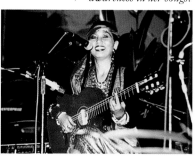

Keroncong and Dangdut

*T*here are many types of fully Western-oriented music in Indonesia, like pop, jazz, rock, and others, but the most prevalent form throughout the Indonesian Archipelago is entertainment music bearing Indonesian characteristics and tastes. This demonstrates the power of adapting a variety of cultural elements to produce new forms of Indonesian (national) culture. The most significant examples of this new Indonesian music are keroncong *and* dangdut.

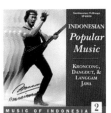

Rhoma Irama on the cover of a compact disc produced by the Smithsonian Institute, New York.

CENTRES OF *KERONCONG* MUSIC

The above map shows the distribution of various centres of *keroncong* music on the island of Java.

Various cassette covers of song albums on dangdut.

An old-fashioned keroncong *band from Tugu in Jakarta. Tugu is the area where the Portuguese once settled.*

Early keroncong *singers did not enjoy the status or respect that can be achieved by today's singers.*

Keroncong and *Dangdut* as Music For Entertainment

Keroncong and *dangdut* are considered music for entertainment, as they possess the following characteristics:
1. they are urban;
2. they have entertaining, commercial and industrial values, and follow market taste;
3. their development is affected by the urban culture;
4. they are Western-oriented with regard to instrumental, melodic and musical structure; but
5. composition and presentation, idioms, style and musical expressions are typically Indonesian.

Keroncong Music

The word *keroncong* or *kroncong* is an onomatopoeia derived from the sound produced by plucking a four-stringed musical instrument that dominates this musical ensemble and resembles the Hawaian ukulele, known in Indonesia as *cukulele, cuk* (pronounced chook), *crung* (chroong), and today *keroncong* (ke-ron-chong).

Rumour has it that *keroncong* originated in a Portuguese genre of music which was popular in the early 16th century, called *moritsku* (*moresco/moresca* in Portuguese). This theory is difficult to prove, because the *keroncong* style of music did not really begin to develop until the beginning of the 20th century. People say that the descendants of the Portuguese

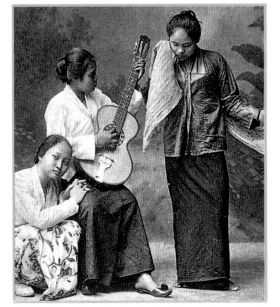

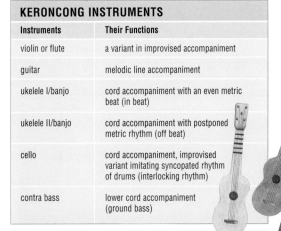

KERONCONG INSTRUMENTS	
Instruments	**Their Functions**
violin or flute	a variant in improvised accompaniment
guitar	melodic line accompaniment
ukelele I/banjo	cord accompaniment with an even metric beat (in beat)
ukelele II/banjo	cord accompaniment with postponed metric rhythm (off beat)
cello	cord accompaniment, improvised variant imitating syncopated rhythm of drums (interlocking rhythm)
contra bass	lower cord accompaniment (ground bass)

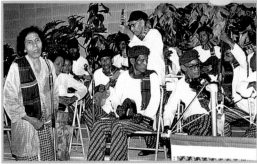

still live in Kampung Tengah, a district of Tanjung Priok, Jakarta, and they have continued the *moritsku* 'keroncong' tradition which they consider to be the original form of this kind of music. The name *keroncong kemayoran,* given to one of the best-loved pieces, derives from the name of an ethnic Betawi village in Jakarta; it is regarded as representing the new genre of *keroncong*. The early *keroncong* music was in fact associated with a particular Javanese stereotype known as the *buaya* (crocodile) or *jago* (rooster).

Keroncong *Today*

In some one hundred years of evolution, the *keroncong* has undergone many alterations. Today, we can identify several different types: *keroncong asli* (original), *keroncong kemayoran, stambul I* (II and III), *langgam keroncong* and even more recently, the *keroncong beat, keroncong pop,* etc. The more important differences lie in the length of the rhythm, changes in patterns and arrangement of harmony, tempo, characterisation and presentation. Nevertheless, *keroncong* does have a standard pattern, called *irama keroncong*. This gives the *keroncong* its specific character, distinguishing it from other kinds of music.

Music and Structure

The pattern of *keroncong* music consists of the melodic line as *cantus firmus* with an accompanying musical ensemble in which each instrument, with its own distinctive character, follows the functional patterns that have been laid down.

The uniqueness of *keroncong* music lies in the different way of playing the cello and bass, which differs from the usual mode: they are plucked. The cello has the same function as the small drum

DANGDUT INSTRUMENTAL ARRANGEMENT

Instruments	Function
Bamboo flute	a melodious instrument functioning as the lead of the main song, the variant-giver and the interlude in improvisation between melodic lines.
Mandolin	a melodic instrument functioning simultaneously as cord accompaniment in *ostinato* (the *plentingan* technique).
Gendang	a percussion instrument and main accompaiment that gives *dangdut* music its individuality; also gives the interlocking variant (*kotekan*) in the *glissandi* (*besutan*) technique.
Guitar	string accompaniment for solo melody which couples with the mandolin to play the soprano, mezzo-soprano or alto voice, or imitate the *gendang*-drum's high pitch by smothering its echo with a handkerchief.
Bass	gives the basic cord in dancing music of any style, like the rhumba, tango, cha-cha-cha, rock and disco.
Various percussion instruments; accordion and keyboard	function as a contra-rhythm and sound-colour *vis-à-vis* the other instruments; accompanying and melodic instruments, and when the piano is used, it functions solely as an harmonious cord accompaniment.

(*kendhang, gendang*) in gamelan music; the plucking of the cello is referred to as *kendhangan* or *gedugan*.

The modern *keroncong* ensemble contains one or more singers, a violin, a flute, a 'melody guitar', a cello, a string bass, and two small plucked lutes — a ukelele and a banjo. The main singer, violin or flute will carry the main melody and the other instruments will decorate or support them.

With its lyrics full of praise for romance, nature, the country and the nation, or political messages, the *keroncong* is very close to the people. It is widely known throughout the country. However it appeals mainly to the older generation, and it has become the nostalgic music of the people who have lived through the revolution.

Dangdut

The term *dangdut, dang dut* or *ndangdut* is also an onomatopoeia originating in the sound produced by one of the percussion instruments used in the music which goes by the name of *gendang*, *konga* (congo), *ketipung*, etc. *Ndut* is an exaggerated accentuation in the *glissandi* technique; it appears at the first beat of a metric rhythm preceded by the sound *ndang* produced by the last accentuated beat (off-beat) of the previous rhythm. The specific characteristics of *dangdut* are affected by manner of presentation, playing technique and instrumental arrangement.

Structure of the Song

1. Introduction: vocal solo or instrumental
2. Main songs: 1-2 themes of main *dangdut* song
3. Interlude: instrumental improvisation as a transition from the theme of the main song to the second theme.
4. Theme of second song called refrain; contains a contra melody of the theme of the main song.
5. Coda: epilogue, either vocal solo and/or instrumental.

Dangdut *and Social Discourse*

Dangdut songs are generally sensual and melancholic. The words concern romance, suffering, misery; they give advice and religious sermons; they criticise and satirise. Unlike *keroncong* music, in which lyrics tend to be poetic, *dangdut* lyrics are bold, to-the-point and appear to avoid biased expressions and allusions. *Dangdut* draws its audience largely from the Muslim youths of the lower and lower-middle class. It expresses the resentment of these youths against the inequities in Indonesian society. Examples of social critique can be found in some of Rhoma Irama's songs, such as *Qur'an dan Koran* in which he laments how progress and development have led people to become materialistic and arrogant. *Dangdut* lyrics touch on issues such as marriage, unemployment, gambling, debt, prostitution and many other social problems.

While the *keroncong* tempo tends to be slow, *dangdut* tempo is dynamic and temperamental. In *dangdut,* the inner rhythm emits a sense of power.

Development of Dangdut

Dangdut came onto the Indonesian music scene much later than *keroncong*. It has developed very quickly since the 1950s, paralleling the spread of entertainment music through the Archipelago. Even so, the cultural resources that built 'modern' *dangdut* can be traced back through the long process of fusion to coastal Malayan music on the east, north and west Sumatran littoral, the north Java coastal regions, east Indian music, Islamic music from the Middle East, Latin-American music and several other kinds of folk music. Yet, the most dominant influence has been that derived from popular east Indian and Malayan (Malaysian) movies which were screened all over the country during the early 1950s. Early *dangdut* from the 1960s sounded mainly like Indian film music sung in Indonesian.

Due to its simple form and its ability to accept new arrangement patterns, *dangdut* music is currently in the process of absorbing elements from pop music and rock forms. The rock elements were added in the 1970s by Rhoma Irama.

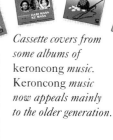

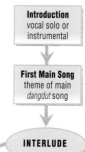

Cassette covers from some albums of keroncong *music.* Keroncong *music now appeals mainly to the older generation.*

Introduction
vocal solo or instrumental

First Main Song
theme of main *dangdut* song

INTERLUDE

| Instrumental improvisation as a transition from the theme of the main song to the second theme | **MUSICAL STRUCTURE OF *DANGDUT*** | **Second Song** called 'refrain' contains a contra melody of the theme of the main song |

Coda
epilogue either vocal solo or/and instrumental

(Below) Rhoma Irama, the king of dangdut *music, performing in front of a crowd of 200,000 people at the Yellow Dynamic Dangdut Fiesta.*

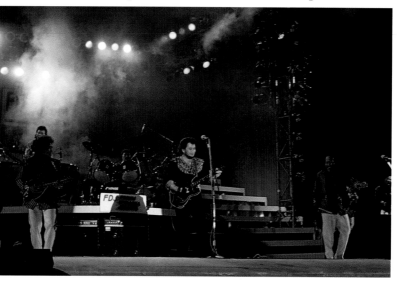

Music in Contemporary Indonesia

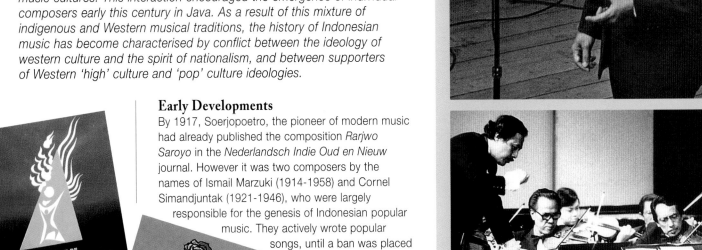

The rise of modern music in Indonesia can be viewed as a result of a dynamic encounter between indigenous music and Western classical music cultures. This interaction encouraged the emergence of individual composers early this century in Java. As a result of this mixture of indigenous and Western musical traditions, the history of Indonesian music has become characterised by conflict between the ideology of western culture and the spirit of nationalism, and between supporters of Western 'high' culture and 'pop' culture ideologies.

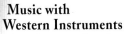

Posters promoting the holding of concerts by young composers at Taman Ismail Marzuki Arts Centre, Jakarta.

Early Developments

By 1917, Soerjopoetro, the pioneer of modern music had already published the composition *Rarjwo Saroyo* in the *Nederlandsch Indie Oud en Nieuw* journal. However it was two composers by the names of Ismail Marzuki (1914-1958) and Cornel Simandjuntak (1921-1946), who were largely responsible for the genesis of Indonesian popular music. They actively wrote popular songs, until a ban was placed on Western popular music by the Japanese Cultural Council during the Japanese Occupation (1942-1945). During this period, two distinct music groups arose, one using the traditional Javanese music system and the other employing Western classical techniques.

Music with Western Instruments

Western-oriented music or *musik seriosa* (serious music) became very popular after 1945. It was strongly influenced by the Romantic Period of Western classical music. Songs in this category, written using the Western classical musical style of 19th-century Europe, became the standard vocal music repertoire in Indonesia in the 1950s and 1960s. Although the lyrics were distinctly Indonesian, the approach was wholly Western-oriented in

The experiment with Western musical instruments had begun much earlier, even in village bands where the violin was used as accompaniments to traditional instruments such as the kendhang *and the* rebana.

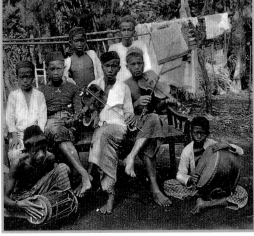

structural forms, harmonisation, arrangement, orchestration and presentation.

Promotion of Musik Seriosa

The government radio station, Radio Republik Indonesia (RRI), became the centre for the encouragement of *musik seriosa*. Annual national music competitions were instituted in 1951 from which the best vocalists in the *musik seriosa*, *keroncong* and *hiburan* music categories were chosen, and they became *bintang radio* (radio stars). *Musik seriosa* enjoyed considerable popularity for two decades, from 1950 to 1970.

Development and Change

European classical and modern music and Western contemporary music continue to have a strong influence on the development of modern Indonesian music. Music institutes in Jakarta, Bandung, Yogyakarta, Surabaya, Medan and other big cities produce musicians trained in Western classical and modern music. The Orkes Simfoni Jakarta, Ensembel Jakarta and Nusantara Chamber Orchestra only perform orchestral arrangements of Western music and modern Western-oriented Indonesian music. The latest works of Indonesian composers have attempted to introduce traditional and ethnic elements in their formulations. Gamelan music and folk songs provide inspiration to contemporary Indonesian music, both of which have either originated from classical Western style or have derived from traditional music. With the use of electronic media and computers, contemporary

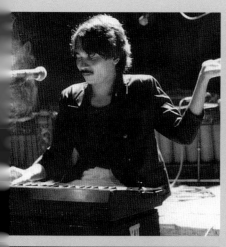

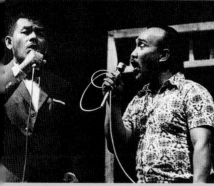

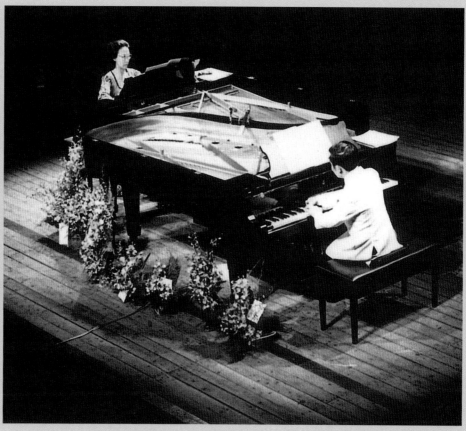

Indonesian experimental music can be made available to the rest of the world.

Institutional Support

While pop music has enjoyed unprecedented growth in the recent years, institutional support was sought to promote the development of modern music composition using Western and traditional instruments and scales. In 1968, the Taman Ismail Marzuki (TIM) Arts Centre was opened in Jakarta by Ali Sadikin, who was Governor of Jakarta at that time. Twenty-five leading personalities in the arts were appointed to the Arts Council to plan and manage programmes. The centre was completed with the opening of the Jakarta Arts Institute in 1970. During this time, musical composition was taught

under a formal curriculum, a movement first developed by the Arts Institute and emulated by AMI/ISI (National Music Academy/Indonesian Arts Institute in Yogyakarta).

By 1974 the Jakarta Arts Council had developed a national competition for musical composition which helped to promote a new generation of young composers. However, since composition programmes were based on a Western music model, composers that emerged were only those who had Western classical music backgrounds. In 1979, the Jakarta Arts Council developed a new programme, the Young Composers' Festival which expanded the scope of performances to include works by young composers with traditional music training.

(From top left, clockwise) Pranajaya in concert, 1970.

Sapto Raharjo performed his composition for keyboard and gamelan at Purnabudaya, Yogyakarta.

Performances on two pianos by Irawati M. Sudiarso and Rudy Laban, April 1977.

Bing Slamet (right) and Sam Saimun, two well-known singers of the 1960s and 1970s.

Orkes Simfoni Jakarta, conducted by F.X. Sutopo in May 1984.

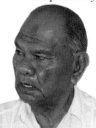

Amir Pasribu, a pioneer of Indonesian modern music.

ART SUMMIT INDONESIA 1995: MUSIC AND DANCE

In early 1993, the Indonesian government (especially the Directorate-General of Culture) decided it was time to hold a landmark event in the dance and music field which would coincide with the 50th anniversary of Indonesian independence. It was the right time. Indonesia's composers and choreographers were already gaining international reputations through participation in festivals abroad. Invitations were sent to the best composers and choreographers around the world to take part in the Art Summit Indonesia 1995 Music and Dance. Prominent music and dance groups from France, Africa, India, Argentina, Germany, USA, Japan and Great Britain were invited. With particular respect to contemporary music, Indonesia was represented by Slamet Abdul Sjukur (*Jawara, Ji-Lala-Ji, Uwek-Uwek, OM*), Rahayu Supanggah (*Garap*), and Paul Gautama Soegijo (*Deprokan, Incantation, Genderan I, Dolanan, Saman Drumming*).

Name of group/Individual	Country
Urban Sax	France
Ghana Dance Ensemble	Africa
Slamet Abdul Sjukur	Indonesia
Chandralekha	India
Nucleodanza	Argentina
Sardono W. Kusumo	Indonesia
Banjar Gruppe Berlin	Germany
The Paul Dresher Ensemble	USA
Rahayu Supanggah	Indonesia
Orchestra Ensembles Kamazawa	Japan
Sankai Juku	Japan
Richard Alston Dance Company	United Kingdom
Kazuo Ohno	Japan
Bagong Kussudiardja	Indonesia
Weimarer Tanztheater	Germany

Glossary

ABBREVIATIONS:

Ar. - Arabic, Bal. - Balinese,
Cir. - Cirebonese, Ind. -
Indonesian, Jav. -
Javanese, Mak. - Makasar,
Mand. - Mandailing, Min. -
Minangkabau, Skr. -
Sanskrit, Sun. - Sundanese

A

adok (Min.): frame-drum.

alau ambek (Min.): dance form based on the art of self-defence.

alus/halus (Ind.): refined.

angklung (Jav.): bamboo idiophone.

Anoman/Hanoman: monkey-warrior who serves Rama in the **Ramayana** epic.

Arjuna: third of the five **Pandawa** brothers in the **Mahabharata** epic. He is skilled, handsome and the spiritual son of the god, Indra.

Arjunawiwaha (Jav.): literally 'the meditation of **Arjuna**'/'the marriage of **Arjuna**'. Original 11th-century Javanese epic.

awiran (Bal.): breast-high cloak-like garment of ribbons worn by *baris* dancers.

B

babad (Jav./Sun.): traditional historical account.

bakaba (Min.): to recite traditional *kaba* verse.

balih-balihan (Bal.): secular.

balungan (Jav.): basic melodic structure in **gamelan** music.

bangsawan (Ind.): nobleman,aristocrat; Malay theatre form with **pantun** delivery.

barangan (Jav.): for entertainment or amusement; travelling theatre.

baris gede (Bal.): 'big' *baris*; *baris* dance with large company.

baris tunggal (Bal.): solo *baris* dance.

barong (Jav., Bal.): extra large; a mythical creature.

basijobang (Min.): to recite *sijobang* ballads in a specific style.

bedhaya (Jav.): dance form, generally with 9 female dancers.

bedhayan (Jav.): in *ludruk* theatre, a chorus line of men in women's dress.

bende (Jav.): small hanging gong.

bersih desa (Ind.): ritual village-cleansing.

berutuk (Bal.): particular mask; also the god represented in the mask in Trunyan, Bali.

besutan (Jav.): *lerok* comedy play featuring the character Besut.

Bharatayudha: literally 'The Great War of the Bharata clan'; it is the concluding portion of the **Mahabharata** epic.

Bima: second of the five **Pandawa** brothers. A powerful character, he is easily identified by the long thumbnail on his left hand. He is the spiritual son of god Bayu.

bintang radio (Ind.): radio star; winner of an annual contest conducted by Radio Republik Indonesia.

blencong (Jav.): oil lamp used to project puppet shadow onto screen.

bonang (Jav.): **gamelan** instrument, 10-14 kettle-gongs in a frame.

bonang barung (Jav.): large **bonang**.

bonang panerus (Jav.): small **bonang**.

bongkel (Jav.): bamboo idiophone with four tubes, *slendro* pitch.

buaya keroncong (Ind.): person with consuming passion for **keroncong** music.

buka tanah (Ind.): 'open' or plough the earth, a ritual in the Malay theatre.

buka panggung (Ind.): 'open' the stage, or the play, in the Malay theatre.

buncis (Jav.): orchestra of several **angklung**, plus a drum, in Banyumas.

C

calung (Jav.): **angklung** orchestra playing **gamelan** music.

capala/cempala (Jav.): knobbed wooden beater held between toes of right foot or in left hand to knock the **wayang** storage box, as a sound effect during a **wayang** show.

canang (Ind.): very small hanging gong.

celempung (Jav.): zither.

ceracap (Jav.): bamboo clappers or a set of round metal plates strung one atop the other, that clack or rattle when struck [used in **wayang** theatre].

D

dabus (Aceh): *debus* in Indonesian; a display of self-mutilation accompanied by frame-drum music.

dalang (Ind.): puppeteer; puppeteer-narrator.

dalang topeng (Jav.): narrator-dancer in Cirebon masked play.

dampeang (Min.): accompaniment (musical).

dangdut (Ind.): romantic, melancholic music with strong Indian and Islamic flavour.

demung (Jav.): large low-toned xylophone.

depok (Sun.): specific position performed in dance and *cikeruhan* martial arts.

didong (Aceh): form of entertainment by men with chanted songs and hand-clapping.

dubalang (Min.): district chief.

dukun (Ind.): indigenous medical practitioner or shaman.

E

embat (Jav.): difference in intervallic structure of a **gamelan**.

emban (Jav.): nursemaid.

enek-enek (Batak): drum; child.

G

galembong (Min.): low-crotched men's trousers.

galombang (Min.): processional dance based on martial arts movements; like waves.

gambang (Jav.): wooden xylophone.

gambus (Ind.): wooden plucked lute.

gamelan (Ind.): traditional percussion orchestra, made mainly of bronze or brass.

gandang (Dayak): double-headed drum.

gandrung (Jav.): besotted (with love); term for certain dancers.

gantar, giring-giring (Dayak): dancer's leg ornament consisting of many small bells.

garebeg (Jav.): important Javano-Muslim ritual celebration in Central Java.

gedebok/gedebog (Jav.): banana bole into which leather puppet figures are staked.

gelluk (Toraja): generic term for dance.

gembyangan (Jav.): in **gamelan** music, high & low notes struck simultaneously.

gendang (Ind.): double-headed membranophone (drum).

gender (Jav./Bal.): xylophone with metal keys.

gender barung (Jav.): large **gender**.

gender panerus (Jav.): small **gender**.

gendhing (Jav.): musical piece, melody, composition.

genrang (Mak.): double-headed drum.

golek (Jav.): wooden figure, doll, puppet; a wooden rod-puppet.

golek menak (Jav.): stage drama based on **Menak cycle** of Persian-based stories in which the dancer-actors imitate wooden rod-puppets, in Yogyakarta.

gondang (Batak): double headed drum; ensemble including two such drums; song, melody.

gong gede (Bal.): big gong; full **gamelan** orchestra.

gongan (Jav.): gong playing cycle.

gordang (Mand.): single-headed drum; a musical ensemble featuring such drums.

gordang sambilan (Mand.): ensemble of nine single-headed drums graded from big to small and consisting of four pairs of mother (larger) and father (smaller) drums plus one 'child'.

gunungan (Jav.): large leaf-shaped object in the shadow-puppet theatre representing the universe, or the beginning and the end.

H

hadrah (Ar.): Muslim religious performance.

huda-huda (Batak): hornbill bird mask that covers the whole body, used in funerary rites.

hudoq (Dayak): Bahau & Modang mask-dance, to contact spirits.

hudoq kita' (Dayak): Kenyah mask-dance, to contact spirits.

I/J

indang (Min.): small frame-drum.

induk (Batak): drum; mother.

irama (Ind.): rhythm.

jaba tengah (Bal.): middle courtyard of temple.

jaipongan (Sun.): recent adaptation of the **ketuk tilu** dance.

jaran kepang (Jav.): hobbyhorse made of plaited bamboo.

jathilan (Jav.): flat hobby-horses made of bamboo matting; a dance.

jejer (Jav.): dance alternating with song, in East Java.

jeroan (Bal.): inner court of temple.

jipae/jipai (Asmat): ritual mask that covers the whole body, representing a spirit.

jipui pokmbu/pokman pokmbi (Asmat): ritual to commemorate or contact spirits.

joget (Mal./Ind.): form of street dance in which a professional entertainer invites male onlookers to partner her.

K

kanjet (Dayak): generic term for a dance genre.

kasar (Ind.): coarse, crude and vulgar.

kaulan (Ar.): thanking God for a wish fulfilled.

kayon (Bal.): large leaf-shaped object in **wayang kulit** performance which marks the end of a scene and can represent forest, mountain, palace or other locations.

kecapi (Ind.): zither.

kedhok (Jav.): mask; representation of face.

kejiman (Jav.): state of trance.

kelir (Jav.): screen used in shadow-puppet theatre.

kemanak (Jav.): hollow bars struck with padded mallet.

kempluk (Sasak): small gong.

kempul (Jav.): small hanging gong.

kempyang (Jav.): pair of small kettlegongs in joined frames.

kendhang (Jav.): double-headed asymmetrical barrel drum.

kenong (Jav.): large kettlegong in frame.

keprak (Jav.): (1) slit wooden signal-box sounded with wooden mallet (pengeprak; *cempala*); (2) rattles of pieces of wood or metal sounded with wooden mallet; used in **wayang** performance.

kepyak (Jav.): three copper plates, struck to make a rattling sound during a **wayang** performance.

keras (Ind.): not refined.

keroncong : hybrid form of popular music known in various forms throughout most of Indonesia.

kesenian barangan (Jav.): comedy show, East Java.

ketek ogleng (Jav.): traditional theatre form, Yogyakarta.

kethuk, ketuk (Jav./Sun): small kettle-drum in a frame.

ketipung, ketimpung (Ind.): small single-headed drum played with the fingers.

ketoprak (Jav.): traditional Javanese folk theatre (comedic).

ketua panjak (Mal.): director of a performance; head of actors.

ketuk tilu (Sun.): dance.

kinthilan (Jav.): **gamelan** playing mode.

klana alus (Jav.): refined prince.

kothak (Jav.): **wayang** puppet storage chest.

kuda kepang (Jav.): hobbyhorse made from plaited bamboo slats; form of dance.

kuntulan (Jav.): type of East Javanese musical ensemble.

L

lagu (Ind.): song, melody.

lakon (Jav.): story, stage play.

langendriyan (Jav.): form of dance-drama in Central Java performing Damar Wulan stories.

laras (Jav.): tuning system (*slendro*, *pelog*).

lerok (Jav.): comedy show in East Java, popular term for **kesenian barangan**.

longser (Sun.): farcical folk theatre from West Java.

ludruk (Jav.): East Javanese drama form, all male cast.

M

Mahabharata: epic about the struggle between the **Pandawa** and Korawa.

mamanda (Banjar): **bangsawan**-influenced folk theatre in Kalimantan.

mantra (Skr./Ind.): magic formulae; sacred sayings recited in ritual.

marwas (Malay): double-headed frame-drum.

masres (Cir.): folk theatre from Cirebon.

memetri desa (Jav.): village-cleansing ritual; lit. to take good care of the village.

Menak cycle: plays dramatising the adventures of the Islamic hero, Amir Hamzah.

mendu (Mal.): folk theatre in Riau; old Malay background.

musik seriosa (Ind.): 'serious' music.

N

nagari (Min.): historical political unit in West Sumatra.

ngamen (Jav.): to perform in the streets, to earn money.

ngremo (Jav.): act of covering shoulders/neck with a stole (*remong/ rimong*).

ninik-mamak (Min.): the elders, highest authority in Minangkabau hierarchy.

O

odalan (Bal.): calendrical temple festival.

omprok (Jav.): form of headdress worn by East Javanese dancers.

oncor (Sun.): oil lamp on top of a bamboo stake.

ondel-ondel (Betawi): huge masked figures (ancestral pair).

P

pajaga (Bugis): dance genre.

pajogek (Bugis): form of dance; the dancer.

pakarena (Mak.): group of secular dances.

panakawan (Jav.): also known as *punakawan*, clown servant-advisor.

Pandawa: literally 'sons of Pandu', the cycle of *lakon* about the five Pandawa brothers.

panggung (Ind.): stage, platform.

panjak (Jav.): **gamelan** musician.

pantun (Ind.): traditional quatrain-versed poetry.

pathet (Jav.): modal pitch in Javanese music.

pawang (Ind.): person with special powers, like a shaman.

peking (Jav.): the small xylophone or **saron panerus**.

pelog (Jav.): five-toned musical octave.

pemaju (Jav.): one who advances/promotes; male dancer in East Javanese dance.

penasar (Jav./Bal.): clown attendant.

pencak silat (Ind.): local form of the art of self-defence.

pencon (Jav.): a single kettlegong.

pengrawit (Jav.): **gamelan** player.

pengudang (Jav.): in East

Javanese ritual, an elderly woman.

pesinden (Jav.): **gamelan** singer(s), female.

pratima (Bal.): wooden effigy into which the deities descend at an *odalan*.

pupuik (Min.): wind instrument.

pura (Bal.): temple of worship.

purwa, parwa (Skr., Kawi): book, volume (**Ramayana** and **Mahabharata** epics); antiquity, the beginning [of time].

Q/R

qasidah (Ar.): Arabic poetry sung by women accompanied by frame drums.

rabab (Min.): two-stringed lute/rebecca.

Ramayana: literally 'the story of Rama', one of the two Indian epics which became really popular in the **wayang purwa** shadow play of Indonesia.

randai (Min.): narrative dance-drama form in West Sumatra.

Rangda (Bal.): witch-figure portrayed in dance.

rebab (Ind.): rebecca or lute with two or three strings.

rebana (Ind.): single-headed frame drum.

rebana biang (Ind.): type of frame-drum music in Betawi (*biang* = mother).

Reog Ponorogo (Jav.): processional performance from East Java.

ronggeng (Mal.): professional female dancer-singer who entices male onlookers to join her.

ruwatan (Jav.): ritual to release from bad luck.

S

sakti (Ind.): inner power; supernatural.

salam (Ind.): salute of

respect; greeting.

salawat, sholawat (Ar.): lit. good wishes; a form of music with sung verses.

sampakan (Jav.): theatre form stressing teamwork, Yogyakarta tradition.

sampe' (Dayak): two- to four-stringed plucked lute.

sandiwara (Ind.): drama.

Sanghyang Dedari (Bal.): ritual dance performed during village cleansing ritual; the characters portrayed in this particular performance are the celestial nymphs.

santiswaran (Ar.): performance of a form of religious (Islamic) music.

saron (Jav.): xylophone.

saron barung (Jav.): large **saron**.

saron panerus (Jav.): high-pitched, small xylophone.

sarunai (Bat.): wind instrument resembling a clarinet.

sekaten (Jav.): Javano-Muslim ritual celebration.

selamatan (Ind.): thanksgiving, communal feast.

selompret (Jav.): trumpet-like instrument.

sendratari (Ind.): dance-drama.

seudati (Aceh): dance form with male singer-dancers and body-music.

silek (Min.): local art of self-defence.

sirih/sirih-pinang (Ind.): the betel quid.

slendro (Jav.): five-toned octave in **gamelan** music.

slenthem (Jav.): xylophone with vertical resonating tubes underneath the metal keys.

soder (Sun.): long scarf played with in dancing.

srandul (Jav.): traditional theatre form, Yogyakarta.

suling (Ind.): flute.

T

tabuik/tabot (Min.):

Muslim miracle play in West Sumatra commemorating the death anniversary of Husein.

talempong (Min.): kettlegongs.

tayuban (Sun.): traditional dance performed indoors.

tembang (Jav.): song, piece of music.

terbang (Jav.): frame-drum.

topeng (Ind.): mask.

topeng babakan (Ind.): masked-play in Cirebon presented as a series of (solo) scenes (*babak*).

topeng dalang (Ind.): masked-play with puppeteer-narrator.

topeng pajegan (Bal.): masked-dance in which all roles are performed by a soloist.

toping-toping (Batak): masks of human figures, used in funerary rites.

tortor (Batak): Batak dance form employing very simple hand movements.

U

ubrug (Sun.): theatre form from Banten, West Java.

W

wali (Bal.): sacred.

wayang (Ind.): form of drama, based on the Hindu epics, their Indonesian adaptations, and several forms of traditional folk literature.

wayang cepak (Cir.): wooden rod-puppets with flattish heads and headdresses.

wayang golek (Jav.): three-dimensional, wooden, rod-puppets.

wayang gong (Banjar): South Kalimantan form of *wayang* play enacted by humans, of Javanese origin and influenced by Malay *bangsawan* theatre.

wayang klitik (Jav.): flat wooden rod-puppet.

wayang kulit (Jav.): leather shadow-puppet theatre; leather shadow-puppet figure.

wayang parwa (Bal.): *wayang* plays based on **Ramayana** and **Mahabharata** epics, and local epics.

wayang purwa (Jav.): *wayang* plays based on **Ramayana** and **Mahabharata** epics.

wayang suluh (Ind.): recently created puppet theatre based on local 20th-century history.

wayang topeng (Jav.): masked-play in the *wayang* theatre style.

wayang wong (Jav.): drama enacted by human actors following the *wayang* style.

Z

zapin (Mal.): Islamic Malayan dance genre.

REGION — NAME OF STORY CYCLES AND THEIR MAIN CHARACTER	JAVANESE	BALINESE	SUNDANESE	SOUTH KALIMANTAN
Ramayana: Rama, Sita, Laksmana, Hanuman, Sugriwa, Subali, Rawana, Kumbakarna, Wibisana, Sarpakenaka, Trijata	wayang kulit purwa langrendmandrawanara wayang wong sendratari	wayang kulit ngramayana kecak sendratari wayang wong	wayang golek sendratari	wayang gong
Mahabharata: The Pandawas: Yudhistira, Bima, Arjuna, Nakula, Sadewa; The Korawas: Suyudana, Dursasana, Drona, Sakuni; Kresna, Baladewa, Subadra	wayang (kulit) purwa wayang wong	wayang kulit parwa wayang wong parwa (without mask, except *punakawan*) arja sendratari preman janner wayang lewat (ruwat)	wayang golek	wayang gong
Panji: Panji Inu Kertapali, Galuh Candrakirana, Gunungsari, Klana Sewandana, Sarag	wayang gedog	wayang kulit gambuh gambuh arja drama gong		
Menak: Wong Agung Menak Amir-Ambyah, Umarmaya, Putri Cina, Kelaswara	wayang golek	gambuh		
Penyalonarangan		barong, wayang kulit calonarang		
Historical Stories (Babad)	wayang krucil wayang klithik	topeng pajegan, topeng panca, prembon, sendratari, drama gong		
Revolution/Modern Historical Stories	wayang suluh wayang pancasila			
Folk Stories (Cerita rakyat): Pan Balang Tamak, Sampek Eng Tai, Jayaprana, Pan Bungking		arja drama gong prembon		
Tantri		prembon wayang tantri (created in 1980s)		

Bibliography

GENERAL WORKS

Bouvier, H. 1990. *Le Arts du Temps et du Spectacle dans la Societé. Madouraise (Madura-est, Indonesie)*. Ph.D. dissertation, L'Ecole des Hautes Etudes en Science Sociales.

Eliade, M. 1959. *The Sacred and the Profane: The Nature of Religion*. New York: Harcourt, Brace & World.

Department of Education and Culture. 1986. *Ensiklopedi Seni Musik dan Seni Tari Daerah* (Encyclopedia of Regional Music and Dance). Report on research and inventory of ethnic cultures of East Java. Surabaya: Department of Education and Culture.

Department of Education and Culture. 1985. *Ensiklopedi Tari Indonesia Seri F-J* (Indonesian Dance Encyclopaedia, F-J). Jakarta: Regional Cultural Inventorization and Documentation Project, Department of Education and Culture .

Department of Education and Culture. *Ensiklopedi Tari Indonesia* (Indonesian Dance Encyclopaedia). Jakarta: Department of Education and Culture.

Mohamad, G. 1991. *Aspects of Indonesian Culture: Modern Drama*. New York: Festival of Indonesia Foundation.

Herbert, E. 1981. "Intrinsic Aesthetics in Balinese Artistic and Spiritual Practice". *Asian Music* Vol. 13, no. 1: 43–52.

Holt, C. 1967. *Art in Indonesia, Continuities and Change*. Ithaca: Cornell University Press.

Kartomi, M. (ed.). *Studies in Indonesian Music*. Victoria: Centre of Southeast Asian Studies, Monash University.

Kusumadilaga, K.P. A. 1839. *Pakem Sastra Miruda*. Sala: de Bliksem

Murgiyanto, S. 1991. *Aspects of Indonesian Culture: Dance*. New York: Festival of Indonesia Foundation Inc.

Prawiroatmojo, S. 1980. *Bausastra Jawa-Indonesia*, 2 parts. Jakarta: Gunung Agung.

Sedyawati, E. (ed.). 1984. *Tari, Tinjauan dari Berbagai Segi* (Dance Viewed from Various Aspects). Jakarta: Pustaka Jaya.

Stutterheim, W.F. 1935. *Indian Influences in Old Javanese Art*. London: India Society.

de Zoete, B., and Spies, W. 1938. *Dance and Drama in Bali*. London: Faber and Faber Limited.

RITUAL AND PROCESSIONAL PERFORMANCES

Bandem, I Made, and de Boer, F.E. 1981. *Kaja and Kelod: Balinese Dance in Transition*. Kuala Lumpur: Oxford University Press.

Jasper, J.E. 1902. 'De Gandroeng Bali', in *Tijd Onder de Baliërs. Eene Reisbeschrijving Met Aanteekeningen Betreffende Hygiène, Land–en Volkenkunde van de Eilanden Bali en Lombok*. Batavia: G. Kolff and Company.

Munardi, A.M. and Murgiyanto, S. 1991. *Seblang dan Gandrung: Dua Bentuk Tari Tradisi di Banyuwangi*. Jakarta: Departemen Pendidikan dan Kebudayaan.

Scholte, J. 1927. 'Gandroeng van Banjoewangi', *Djawa* 7: 144-153.

Soekawati, T.G.R. 1925. 'De Sanghyang op Bali', *Djawa* 5: 320-325.

Soelarto, B. 1993. *Garebeg di Kesultanan Yogyakarta*. Yogyakarta: Penerbit Kanisius

Timoer, S. 1978. *Reog di Jawa Timur*. Jakarta: Departemen Pendidikan dan Kebudayaan.

Wolbers, P. A. 1986. 'Gandrung and Angklung from Banyuwangi: Remnants of a Past Shared with Bali', *Asian Music* Vol. 18, no. 1:71-90.

TRADITIONAL MUSICAL ENSEMBLES

Becker, J. 1980. *Traditional Music*

in Modern Jawa: Gamelan in a Changing Society. Honolulu: University of Hawaii Press.

Devale, S. C. 1992. 'Lions and Tigers and Trees, Om eye: Cosmological Symbolism in the Design and Morphology of Gamelan in Java', Foley, K. (ed.) Local Manifestations and Cross–Cultural Implications. Berkeley: Center for South and Southeast Asia Studies.

Fagg, W. 1970. The Raffles Gamelan, a historical note. London: British Museum.

Hood, M. 1963. 'The enduring tradition: music and theatre in Java and Bali', in McVey, R.T. (ed.) Indonesia. New Haven: Southeast Asia Studies, Yale University; by arrangement with HRAF Press.

Kunst, J. and Kunst- van Wely, C.J.A. 1922. 'Over Bali'sche Muziek', Djawa 2: 117-146; 194-196.

Kunst, J. 1968. Hindu-Javanese Musical Instruments. The Hague: Martinus Nijhoff.

—. 1973. Music in Java: Its History, Its Theory and Its Technique. 2 vols. Heins, E.L. (ed.) The Hague: Martinus Nijhoff.

Lindsay, J. 1992. Javanese Gamelan: Traditional Orchestra of Indonesia. Singapore: Oxford University Press.

McPhee, C. 1937. 'Angkloeng Gamelans in Bali', Djawa 17: 0322-66.

—. 1949. 'The Five-Tone Gamelan Music of Bali', Musical Quarterly 35: 250-281.

—. 1966. Music in Bali. New Haven and London: Yale University Press.

Lentz, D. A. 1965. The Gamelan Music of Java and Bali. Lincoln: University of Nebraska Press.

Sumarsam. 1988. Introduction to Javanese Gamelan. Middletown: Wesleyan University Music Department.

THE MASK IN PERFORMANCE

Dananjaya, J. 1985. Pantomim Suci Betara Berutuk dari Trunyan Bali (Betara Berutuk Sacred Pantomime from Trunyan, Bali). English and Indonesian. Jakarta: PN Balai Pustaka

Emigh, J. 1979. 'Playing with the Past: Ancestral Visitation in the Masked Theater of Bali', Drama Review, 82: 11-36.

Lommel, A. 1972. Masks: Their Meaning and Function. New York: McGraw-Hill.

Noosten, H.H. 1936. 'Maskers en Ziekten op Java en Bali', Djawa 16: 311-17.

Onghokham. 1972. 'The Wayang Topeng World of Malang', Indonesia, vol. 14:111-24.

Poerbatjaraka, R. M. Ng. 1968. Tjerita Pandji dalam Perbandingan. Jakarta: Gunung Agung.

Schneebaum, T. 1985. Asmat Images. Agats, Irian Jaya: Asmat Museum of Culture and Progress.

Sedyawati, E. 1993. 'Topeng dalam Budaya', in Seni Pertunjukan Indonesia. Jakarta: PT Gramedia Widiasarana Indonesia

Slattum, J. 1992. Masks of Bali: Spirits of an Ancient Drama. San Francisco: Chronicle Books.

Soedarsono. 1980. 'Masks in Javanese Dance–Dramas', Journal of the International Institute for Comparative Music Studies and Documentation, vol. 22, no. 1:5-22.

Suanda, E. 1981. 'The Social Context of Cirebonese Performing Artists', Asian Music XIII no. 1: 27-42.

Suanda, E. 1985. 'Cirebonese Topeng and Wayang of the Present Day', Asian Music Vol. 16, no. 2: 84-120.

Taylor, P. M. and Aragon, L. 1991. Beyond the Java Sea: Art of Indonesia's Outer Islands. Washington D.C.: Smithsonian Institution, National Museum of Natural History.

WAYANG THEATRE

Amengkunegara II, K.B.P.A.A. 1986. Serat Centhini (Suluk Tambang Raras). Part 2. Kaltinaken Miturut Aslinipun dening Kamajaya, Yogyakarta: Yayasan Centhini.

Anderson, B. R.O.G. 1965. Mythology and the Tolerance of the Javanese. Ithaca, New York: South East Asia Program, Department of Asian Studies, Cornell University.

Brandon, J.G. 1966. 'Indonesia's Wayang Kulit', Asia, 5 (Spring 1966), pp. 51-61.

—. (ed.). 1970. On Thrones of Gold: Three Javanese Shadow Plays. Cambridge, Massachussetts: Harvard University Press.

deBoer, F. 1987. 'Functions of the Comic Attendants (Penasar) in a Balinese Shadow Play', in Dina and Sherzer, J. (eds.) Humor and Clowning in Puppetry. Athens, Ohio: Popular Press.

Juynboll, H.H. 1915. Het Javaansche Toneel. Baarn: Hollandia Drukkerij.

Kats, J. 1923. Het Javaansche Toneel: Wajang Poerwa. 2 vols. Weltevreden: Commissie voor de Volkslectuur.

Keeler, W. 1982. Father Puppeteer. PhD Thesis Chicago, Committee on Social Thought, University of Chicago.

de Kleen, T. 1947. Wayang (Javanese Theatre). Stockholm: Gothia Ltd.

Kusumadilaga, K.P.A. 1839. Pakem Sastra Miruda. Sala: de Bliksem.

Mangkunegara VII of Surakarta. 1957. On the Wayang Kulit (Purwa) and Its Symbolic and Mystical Elements. Trans. by Claire Holt. Ithaca, New York: Cornell University Southeast Asia Program.

McPhee, C. (1936) 1970. 'The Balinese Wayang Kulit and Its Music', in Belo, J. (ed.) Traditional

Balinese Culture. New York: Columbia University Press.

Mellema, R.L. 1954. *Wayang Puppets: Carving, Colouring and Symbolism.* Trans. by Mantle Hood. Amsterdam: Royal Tropical Institute.

Moebirman. 1960. *Wayang Purwa: The Shadow Play of Indonesia.* The Hague: van Deventer-Maasstichting.

Pigeaud, Th.G.Th. 1938. *Javaanse Volksvertoningen.* Batavia: Volkslectuur.

Prawiroatmojo, S. 1980. *Bausastra Jawa-Indonesia,* 2 parts. Jakarta: Gunung Agung.

Sutaarga, M. A. 1955. 'De wajang golèk in West Java', *Indonesië* 8: 441-56.

Ulbricht, H. 1979. *Wayang Purwa: Shadows of The Past.* Kuala Lumpur: Oxford University Press.

Widjojo, R. 1941. *Serat Menak.* Jakarta: Gunung Agung.

ISLAMIC PERFORMANCES

Nor, Moh. A. Md. *Zapin: Folk Dance of the Malay World.* Singapore: Oxford University Press, 1993.

Widjojo, R. 1941. *Serat Menak.* Batavia: Balai Poestaka.

NON-REPRESENTATIONAL DANCE

Bandem, I M. 1975. 'The Baris Dance', *Ethnomusicology* 19: 259-66.

Department of Education and Culture. *Buku Acara Festival Tari Tradisional Tingkat Nasional 1988/89.* Jakarta: Departemen Pendidikan dan Kebudayaan.

Department of Education and Culture. *Ensiklopedi Tari Indonesia 1995-1996.* Jakarta: Departemen Pendidikan dan Kebudayaan.

van Helsdingen–Schoevers, B. 1925. *Het Srimpi Boek.* Weltevreden: Volkslectuur.

Hinzler, H.I.F. 1980. 'The Balinese

Baris Dadap: Its Tradition and Texts (A Preliminary Study)', in Voight, M. (ed.), *XX deutscher Orienta-listentag vom 3. bis 8. Oktober 1977 in Erlangen: Vorträge.* Wiesbaden: Steiner.

Holt, C. and Bateson, G. (1944) 1970. 'Form and Function in the Dance in Bali', in Belo, J. (ed.), *Traditional Balinese Culture.* New York: Columbia University Press.

—. 1976. 'The Barong Dance', *World of Music* 18. (3): 45-52.

—. 1984. 'Evolusi Legong dari\ Sakral Menjadi Sekuler dalam Tari Bali', in Sedyawati, E. (ed.) *Tari.* Jakarta: Pustaka Jaya.

de Kleen, T. 1936. *The Temple Dances of Bali.* Stockholm: Bokforlags Aktiebolaget Thule.

Sedyawati, E. 1984. 'Gambyong Menurut Serat Cabolang dan Serat Centini', in Sedyawati, E. (ed.) *Tari.* Jakarta: Pustaka Jaya.

Soedarsono (ed.). 1976. *Mengenal Tari-tarian Rakyat di Daerah Istimewa Yogyakarta (Introduction to Folk Dances in the special Territory of Yogyakarta).* Yogyakarta: Indonesian Art Academy of Dance (ASTI).

Surharto, B. 1979-80. *Tayub: Pengamatan Dari Segi Tari Pergaulan Serta Kaitannya dengan Unsur Upacara Kesuburan.* Jakarta: Proyek Pengembangan Institut Kesenian Indonesia, Departemen Pendidikan dan Kebudayaan.

TRADITIONAL THEATRE

Bandem, I M. 1976-77. *Panitihalaning Pêgambuhan.* Denpasar: Proyek Sasana Budaya Bali.

Bandem, I M. and de Boer, F. 1978. 'Gambuh: a Classical Balinese Dance–Drama', *Asian Music* X: 115-127.

Bujang, R. 1989. *Seni Persembahan Bangsawan.* Kuala Lumpur: Dewan

Bahasa dan Pustaka.

Dananjaya, J. 1991. 'Fungsi Teater bagi Kehidupan Masyarakat', in Sedyawati, E. & Damono, S. D. (eds.). *Seni dalam Masyarakat Indonesia, Bunga Rampai.* 2nd ed. Jakarta: P.T. Gramedia Pustaka Utama

Dibia, I W. 1978-79. *Dramatari Gambuh dan Tari-tarian Yang Hampir Punah.* Denpasar: Proyek Pusat Pengembangan Kebudayaan Bali.

—. 1993. *Arja: a Sung dance–drama of Bali; a study of Change and Transformation.* Ann Arbor, Michigan: University Microfilms International.

Department of Education and Culture. *Ensiklopedi Nasional Indonesia.* 1991. Jakarta: P.T. Cipta Adi Pustaka.

Esten, M. 1991. 'Randai dan Beberapa Permasalahannya', in Sedyawati, E. & Damono, S.D. (eds.) *Seni dalam Masyarakat Indonesia, Bunga Rampai.* 2nd ed. Jakarta: P.T. Gramedia Pustaka Utama

Hatley, B. 1979. *Ketoprak Theatre and the Wayang Tradition.* Centre of Southeast Asian Studies Working Paper No. 19. Melbourne: Monash University.

Hood, M. 1963. 'The Enduring Tradition: Music and Theatre in Java and Bali', in McVey, R. (ed.) *Indonesia.* New Haven, Connecticut: Human Relations Area Files.

Kristanto, J.B. 1991 'Srimulat, Kesenian Kota', in Sedyawati. E. & Damono, S.D. (eds.) *Seni dalam Masyarakat Indonesia, Bunga Rampai.* 2nd ed. Jakarta: P.T. Gramedia Pustaka Utama

Soedarsono. 1984. *Wayang Wong: The State Ritual Dance Drama in the Court of Yogyakarta.* Yogyakarta: Gadjah Mada University Press

Spies, W. and Goris, R. 1937. 'Overzicht van Dans en Tooneel in Bali', *Djawa* 17:444-447.

Sucipto, F.A. and Wijaya. 1978. *Kelahiran dan Perkembangan Ketoprak*. Jakarta: Departement Pendidikan dan Kebudayaan.

Supriyanto, H. 1994. 'Sandiwara Ludruk di Jawa Timur', in *Seni Pertunjukan Indonesia*. Jakarta: PT Gramedia Widiasarana Indonesia

—. 1992. *Lakon Ludruk Jawa Timur*. Jakarta: P.T. Gramedia Widiasarana Indonesia.

MODERN INDONESIAN THEATRE

Rafferty, E. (ed.). 1989. *Putu Wijaya in Performance: a Script and Study of Indonesian Theatre*. Madison, Wisconsin: Center for Southeast Asian Studies, University of Wisconsin-Madison.

CONTEMPORARY INDONESIAN DANCE

Hough, B. 1992. *Contemporary Balinese Dance Spectacles as National Ritual*. Clayton, Victoria: Centre of Southeast Asian Studies, Monash University.

MODERN INDONESIAN MUSIC

Becker, J. 1976. 'Keroncong, Indonesian Popular Music', *Asian Music* VII: 14–38.

Frederick, W. H. 1982. 'Rhoma Irama and the Dangdut Style: aspects of contemporary Indonesian popular culture', *Indonesia* 34: 103-130.

Hatch, M. 1989. 'Popular Music in Indonesia (1983)', in Firth, S. (ed.) *World Music, Politics and Social Change*. Manchester: Manchester University Press.

Kornhauser, B. 1978. 'In Defence of Kroncong', in Kartomi, M. (ed.). *Studies in Indonesian Music*. Victoria: Centre of Southeast Asian Studies, Monash University.

Kunst, J. 1973. *Music in Java*. The Hague: Martinus Nijhoff.

Kusbini. 1972. 'Kroncong Indonesia', *Musica* I: 19-43.

Lohanda, Mona. 1991. 'Dangdut, Sebuah Pencarian Identitas', in Sedyawati, E. & Damono, S. D. (eds.) *Seni dalam Masyarakat Indonesia, Bunga Rampai*. 2nd ed. Jakarta: P.T. Gramedia Pustaka Utama

Matursky, P. 1985. 'An Introduction to the Major Instruments and Forms of Traditional Malay Music', *Asian Music* XVI. (2): 121-182.

McPhee, C. 1955. 'Children and Music in Bali', in Mead, M. and Wolfenstein, M. (eds.) *Childhood in Contemporary Cultures*. Chicago: University of Chicago Press.

Muchlis, B.A. and Azmy, B.A.. (compilers) 1992. *Lagu-Lagu untuk Sekolah Dasar dan Lanjutan: I Lagu Wajib*. Jakarta: Penerbit 'Musika'.

Muchlis, B.A. and Azmy, B.A. (compilers) 1995. *Lagu-Lagu untuk Sekolah Dasar dan Lanjutan: II Lagu Wajib*. Jakarta: Penerbit 'Musika'.

Soewito M, D.S. and Pardede, G.S. (compilers) 1985. *Lagu Lagu Pilihan: Ismail Marzuki: dilengkapi not balok dan not angka*. Jakarta: Titik Terang.

Subagio, G. (ed.). 1989. *Apa Itu Lagu Pop Daerah*. Bandung: PT Citra Aditya Bakti.

Sylado, R. 1991. 'Musik Pop Indonesia, Suatu Kekebalan Sang Mengapa', in Sedyawati, E. & Damono, S.D. (eds.) *Seni dalam Masyarakat Indonesia, Bunga Rampai*. 2nd ed. Jakarta: P.T. Gramedia Pustaka Utama.

Yampolsky, P. 1989. 'Hati Yang Luka, an Indonesian Hit', *Indonesia* 47:1-18.

Yampuger. 1995. *Suburlah Tanah Airku*. Jakarta: Yayasan Musik Gereja.

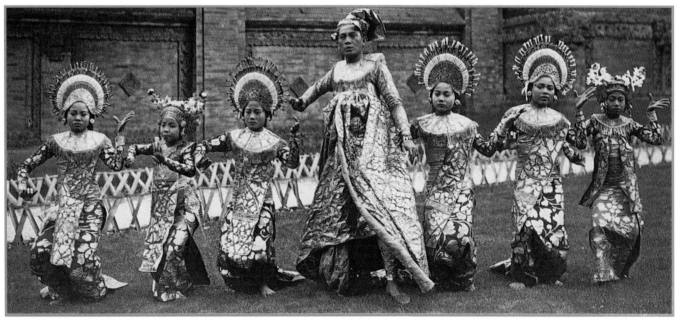

A Balinese traditional dancemaster and his entourage of performers, two were legong *dancers and the others were* janger *dancers with their halo-like headdresses.*

Photo Credits

Unless otherwise specified, pictures have been taken from Editions Didier Millet's private collection.

The Publisher acknowledges the kind permission of the following for the reproduction of photographs.

Chapter Openers:
Ritual and Processional Performances, *reog ponorogo* and *tabuik* by Jill Gocher; *garebeg* procession by Luca Tettoni; *rejang* dancer by Jack Vartoogian; *hudoq* dancer by Alain Compost; and *galombang* by Julianti Parani.
Traditional Musical Ensembles, all pictures from EDM's collection.
The Mask in Performance, *hudoq* mask, and *wayang topeng* dancers by Luca Tettoni, *reog ponorogo* and Jero Luh by Tara Sosrowardoyo; and Hanoman by Jill Gocher.
Wayang Theatre, *wayang kulit* puppets and Balinese *wayang* by Luca Tettoni; *wayang golek* and *wayang cepak* puppets by John Miksic.
Islamic Performances, *seudati, remplis mude* and *beksa golek menak* by Jack Vartoogian; *salawat* by TAP; *zapin* by Yudi Trisnahadi; and *terbang* player by Sri Hastano.
Non-representational Dance, Javanese and Toraja dancers by Luca Tettoni; *baris tunggal* by Jill Gocher; Flores dance by Alain Compost; Makassarese dancer by TAP; Covarrubias' *baris gede* dancer by John Falconer; *randai* by Julianti Parani; and *bedhaya* dance by Yayasan Nusantara Jaya/ Rachel Cooper.
Traditional Theatre, Javanese *topeng* by TAP; *wayang wong* by Luca Tettoni; Nyai Bei Mardusari from Iwan Tirta; *arja* by Leo Haks; Balinese *sendratari* (bottom) by Rio Helmi; and *ramayana sendratari* (3) by Amir Sidharta.
Modern Indonesian Theatre, *Oidipus* tryout by TAP; *Jayaprana* by Teater Populer; Rendra by Hadi Purnomo; and White Snake by Teater Koma.
Contemporary Indonesian Dance, Sulistyo, *One Way Ticket to Bosnia* and *Panji Sepuh* by Republika/Ali Said; *Passage through the Gong* and Sardono Kusumo by Jack Vartoogian; new dance by Julianti Parani; and *Areinam* by Kompas.
Modern Indonesian Music, composers by Anuar bin Abdul Rahim; all posters by Jaulam Hutasoit; and all photographs by Sunarya, B.A.

Reproduced by kind permission of the British Library, p. 72, Serat Menak, ADD. 12309, f.4R.
Reproduced by kind permission of the New York Public Library, p. 41, *huda-huda* dancer, MGZEB 87-288.
Reproduced by kind permission of the National Museum of Jakarta, p. 5, *wayang* puppets; p. 6, Gunungsari mask; p. 30, gamelan treatise; and p. 43, Candra Kirana. (Photographs by Tara Sosrowardoyo).

A.S. Achjadi, p. 126, *keroncong* singers.
Judi Achjadi, p. 67, a combined frame-drum and *zapin* performance.
Catherine Basset, p. 92, the refined prince and one of his servants; and p. 93, the king pushing his servant, the king and the beautiful princess, a pair of royal couples, and the angry king.
Beck Tohir (Secretariat Negara), p. 23, *singabarong*'s followers.
Buku Antar Bangsa, p. 61, *wayang revolusi* (6).
Butet Kertarajasa, p. 112, Semar.
Peter Buurman, p. 56, *patih, djinn*, Panji, Menak Jingga, and soldier; p. 57, prince, king on horse, and king on throne; and p. 58, *wayang klithik* (5 pictures).
Christie's, p. 57, *wayang cepak* puppets painting; p. 58, painting of *wayang golek* puppets; and p. 92, painting of *arja* dancer.
Alain Compost, p. 7, Minangkabau dancers; p. 13, hudoq dancer; p. 34, Asmat man, p. 40, *momie* and Asmat skulls; p. 67, *indang* dance; p. 86, dancers at wedding ceremony; and p. 101, *pencak silat* movements.
Danny Tumbelaka (EDM), p. 81, *ketuk tilu* dance(4 pictures); p. 85, *serampang dua belas* dance (2 pictures), *senandung* dance, male dancer *mengebeng* and Mak Inang dance; p. 86, *pakarena* dancers (6 pictures) and *pajaga* dancer; p. 87, *pajaga* dancer (8 pictures).
Deddy Luthan, p. 21, old *gandrung* dancer.
Department of Education and Culture, p. 83, *gending sriwijaya*.
Departemen Penerangan, p. 84, *kanjet temengan*.
Dewan Kesenian Jakarta, p. 32, *saron* player; p. 41, Rangda (3 pictures); p. 46, poster; p. 77, *jathilan* musical ensemble and flame-throwing; p. 84, *kanjet pepatai* dancer; p. 90, transvestites in *ludruk*; p. 91, *longser* performance; p. 95, *mamanda* theatre; p. 99, *topeng prembon*, p. 100, masked *makyong* and Mak Timah; p. 101, *randai* ring, musical ensemble, poster and marital arts movement; p. 107, *zat*; p. 108, *ketoprak ongklek* (2 pictures); p. 113, Kris Mpu Gandring; p. 116, Julianti and Sentot; p. 130, Pranajaya; p. 131, piano duet and Bing Slamet and Sam Saimun.
Endo Suanda, p. 47, *topeng cirebon* dancer.
Enoch Atmadibrata, p. 46 47, all masks and topeng headdress.
Eri Ekawati, p. 20, *seblang olihsari*.
Farida Oetoyo, p. 118, Putih Kembali.
Femina, p. 14, *hudoq* mask of the bird pest; and p. 84, man playing *sampe'*.
Fendi Siregar, p. 58, *golek* carver.
Franki Raden, p. 127, Trisutji Kamal and Harry Rusli in Jakarta; and p. 131, Sapto Raharjo and Amir Pasribu.
Jill Gocher, p. 36, man with drum, Kalimantan; p. 47, village *topeng* Cirebon; and p. 78, *gong gede*.
Hadi Purnomo, p. 73, *menak cina*; p. 116, a blend of dance techniques and cultural ideas; p. 117, I Wayan Diya; and p. 118, young choreographers.
Leo Haks, p. 18, *baris gede*; p. 33, Balinese gamelan; p. 80, *ronggeng*; p. 90, *tari beskalan*; p. 92, prince and princess; p. 93, *gong kebyar*; p. 94, *sandiwara sunda*; p. 96-97, *wayang wong*; p. 98, rangda; and p. 128, female singers.
Halilintar Lathief, p. 86, Mamasa's dancers.
Kunang Helmi, p. 11, Statue of dancer.
Rio Helmi, p. 8, *topeng prembon*; p. 17, *gamelan sekaten* in Yogyakarta; p. 18, *memendet* and *rejang* from Bangaya; p. 19, *gabor* and *rejang* from Asak, and *mendet*; p. 32, sanctifying *gong*; p. 35, *gamelan gambuh*; p. 42, monkey troupes, Rawana and harelipped mask; p. 43, *penasar* character; p. 44, *sidhakarya* performer; p. 45, *topeng keras* and *bondres* masks; p. 54, rangda and barong; p. 55, Rama, Bima, and musical accompaniments and *dalang* behind the *wayang* screen; p. 79, *sanghyang dedari*; p. 98-99, the *tua*; and p. 99, *gambuh* dancer.
I Ketut Gede, p. 92, a manuscript on the *arja*.
Institut Kesenian Jakarta, p. 25, *pencak silat*; and p. 127, student practising.
Irwan Holmes/William Woodruff, p. 58, Bhatara Guru.
I Wayan Dibia, p. 45, Dalem; and p. 79, *gabor* dancers.
Jakarta Post, p. 126, a Yogyakarta musician.
Jaulam Hutasoit, p. 21, *gandrung*; p. 48, *wayang topeng*; p. 90, *ludruk* at Gema Tribrata; p. 108, Dor; p. 109, Dagelan Ketoprak Mataram; and p. 130, Orkes Simfoni Jakarta and two posters.
Julianti Parani, p. 24, Sumatran wedding and *penghulu*; p. 25, *galombang* (4 pictures); p. 67, Minang with drum; p. 68, poster and dancers; p. 70, *saman lo hoyan*; p. 71, the *syech*; p. 82, two authorities on *alang suntiang* and *alau ambek*; p. 83, *alang suntiang* (7 pictures); p. 93, Aji Saka; p. 100, garuda and *makyong*; p. 101, *randai* (3 pictures); p. 107, Ozone; p. 109, Dhemit and Isyu; p. 117, Plesiran-Cokek; p. 118, young choreographers box; p. 122, Ismail Marzuki; p. 124, children choir; p. 125, Pak Kasur at his playschool, children concert, and Ibu

Photo Credits

Kasur with children (2 pictures); p. 128, *keroncong* singers; and p. 129, Rhoma Irama.

Ibu Kasur, p. 124, book cover; and p. 125, Pak Kasur on his birthday.

Kompas, p. 91, *srimulat* performance in Jakarta.

Leo Kristi, p. 127, Leo Kristi in concert.

Marcus Lindenlaub, p. 37, Asmat with drum.

John Miksic, p. 10, dancing figures from Padang Lawas, Sumatra, and the temptation of Buddha by Mara's daughters; p. 11, hunting scene from Lara Jonggrang, dancing *apsara*, turned-out leg stance, Krsynayana relief, Candi Tegawangi reliefs (2 pictures), *gandarwa* from Borobudur, Kumbakarna killed by the monkey troops and Arjuna Bertapa from Candi Surawana; p. 27, *tabuik* procession and transvestite with lion; p. 30, stained glass showing gamelan players; p. 37, Tegawangi relief depicting drummers; p. 40, prehistoric gold mask; p. 43, Klana and servant; p. 56, *wayang cepak* puppets of a princess and two ladies-in-waiting; p. 59, *wayang golek* illustrations (6 pictures); p. 64, *salawatan* and religious chant; p. 80, earlier form of *tayuban*; p. 81, *tari jaipongan*; p. 82, *tari piring*; p. 99, *condong* and *gambuh*; p. 122, cassette; p. 126, cassette; p. 128, Rhoma Irama; and p. 129, *keroncong* cassettes.

Rafli Lindaryadi, p. 61, *wayang kancil*.

Republika/Ali Said, p. 107, Arifin C. Noer; p. 117, Panji Sepuh; and p. 118-119, One Way Ticket to Bosnia.

Vicki Salisbury, p. 26, *tabuik* tower.

Seti-Arti Kailola, p. 112, Seti-Arti and Martha Graham, Martha Graham, and the Shell dance; and p. 113, three pioneers and Seti-Arti Kailola dancing.

Mahendra Singh, p. 123, marching schoolgirls.

Sri Hastanto, p. 65, *kendhang* player, *santiswaran*, *kemanak* player, female *santiswaran* and *terbang* player.

Soedarsono, p. 43, Gunungsari, Panji, and Klana; and p. 49, topeng dalang malang.

Suyatna Anirun, p. 104, *Karto Loewak (Volpone)* (2 pictures), and scene from Shakespeare's *King Lear*; p. 105, *Don Carlos* (2 pictures), *Sang Naga*, and *Lingkaran Kapur Putih*, a masked drama.

Taman Ismail Marzuki, p. 41, *ondel ondel*; p. 90, male *ngremo*; p. 126, TIM centre; and p. 127, Harry Rusli and Paul Gautama.

TAP, p. 19, *sanghyang dedari*; p. 22, *reog ponogoro*; p. 37, *gordang sabangunan* (2 pictures); p. 44, I Made Djimat; p. 45, *bondres* character; p. 46, *topeng cirebon* with no mask; p. 47, Klana; p. 65, *salawat* at Bukitinggi; p. 67, *rebana* and frame-drum ensemble; p. 86, *pagelluq*; p. 105, Romeo and Julia; p. 106, Oidipus, posters and Rendra; p. 107, Burisrawa; and p. 123, Ismail Marzuki's bust.

Tara Sosrowardoyo, p. 17, gamelan; p. 23, Kelana; p. 30, gamelan maker; p. 47, Panji; p. 48, *topeng* dancers; p. 52, *dalang*; p. 53, making *wayang kulit*; p. 72, Sultan; p. 117, Sulistyo; and p. 123, flag and children.

Teater Populer, p. 106, Inspektur Jenderal.

Tempo, p. 66, *indang* dance; p. 91, Teguh; p. 122, Kusbini; and p. 124, Ibu Soed.

Luca Tettoni, p. 14, *hudoq* dancer holding mask and *hudoq* dancers in a file; p. 15, Kenyah Dayak masked dancers; p. 16, *garebeg* procession; p. 19, *baris tumbak* dance and dancer; p. 31, *gong* player; p. 40, *jipae* mask; p. 41, *barong landung*; p. 42, mask of a comical and mythical figure and *barong ket* mask; p. 44, mask of *tua*; p. 45, *sidhakarya* mask; p. 52, gamelan players and shadow of a *gunungan*; p. 54, puppet of a *rsi*; p. 55, Hanoman, Acintya, *dalang* performing Balinese *wayang* and shadow-play; p. 79, *legong* and *baris tumbak*; p. 97, Hanoman; p. 98, *barong* and rangda and the *leyak-leyakan*; and p. 123, marching.

Jack Vartoogian, p. 7, gamelan; p. 8, Sardono at Candi Plaosan, and *wayang wong* character; p. 66, *gayo* of Aceh (2); p. 72, *beksa golek menak* dancers, p. 73, Widaninggar, and Garuda; p. 114, Sardono at Plaosan (2 pictures); p. 115, Siegel on Passage Through the Gong, Eko Kadarsih, Sony Suharsono, Dutch soldiers, masked woman, and Eko Kadarsih as Ratu Kidul.

Linda Vartoogian, p. 6, *baris tunggal* dancer.

William Woodruff, p. 6, mask of Srikandi.

Mike Yamashita, p. 64, *cakepung* performance in Lombok and p. 65, another form of Islamic performance.

Philip Yampolsky, p. 128, cassettes on *dangdut*; and p. 129, cassettes on *keroncong*.

Yayasan Garuda Nusantara, p. 127, Ully Sigar.

Yayasan Budaya, p. 68, *zapin* dance Mak Inang and Kasih dan Budi.

Yayasan Nusantara Jaya, p. 15. *hudoq* mask-maker (Arwah S.); p. 48, *topeng madura* performance(Sal Murgiyanto); p. 73 and 97, *beksa golek menak* performance (Terry Stark).

Yudi Trisnahadi, p. 69, zapin.

Anuar Bin Abdul Rahim, p. 23, *reog ponorogo* procession; p. betel sirih container; p. 26, *tabuik* structures, p. 31, *kendhang* drum and *suling* flute; p. 34, Apo Kayan woman playing the *kledi* mouth organ; p. 37, assemblage of drums and boy holding *moko* drum; p. 53, *wayang kulit* puppet eyes; p. 57, anatomy of *wayang cepak* puppet; p. 59, 3 *wayang golek* headdresses; p. 60, *wayang suluh* puppets (Asia-African Confer-ence); p. 64, *sholawat dulang*; p. 66, *rebana biang* player; p. 67, *rebana burdah* entourage; p. 68, modern variation of *zapin* using ribbons; p. 69, *zapin* instruments; p. 79, *legong* dancers and their movements; p. 84, *kanjet teweg* dancer on *gong*;

p. 94, *bangsawan* backdrops; p. 95, *wayang gong*, Malay *bangsawan* and Javanese *bangsawan*; p. 96-97, 3 group of *wayang wong* characters; p. 122, Bagimu Negeri music score and Indonesian flag; p. 123, symbols; and p. 127, Iwan Fals.

Bruce Granquist and his team of illustrators, p. 15, *hudoq kiba'* dancers in their beadworked masks; p. 20, teenage *seblang olihsari* dancer; p. 21, *gandrung* dancer and detail of dancer and crown; p. 32-33, Balinese *gamelan gong gede*; p. 33, *gamelan gede*; p. 33, *gamelan gambang*, *gamelan gender* and archaic *gender*; p. 48, two Madurese masks; p. 49, Malang masks; p. 60, *gunungan pancasila*; p. 61, *wayang sadat* puppets of Sunan Bonang and Sunan Gunung Jati; p. 64, frame-drum player; p. 70, *bak saman* illustration; p. 71, seudati illustrations (5 illustrations); p. 77, *jathilan* dancer; p. 78, Balinese temple; p. 80-81, *ibing keurseus monggawa* dance; p. 90, female *ngremo* dancer; and p. 91, male *ngremo* dancer.

The following illustrators have also made contributions to the book:
Kyaw Han
Loh Choi Ying
Pan Dongli
Mallika Sririaman

EDM would like to thank the following for their kind assistance in the preparation of this volume:
A.S. Achjadi, Alex Dea, Ibu Asni, Ayu Bulantrisna Jelantik, A Kasim Achmad, Barbara Johnson, Bagong Kussudiardjo, Elly Rudatin, Sunaryo, B.A., I Wayan Diya, Ibu Kasur, James Danandjaja, Marusya Nainggolan, Noerdin Daud, Poppy Sawitri, Rachel Cooper, Radjito, Retno Maruti R., Soetardjo and staff of the Museum Wayang, Wiwiek Sapala and Yuni Trisapto.

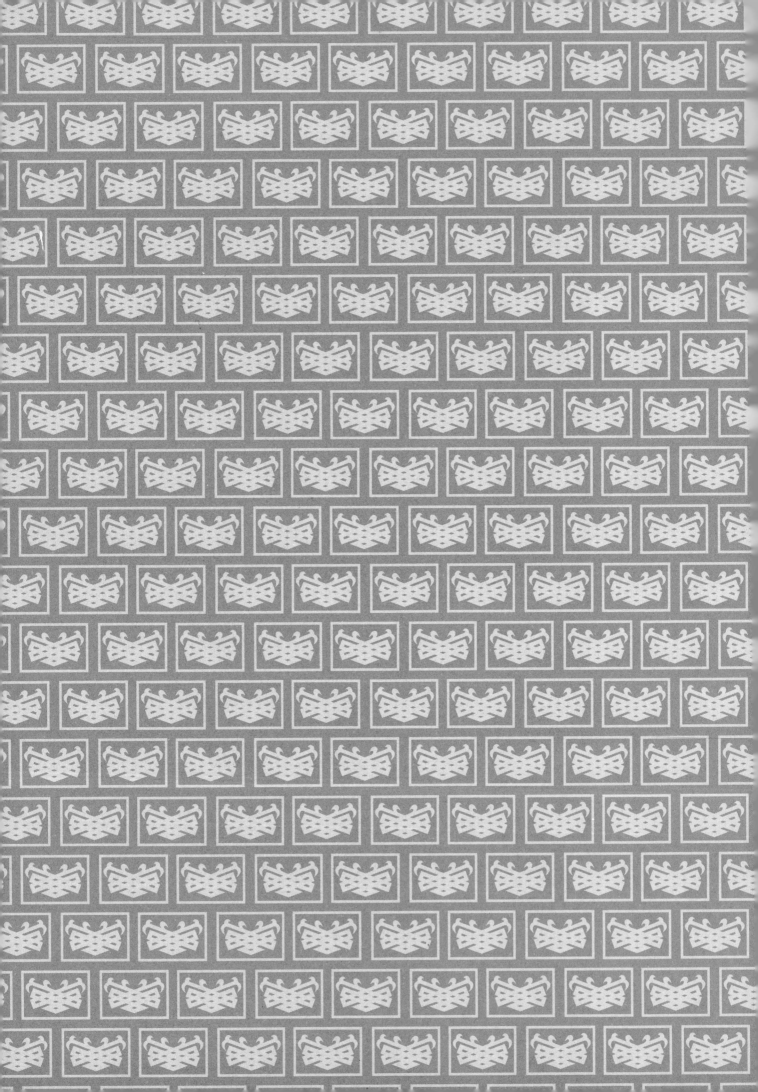